Journal of Semitic Studies Supplement 39

Syriac Medicine and Ḥunayn ibn Isḥāq's Arabic Translation of the Hippocratic *Aphorisms*

by

Samuel Chew Barry

Published by Oxford University Press
on behalf of the University of Manchester
2018

OXFORD
UNIVERSITY PRESS

Great Clarendon Street, Oxford OX2 6DP

Oxford University Press is a department of the University of Oxford. It furthers the University's objective of excellence in research, scholarship, and education by publishing worldwide in

Oxford New York

Athens Auckland Bangkok Bogotá Buenos Aires Cape Town Chennai Dar es Salaam Delhi Florence Hong Kong Istanbul Karachi Kolkata Kuala Lumpur Madrid Melbourne Mexico City Mumbai Nairobi Paris São Paulo Shanghai Singapore Taipei Tokyo Toronto Warsaw

with associated companies in Berlin Ibadan

Oxford is a registered trade mark of Oxford University Press in the UK
and in certain other countries

Published in the United Kingdom
by Oxford University Press, Oxford

First published 2018

A catalogue for this book is available from the British Library

Library of Congress Cataloguing in Publication Data
(Data available)

ISSN 0022-4480

ISBN 978-0-19-882808-2

Subscription information for the *Journal of Semitic Studies* is available at the journal website:
jss.oxfordjournals.org

Printed in Great Britain by Bell & Bain Ltd, Glasgow

For my Father

The cover shows text from the only surviving copy of the Syriac translation of the Hippocratic *Aphorisms* written alongside Ḥunayn ibn Isḥāq's Arabic translation of the same work. Bibliothèque nationale de France MS arabe 6734 68v.

Table of Contents

Acknowledgments vii

Preface ix

Introduction. Syriac Scholarship in the History of Greek-to-Arabic Medical Translation xi

Part One: The Syriac Lexicon of bar Bahlul and the Syriac and Arabic translations of the Hippocratic *Aphorisms*

Chapter 1. On the General Relationship Between Bar Bahlul's Lexicon and the Syriac and Arabic translations of the *Aphorisms* 1

Chapter 2. Greek Loan-words in the Syriac *Aphorisms* and Ḥunayn's Arabic Translation Techniques 51

Part Two: Comparing the Syriac and Arabic Translations of the Hippocratic *Aphorisms*

Chapter 3. The Early Syriac Version of the *Aphorisms* Attributed to Sergius of Reš ʿAynā and ʿAbbāsid-era Syriac and Arabic Medical Translation: A Comparative Study 93

Chapter 4. The ʿAbbāsid-era Syriac and Arabic Translations of the *Aphorisms* and their Scholarly Background 135

Chapter 5. Conclusion 173

Bibliography 185

Appendix: Greek Words 189

Appendix: Latin Words 277

Appendix Unknown Greek Words 279

Indices 283

Acknowledgments

I am deeply grateful for the support provided to me by numerous people over the course of this project. Without the constant help and indulgence of my family, in particular my wife Marie, this book would never have come to fruition. Special thanks is due to my supervisor Peter E. Pormann, whose wide-ranging knowledge and scholarly acumen were guiding lights in every stage of the production of this work. I am also very thankful to the other members of my doctoral panel, John Healey and David Langslow, for their close attention to my work and their continual interest and encouragement. The patience, wisdom and friendship of the team of scholars and students working on the Aphorisms project has been of immense benefit. Of these I should mention specifically Taro Mimura and Kamran Karimullah, whose mentorship over the course of this project I value greatly. I would be remiss if I did not mention the immense debt of gratitude I owe to my M.A. supervisor, Kenneth Honerkamp, for his sustained instruction and encouragement. I must also thank Professor Hinrich Biesterfeldt, Grigory Kessel, Oliver Overwien and David Bertaina for their willingness to supply invaluable resources. In so doing they presented models of professionalism and collegiality.

ܥܠ ܣܒܪܐ ܘܬܘܟܠܢܐ ܫܪܪܐ ܕܚܕ ܐܠܗܐ
به أستعين
ܘܬܫܒܘܚܬܐ ܠܐܠܗܐ ܠܥܠܡ ܥܠܡܝܢ

Preface

Concerning the transliteration of Syriac and Arabic characters, I have adopted the following approaches. For Syriac, I have used the system found in Wheeler M. Thackston’s *Introduction to Syriac* (1999), which renders the Syriac consonants like this: *’ b g d h w z ḥ ṭ y k l m n s ʿ p ṣ q r š t* and the vowels like this: *a ā e ē ê i o u*. For the spirantized begadkepat consonants, an underscore is used: *ḇ g̱ ḏ ḵ ṯ*. Due to the fact that this work concerns East Syriac exclusively, following Nöldeke I have omitted to underscore the letter pē throughout. In part minimally to distinguish between the transcriptions of the two languages, I have used a rather different approach to tranliterating Arabic. I have rendered the consonants thus: *’ b t th j ḥ kh d dh r z s sh ṣ ḍ ṭ ẓ ʿ gh f q k l m n h w y* and the vowels thus: *a ā i ī u ū*.

Introduction

Syriac Scholarship in the History of Greek-to-Arabic Medical Translation

The relative importance of Syriac scholarship for the ʿAbbāsid-era Arabic translations of Greek works has been a question of central concern since the inception of the field of Graeco-Arabic studies. Consider the following passage in Amable Jourdain's classic work *Recherches critiques sur l'age et l'origines des traductions d'Aristote et sur des commentaires grecs ou arabes employés par les docteurs scolastiques*:

> (J)e me livrerai à quelques remarques sur un point d'histoire littéraire souvent agité et jamais résolu. On s'est demandé fréquemment si les traductions arabes d'auteurs grecs étaient faites d'après le texte grec même, ou d'après des versions syriaques… Pour juger avec certitude du mérite des versions arabes, il faudrait donc s'assurer: 1°. si elles sont faites du grec ou du syriaque; 2°. si c'est une simple interprétation, ou une révision, ou une transcription.[1]

In the course of close and intensive study of the Arabic translations of the great translator Ḥunayn ibn Isḥāq in particular, the quality of the finest products of the so-called Greek-to-Arabic translation movement has been judged to be very high, and to represent faithfully the original Greek sources.[2] Yet in certain key respects, questions such as Jourdain's that concern the part of preceding Syriac scholarship in the production of these translations still remain unanswered.

In the earlier stages of the development of Graeco-Arabic studies, a certain reticence to treat these questions perhaps would have been understandable. In the absence of critical studies on the viability of the Greek-to-Arabic

1 A. Jourdain, *Recherches critiques sur l'age et l'origine des traductions latines d'Aristote et sur des commentaires grecs ou arabes employés par les docteurs scolastiques* (Paris 1843), 86–7.

2 At present, the standard reference work on the Arabic scientific tradition is Gerhard Endress' extended essay 'Die wissenschaftliche Literatur', in *Grundriss der arabischen Philologie* vols. II and III, Wolfdietrich Fischer ed. (Wiesbaden 1987–92). Also important are Manfred Ullmann's technical studies of specific translations of Greek works, such as for example his *Die Nikomachische Ethik des Aristoteles in arabischer Überlieferung* (Wiesbaden 2011–12). Recent articles on the subject include for example O. Overwien, 'The Art of the Translator, or: How did Ḥunayn ibn Isḥāq and his school translate?' in P.E. Pormann (ed.), *Epidemics in Context. Greek commentaries on Hippocrates in the Arabic tradition* (Berlin 2012); P.E. Pormann, 'The Formation of the Arabic Pharmacology: Between Tradition and Innovation', *Annals of Science* 68:4 (2011); and U. Vagelpohl, 'In the Translator's Workshop', *Arabic Sciences and Philosophy* 21:2 (September 2011).

translations, too-strong emphasis on their potential Syriac mediation could have undermined nascent scholarship by suggesting that the Arabic translations were mere translations-of-translations, and thus were in some way inferior products unworthy of serious attention. Now, however, as the field approaches a more mature state, it seems possible to return to the question of Syriac mediation without impugning the quality of the translation movement's products in the process. In doing so, we may hope to gain an understanding of the ways in which Syriac-language scholarship contributed to Greek-to-Arabic translation. This in turn may be expected to open passage to a clearer understanding both of the social and cultural history of these translations and of the detailed contents of the translations themselves.

A good deal more attention has been given to the importance of Syriac mediation in the studies of Arabic philosophy than in other fields.[3] Yet, while Syriac medical translation lacks a rich body of surviving primary texts, important secondary sources in the field remain underexploited. Some of these are found in the form of the famous translator Ḥunayn ibn Isḥāq's descriptions of his numerous translations into Syriac and Arabic of the works of Galen, as well as sizable Syriac-to-Arabic lexicons that contain the philological notes of Ḥunayn and his students and successors. In the following pages, I undertake extensive comparisons of this material with an important surviving example of ʿAbbāsid-era Syriac medical writing, the Syriac translation of the Hippocratic *Aphorisms*. Deploying these resources will deepen understanding of the part played by Syriac scholarship in the development of the Arabic medical tradition, and by extension of ʿAbbāsid-era intellectual life more generally.

As Jake Tannous has argued clearly in a recent study, Syriac intellectual history forms an important bridge between the Greek and Arabic philosophical traditions, and thus between the traditional historical categories 'late Antique' and 'early Medieval'.[4] Viewed from the present, the study of Syriac intellectual history allows for an unbroken chain of transmission to be established that runs

---

3 See the contributions collected in H. Hugonnard-Roche, *La logique d'Aristote du grec au syriaque: études sur la transmission des textes de l'Organon et leur interpretation philosophique* (Paris 2004). For natural philosophy and the sciences more generally, including mathematics and astronomy, see H. Takahashi, 'The Sciences in Syriac from Serverus Sebokht to Barhebraeus' in H. Kobyashi and M. Koto (eds), *Transmission of Sciences: Greek, Syriac, Arabic, and Latin* (Tokyo 2010).

4 J. Tannous, 'Syria Between Byzantium and Islam: Making Incommensurables Speak', (Ph.D. diss., Princeton University, 2010), 60.

from Classical Greek to Classical Arabic to scholastic Latin, and thus to the development of modern intellectual notions. Viewed from its own time, such a study clarifies the debt of Islamicate cultural forms to pre-Islamic and specifically eastern Christian adaptations of Hellenic intellectual life. At the same time it shows the extent to which the establishment of Arabic as the pre-eminent language of thought and culture in western Asia transformed that heritage and further integrated it with Greek, Jewish, Persian, Indian and native Arab traditions into a broader cultural and scientific edifice that has exerted global influence for centuries.

Secular Greek Scholarship in Syriac up to the Time of Ḥunayn

The first serious attempts to carry works of pagan Greek philosophy into Syriac were undertaken by the seminal translator Sergius of Reš ʿAynā during the first half of the sixth century of the Christian era.[5] Sergius' Greek learning derived largely from the Alexandrian curricula of Galenic medicine, Aristotelian logic, and the pseudo-Dionysian corpus of neo-Platonic Christian theology.[6] These initial efforts to establish a corpus of secular Syriac literature were conserved in monastic institutions across Mesopotamia and the Levant during the final centuries of Byzantine and Sassanid rule in these regions and through the initial centuries of Muslim rule.[7]

The decades following the assumption of the caliphate by the ʿAbbāsid dynasty in the middle of the eighth century witnessed an efflorescence of intellectual effort prompted in large part by the patronage of the ruling classes.[8] The heirs of several great pre-Islamic traditions of learning were recruited to contribute their expertise to this endeavour. Syriac-speaking families of scholars

5 For Sergius' biography, see Hugonnard-Roche, 'Aux origines de l'exégèse orientale de la logique d'Aristote: Sergius de Reshʿayna (d. 536), médecin et philosophe', *Journal Asiatique* 277 (1989). For the part played by Sergius' translations in the development of Syriac and Arabic medicine, see P.E. Pormann, 'The Development of Translation Techniques from Greek into Syriac and Arabic: The Case of Galen's On the Faculties and Powers of Simple Drugs, Book Six' in R. Hansberger et al. (eds), *Medieval Arabic Thought: Essays in Honour of Fritz Zimmermann* (London 2012), 143–62.

6 H. Hugonnard-Roche, *La logique d'Aristote*, 123–4.

7 D. Gutas, *Greek Thought, Arabic Culture* (London 1998), 14.

8 Gutas, *Greek Thought*, passim.

deriving from the Persian intellectual centre at Gundeshapur were of particular importance for the study of medicine at the caliphal court.[9]

It has been claimed that Arabic translations of Greek works were produced as early as the Umayyad period.[10] However, the accession of the ʿAbbāsid dynasty to the caliphate marks an inflection point in the attitude of the Muslim elites toward secular Greek learning. Important Arabic translations of Greek medicine and philosophy were performed during the reign of al-Manṣūr in the second half of the eighth century.[11] Al-Manṣūr's successors, especially the caliph al-Ma'mūn, sustained and consolidated the translation movement through the first half of the ninth century.[12] In medicine, the key figure in this latter stage of development was the translator/physician Ḥunayn ibn Isḥāq al-ʿIbādī. An Arab Christian and a native of the city of Ḥīra,[13] Ḥunayn gained access to the elite circle of Syriac physicians after a period of studying the Greek language in Byzantium.[14] As evidenced in his *Epistle on what has been Translated of the Works of Galen and what has not been Translated* (hereafter called the *Risālā*), Ḥunayn renovated and significantly broadened the corpus of Syriac translations of the writings of Galen while at the same time producing Arabic translations of many of these same works.[15] Ḥunayn's translations went on to form the

---

9 Gutas, *Greek Thought,* 118. For the history of this city, see L. Richter-Bernburg, 'Gondēšāpur', *Encyclopedia Iranica* 11:2 (2002–12), 131–5.

10 G. Saliba, *Islamic Science and the Making of the European Renaissance*, (Cambridge MA 2007), passim. For a critical reception of these claims, see P.E. Pormann, 'Arabic Astronomy and the Making of the European Renaissance', review of *Islamic Science and the Making of the European Renaissance*, by George Saliba, *Annals of Science* 67 (2010), 243–8.

11 Gutas, *Greek Thought*, 28.

12 Gutas, *Greek Thought*, 75.

13 G. Strohmaier, 'Ḥunain ibn Isḥāq- an Arab Scholar Translating into Syriac', *ARAM* 3 (1991[1993]), 63–4.

14 G. Strohmaier, 'Ḥunayn b. Isḥāk as Philologist', in *Ephrem-Ḥunayn Festival* (Baghdad 1974), 543.

15 G. Bergsträsser (ed.), *Ḥunain ibn Isḥāq über die syrischen und arabischen Galen-Übersetzungen* (Leipzig 1925). This edition of the *Risāla* has been supplemented on the basis of newly-discovered manuscripts in *idem.* ed., *Neue Materialien zu Ḥunain ibn Isḥāq's Galen-Bibliographie*, Abhandlungen für die Kunde des Morgenlandes vol. 19, no. 2 (Leipzig 1932), and more recently in F. Käs, 'Eine neue Handschrift von Ḥunayn ibn Isḥāqs Galenbibliographie', *Zeitschrift für Geschichte der arabisch-islamischen Wissenschaften* 19 (2010–11), 135–93. Furthermore, a new edition of the *Risāla* has recently been published. See J. Lamoreaux, *Ḥunayn ibn Isḥāq on His Galen Translations* (Provo 2015).

foundation of the Arabic medical tradition, which includes the writings of monumental figures like al-Rāzī, ibn Sīnā, ibn Rushd and Maimonides.[16]

The survival of several of his Arabic translations and their profound historical significance has made Ḥunayn best known as an Arabic translator. Yet the emphasis the translator placed on the Syriac translations in the *Risāla*, combined with the much longer extent of the Syriac translation tradition when compared with the Arabic tradition at the time of his career, gives the impression that an understanding of the specific character of the Syriac translations is necessary for a full account of Ḥunayn's contribution to Greek-to-Arabic translation. Yet despite the importance of Syriac for Ḥunayn's profoundly significant translation activity, few if any of his voluminous Syriac translations survive.[17] The descriptions given in the *Risāla* combined with the numerous extant Arabic translations of Ḥunayn's give the historian a window into the translator's praxis. Utilization of these sources in the process of close study of those Syriac medical texts that are extant and that may be linked to Ḥunayn or his students should provide even more valuable context.

Again, the Syriac material is very limited. The most promising text available to us, and the work which has received the most scholarly attention to date, is the Syriac version of the Hippocratic *Aphorisms* extant in a bilingual Syriac-Arabic manuscript,[18] an edition of which was published with a French translation by Henri Pognon in 1903.[19] In part of this manuscript, a Syriac translation of the *Aphorisms* is found facing a copy of Ḥunayn's Arabic translation of the work.

Furthermore, the text of the *Aphorisms* lends itself well to this type of comparative study. Intended as a sort of overview of the art of medicine as understood by the fifth-century BCE Greek physician Hippocrates, the *Aphorisms* covers a variety of material, ranging across subjects like medical

16 For an overview of Arabic medical writing see M. Ullmann, *Islamic Medicine* (Edinburgh 1978). Ullmann's findings are updated on the basis of more recent scholarship in P.E. Pormann and E. Savage-Smith's *Medieval Islamic Medicine* (Washington, D.C. 2007).

17 S. Brock, 'The Syriac Background to Ḥunayn's Translation Techniques', *ARAM* 3 (1991[1993]), 139–42. For a detailed account of the extant Syriac sources, see R. Degen, 'Galen im Syrischen. Eine Übersicht über die syrische Überlieferung der Werke Galens', in V. Nutton (ed.), *Galen: Problems and Prospects* (London 1981).

18 MS Arabe 6734, Bibliothèque nationale Française, Paris, hereafter BnF 6734.

19 H. Pognon (ed.), *Une version syriaque des Aphorismes d'Hippocrate* (Leipzig 1903). All references to the Syriac version of the *Aphorisms* herein refer to this edition unless otherwise noted.

theory, diet, purging, prognostics, diagnostics, gynaecology, and the influence of weather and geography upon health, to name a few. The wealth of the subject-matter is accompanied by a corresponding wealth in terminology, allowing for a large number of Syriac medical terms to be considered. Another element tending to make the *Aphorisms* a suitable entry-point for the study of Syriac and Arabic translations of Greek medicine is the fact that portions of earlier translations of the Hippocratic work in these languages exist alongside the better-known later versions. In total, portions deriving from at least four different classical Syriac and Arabic versions are available. Each of these translations will be described in detail below.

Beyond the texts themselves, important material deriving from the scholarly background of the translations exists in the form of Syriac-Arabic lexicons. Two examples important for the present study are the lexicons of Ḥasan bar Bahlul and Išoʿ bar ʿAli, both of which consist largely of entries originating from Ḥunayn's own lexicographical work. Although I will give a more thorough description of these below, suffice it to say here that they provide resources that greatly enrich the study of the surviving Syriac medical translations.

The **Aphorisms** *of Hippocrates*

As one of the central authorities of classical Ionic medicine, the figure and school of Hippocrates of Kos played a key role in the transmission and development of medical knowledge in antiquity.[20] A leading proponent of humoural theory, Hippocratic contributions ranged from diet to prognosis to surgery to the professionalization of the medical art. Hippocrates and his students promulgated a school of medical theory and practice that exerted great influence from India to Europe up unto the establishment of modern European medicine in the nineteenth century.

It is important to note that the influence of the Hippocratic authors largely came to be mediated by the work of the famous medical theorist Galen of

20 The attribution of the entirety of the Hippocratic corpus to the person of Hippocrates was disputed even in ancient times. The attribution of specific works from the corpus to any given member of the Hippocratic school can at times be difficult. For background on the person and school of Hippocrates, see J. Jouanna, *Hippocrate* (Paris 1992), as well as his article, co-authored with C. Magdelaine, 'Hippocrate de Cos' in R. Goulet (ed.), *Dictionnaire des Philosophes antiques, III: d'Eccélos à Juvenal* (Paris 2000), 771–90.

Pergamon.[21] In claiming to revive the true Hippocratic doctrine, this physician of the second century CE penned highly influential commentaries that gave their own cast to the often ambiguous language of the Hippocratic corpus. Galen's interpretation of Hippocratic doctrine was particularly important for the development of Islamicate conceptions of natural philosophy.[22]

The *Aphorisms* consists of brief statements regarding a wide range of medical concerns, and the text was often viewed as propaedeutic to the body of Hippocratic medical works.[23] For this reason it received a great deal of attention both from commentators and from translators in Arabic. Close to a dozen Arabic commentaries on the *Aphorisms* survive, some of which are quite extensive. The entire extant corpus of Arabic commentaries on the *Aphorisms* is in the process of being edited by a team led by Peter E. Pormann at the University of Manchester, and reference to these editions will be made in this work where relevant. Very strong scholarship on the Greek text also exists. In this book Caroline Magdelaine's edition of the Greek text will generally provide the key point of reference for the Greek tradition of the *Aphorisms*.[24]

The Extant Syriac Translations of the **Aphorisms**

As mentioned above, a largely complete Syriac translation of the Hippocratic *Aphorisms* exists in the Paris manuscript BnF 6734. This text was edited by Henri Pognon in the early twentieth century. Since then, several articles discussing this work have been published.[25] Degen, Brock and Overwien

---

21 For the person and works of Galen, see V. Boudon-Millot, *Galien de Pergame: Médecin et Philosophe* (Paris 2012), as well as her article 'Galien de Pergame' in R. Goulet (ed.), *Dictionnaire des Philosophes*, 440–66.

22 This can be seen in the tendency of Hippocratic works to be transmitted as lemmas in Galenic commentaries, and by the tendency of translators like Ḥunayn to interpret and translate ambiguous Hippocratic texts according to Galen's interpretation of them. Cf. Overwien, 'The Art of the Translator', 165–77.

23 A.Z. Iskandar, 'An Attempted Reconstruction of the Late Alexandrian Medical Curriculum', *Medical History* 20:3 (1976), 258.

24 C. Magdelaine, 'Histoire du texte et édition critique, traduite et commentée, des *Aphorismes* d'Hippocrate', Ph.D. diss. (Université de Paris-Sorbonne, 1988). All references in this work to the Greek text of the *Aphorisms* refer to this edition unless otherwise noted.

25 Four articles in particular should be mentioned: Brock, 'Syriac Background' (already noted in note 17 above); R. Degen, 'Zur syrischen Übersetzung der Aphorismen des Hippokrates', *Oriens Christianus* 62 (1978), 36–52; O. Overwien, 'The Paradigmatic Translator and His Method: Ḥunayn ibn Isḥāq's Translation of the Hippocratic *Aphorisms* from Greek via Syriac into Arabic', *Intellectual History of the Islamicate World* 3 (2015), 158–87 and T. Mimura,

attribute the authorship of the work to Ḥunayn on more or less tentative grounds. Many of the examples found in each of these articles make useful contributions. Brock's article is valuable in particular because of the strong evidence it presents for dating the work in question to the early ʿAbbāsid period. This reduces the urgency of the question of the specific authorship of the work, since a philological study will still provide valuable information about the state of Syriac medicine in an era broadly contemporaneous to Ḥunayn. Along with Mimura, however, it is my view that the attribution of the Syriac *Aphorisms* to Ḥunayn remains problematic for several reasons.

In dating the work to the ʿAbbāsid period, Brock's article makes even more germane Ḥunayn's account of the translations of Galen's *Commentary on the Aphorisms* in the *Risāla.* This account reads as follows:

فح. تفسيره لكتاب الفصول. هذا الكتاب جعله في سبع مقالات. وقد كان ترجمه أيّوب ترجمةً رديئةً ورام جبريل بن بختيشوع أصلاحه فزاده فساداً فقابلتُ به اليونانيّ وأصلحتُه إصلاحاً شبيهاً بالترجمة وأضفتُ إليه فصّ كلام بقراط على حدته وقد كان سألني أحمد بن محمّد المعروف بابن المدبّر ترجمته له فترجمتُ منه مقالة واحدة إلى العربيّة ثمّ تقدّم اليّ ألّا أبتدئ بترجمة مقالة أخرى حتّى يقرأ تلك المقالة التي كنتُ ترجمتها و شُغِل الرجل وانقطعت ترجمة الكتاب فلمّا رأى تلك المقالة محمّد بن موسى سألني استتمام الكتاب فترجمتُه آخره.[26]

88. His commentary on the Book of Aphorisms. He rendered this book into seven chapters. Job made a bad translation, and Jibrīl ibn Bukhtīshūʿ sought to improve it, but corrupted it further. I then compared it with the Greek and improved it in a way similar to translation. I then added to it the lemmas of Hippocrates' words separately. Aḥmad ibn Muḥammad, known as ibn al-Mudabbir, had asked me to translate it for him, so I translated for him one chapter of it into Arabic. He then directed me not to begin translating another chapter until he had read that chapter that I had translated. Then the man became busy, and the translation of the book was cut off. But when Muḥammad ibn Mūsā saw that chapter, he asked me to complete the book, and so I translated it until the end of it.

Here, we learn that two of Ḥunayn's contemporaries, Job of Edessa and Jibrīl ibn Bukhtīshūʿ, had produced Syriac versions of Galen's *Commentary on the Aphorisms* that Ḥunayn found inferior. In discussing these other ʿAbbāsid-era translators of the *Aphorisms* into Syriac, Overwien supposed that Ḥunayn's work represented a significant-enough advance over that of his contemporaries

---

'Comparing Interpretative Notes in the Syriac and Arabic Translations of the Hippocratic *Aphorisms*', *Aramaic Studies* (forthcoming). I am grateful to Mimura for the use of his personal copy.

26 Bergsträsser, *Syrische und arabische Galen-Übersetzungen*, ٤٠.

to have rendered their work obsolete, resulting in the latter's disappearance.[27] It seems clear to me, however, that Ḥunayn's disparaging remarks concerning his contemporaries' translations of Galen's *Commentary* should not be considered sufficient to prove that only Ḥunayn's version could have survived.

Furthermore, it is easy to imagine scenarios that resulted in the loss only of Ḥunayn's Syriac translations while those of his competitors continued to exist. Although the events surrounding Ḥunayn's inquisition and the loss of his library at the hands of the Caliph al-Mutawakkil remain unclear to a significant degree, they do present at least one other plausible avenue for the disappearance of the translator's Syriac works alongside the normal processes of physical attrition.[28] I see no reason to presume solely on the basis of the historical evidence that the extant Syriac translation is the work of any one of the three known ʿAbbāsid-era Syriac translators of the *Aphorisms* to the exclusion of the others. For this reason, the question of the authorship of the Syriac *Aphorisms* must rest on analysis of the text itself.

Textual arguments for and against Ḥunayn's authorship of the Syriac *Aphorisms* exist in this literature. Perhaps most importantly, in the introduction to his edition of the work Pognon asserted that the author of the Syriac *Aphorisms* was a different person from the translator of the Arabic version contained in the manuscript BnF 6734.[29] In agreement with Mimura I hold that these arguments have not been sufficiently considered in the literature to date.[30]

Pognon cited two points against Ḥunayn's authorship of the Syriac *Aphorisms*. First, in the editor's judgment the Syriac translation is overly literal, reducing its serviceability to readers who lack knowledge of Greek. This contrasts with the more reader-oriented approach adopted in Ḥunayn's Arabic translation.[31] Second, a note consisting of several lines criticizing Galen's commentary on aphorism iv. 47 exists in the Syriac text, without corresponding text in the Arabic. Pognon deduced from this that the Syriac and Arabic texts

27 Overwien, 'Paradigmatic Translator', 162.

28 For further details on this episode, see M. Cooperson, 'Two ʿAbbāsid Trials: Aḥmad ibn Ḥanbal and Ḥunayn ibn Isḥāq', *Al-Qantara. Revista de estudios árabes,* 22:2 (2001), 375–93. In several places in the *Risāla* Ḥunayn mentions a disruption of his library. See e.g. Bergsträsser, *Syrische und arabische Galen-Übersetzungen*, ١.

29 Pognon, *Une version syriaque*, ii–iii.

30 Mimura, 'Comparing Interpretative Notes', 2–4.

31 Pognon, *Une version syriaque*, ii.

represent two different works, and thus should be considered to have been written by two different translators.

Mimura has shown that a note ascribed to Ḥunayn in the translator's version of the physician's *Commentary on the Aphorisms* presents largely the same criticism as that found in the exceptional note in the Syriac translation.[32] Although there are some important differences between these two texts, this new evidence is likely sufficient to vitiate Pognon's second argument. To confirm or deny Pognon's first line of argumentation regarding perceived discrepancies between the translation techniques of these two versions of the *Aphorisms*, an extensive if not systematic comparison of the two translations is required. Although the provision of a definite answer to the question of the authorship of the *Aphorisms* is not the primary end of the present work, the material presented herein will make a significant contribution to the debate.

Beside the complete text of the Syriac *Aphorisms* as edited by Pognon, fragments of an earlier Syriac translation of the *Aphorisms* also exist. Grigory Kessel has discovered and extracted seven of the Hippocratic aphorisms from the text of the so-called 'Syriac *Epidemics*', a Syriac version of a commentary on the Hippocratic *Epidemics*.[33] Kessel tentatively attributes the authorship of these translations to Sergius of Reš ʿAynā. Kessel's comparisons of this version with the later ʿAbbāsid-era translation show significant differences between the two.[34]

The Major Arabic Translations of the Aphorisms

As the standard Arabic version of the *Aphorisms,* Ḥunayn's translation of the work exists in a large number of manuscripts. Three broad categories for the transmission of this translation may be noted. They may be transmitted along with Galen's *Commentary on the Aphorisms*, or along with one of the dozen or so independent Arabic commentaries on the work, or in one of the numerous manuscripts which contain only the Hippocratic work itself, separate from any

32 Mimura, 'Comparing Interpretative Notes', 15–18.

33 G. Kessel, 'The Syriac Epidemics and the Problem of its Identification' in P.E. Pormann (ed.), *Epidemics in Context* (Berlin 2012), 118.

34 G. Kessel, 'Sergius ar-Ra'sī has Translated it into Syriac, but Poorly' (paper presented at the conference *Medical Translators at Work*, Humboldt University, Berlin, March 20–1, 2014). All citations of the early Syriac translations refer to this presentation.

commentary. Generally the latter should be considered to have been extracted from Galen's *Commentary* rather than to be fully independent transmissions.

The first modern edition of Ḥunayn's translation was performed by John Tytler and published in Calcutta in 1834.[35] This edition was produced from a few Indian manuscripts, which necessarily are less than representative of the broader textual tradition of the work. Tytler's edition has now been superseded by Taro Mimura's edition of the Arabic translation of Galen's *Commentary on the Aphorisms*, which derives the texts of the lemmas from a diverse set of copies of Ḥunayn's version of Galen's work.[36] Further variations on the texts did occur in the process of the transmission of the several commentaries. Although not represented in Mimura's edition, these tend to be relatively minor, and will only be noted where necessary.

Al-Biṭrīq's Arabic Translation of the **Aphorisms** *and the Arabic Palladius*

A different Arabic translation of the *Aphorisms* has been known to European scholarship at least since the late nineteenth century. A few score aphorisms derived from this translation are reproduced in the *History* of Aḥmad al-Yaʿqūbī.[37] Manfred Ullmann attributes this translation to a late eighth-century scholar named al-Biṭrīq, whose work is known from a few other sources.[38]

---

35 J. Tytler (ed.), *Kitāb al-Fuṣūl li-Abuqrāṭ* (Calcutta 1832).

36 T. Mimura (ed.), *Tafsīr Jālīnūs li-Fuṣūl Abuqrāṭ* (ARABCOMMAPH/editions/Ḥunayn ibn Isḥāq (tr. Galen)/Galen commentaries books 1–7). For the final versions of the editions produced as part of the *Aphorisms* project see www.research.manchester.ac.uk/portal/en/researchers/peter-pormann(3822b0ae-23ba-4b2b-adcf-e635c052319a)/publications.html

37 M.T. Houtsma (ed.), *Ta'rīkh ibn abī Ya'qūb* (Leiden 1883), 107–16. Also see M. Klamroth, 'Über die Auszüge aus griechischen Schriftstellern bei al-Jaʿqūbī', *Zeitschrift der deutschen morgenländischen Gesellschaft* 40 (1886), 189–233 for some terminological comparisons between the versions of al-Biṭrīq and Ḥunayn. All citations herein of the early Arabic version of books three through seven of the *Aphorisms* derive from al-Yaʿqūbī's *History*.

38 Al-Biṭrīq is believed to have worked under the patronage of the ʿAbbāsid Caliph al-Manṣūr (d. 775). His better-known son Yaḥyā ibn al-Biṭrīq was responsible for some early philosophical translations into Arabic. See H. Biesterfeldt, 'Palladius on the Hippocratic Aphorisms' in C. d'Ancona (ed.), *Libraries of the Neoplatonists* (Leiden 2007), 388–9, as well as D.M. Dunlop, 'The Translations of al-Biṭrīq and Yaḥyā (Yuḥannā) b. al-Biṭrīq', *Journal of the Royal Asiatic Society* 91:3–4 (1959), 140–50 and C. Magdelaine, 'Le commentaire de Palladius aux *Aphorismes* d'Hippocrate et les citations d.al-Yaʿqūbī', in J. Jouanna and A. Garzya (eds), *Storia e Ecdotica dei testi medici* (Naples 2003), 321–34. Manfred Ullmann attributes the authorship of the early translation of the *Aphorisms* to al-Biṭrīq in the intial volume of his *Wörterbuch zu den griechisch-arabischen Übersetzungen des 9. Jahrhunderts* (Wiesbaden 2002–7), 52–3. See also idem., 'Die Tadhkira des ibn as-Suwaidi, eine wichtige Quelle zur

A second source for this translation appeared in the late twentieth century upon Hinrich Biesterfeldt's discovery of an Arabic translation of a late-Alexandrian commentary on the *Aphorisms* by a scholar of medicine named Palladius.[39] Given the identity between the translations of the lemmas in this text and those found in al-Yaʿqūbī's *History*, it is clear that the translator of this commentary and al-Yaʿqūbī at the least drew upon a common source. Although the manuscript presents some difficulties that have delayed its publication, for the purposes of this work it provides al-Biṭrīq's translation of the lemmas of the entire first book of the *Aphorisms* and some of the second.[40]

The Syriac-Arabic Lexicons

In the middle of the tenth century of the Christian era, Ḥasan bar Bahlul, a scholar and priest who wrote in Syriac and Arabic, composed a Syriac-Arabic lexicon compiled from the work of several older authorities. Edited and published by Rubens Duval in 1901 from several manuscripts, this tome represents one of the main sources for Syriac lexicography in general.[41] Beyond this general significance for Syriac studies, bar Bahlul's *Lexicon* is of specific importance for the history of the translation of Greek philosophy into Syriac and Arabic as well. This is due to several characteristics of the *Lexicon*, first among them bar Bahlul's extensive utilization of Ḥunayn ibn Isḥāq's Greek-Syriac-Arabic and Syriac-Arabic glossography and translations.[42] Furthermore, bar Bahlul's work preserves very many definitions of key philosophical terms of art that extend well beyond the mere listing of synonyms. At times these resemble

Geschichte der griechisch-arabischen Medizin und Magie', *Der Islam* 54 (1977), 33–65. This work is particularly important for the study of the *Aphorisms*. In it Ullmann considers several Arabic versions of the *Aphorisms*, including fragments and later *ad hoc* renditions outside of those that figure in the present work.

39 Biesterfeldt, 'Palladius on the Hippocratic Aphorisms', 388–9. This text is lost in the original Greek.

40 H. Biesterfeldt (ed.), *Sharḥ Kitāb al-Fuṣūl l-Aflidhus* (ARABCOMMAPH/ Hinrich Biesterfeldt Palladius Transcription/Palladius.pdf). This unpublished transcription was kindly provided to the Aphorisms project by the editor. Citations of the early Arabic versions of *Aphorisms* books one and two derive primarily from this source.

41 R. Duval (ed.), *Lexicon Syriacum auctore Hassano Bar-Bahlule* (Paris 1901).

42 Duval, *Lexicon*, xi. For a preliminary consideration of the relationship between bar Bahlul's *Lexicon* and Syriac and Arabic philosophical translation, see H. Hugonnard-Roche, 'L'intermédiaire syriaque dans la transmission de la philosophie grecque à l'arabe: le cas de l'*Organon* d'Aristote', *Arabic Sciences and Philosophy* 1:2 (September 1991), 198–200.

the entries of an encyclopaedia rather than the definitions of a dictionary. These longer entries are regularly written in Syriac, and so are valuable for the study of ʿAbbāsid-era Syriac intellectual life.

The *Syriac Lexicon* of Išoʿ bar ʿAli is also very important for the study both of the Syriac language and of the Greek-to-Arabic translation movement. The author of this lexicon was in all likelihood a student of Ḥunayn's who flourished in the late ninth century.[43] In his preface, the author mentions his reliance on the work of Ḥunayn and another scholar named al-Marwazī, who was himself also a student of Ḥunayn's.[44] The first volume, comprising the glosses for the letters *alep* to *mim*, was printed from a hand-written transcription prepared by the editor Georg Hoffmann in 1874.[45] The second half of the work was subsequently edited and published in two typeface volumes by Richard J.H. Gottheil.[46]

Due to its more abridged quality, bar ʿAli's *Lexicon* is of somewhat less significance for the Syriac intellectual history than is bar Bahlul's work. However, as will be shown below, the entries of bar ʿAli's *Lexicon* may be shown from time to time to represent Ḥunayn's Arabic translation choices more accurately even than do bar Bahlul's. Other points of interest may be made by citing it in various contexts.

Aims of the Work

On the basis of this material I undertake an extensive comparison of the terminology of the Syriac and Arabic translations of the *Aphorisms*. I do so from several perspectives in four chapters. In Chapter One, I consider the relationship between the Greek and Syriac lexicography in bar Bahlul's *Lexicon* on the one

43 A.M. Butts, 'The Biography of the Lexicographer Ishoʿ bar ʿAli', *Oriens Christianus* 93 (2009), 60–71.

44 Butts, 'Biography of the Lexicographer', 59–63. Although as Butts remarks 'it cannot be assumed that any given lemma found in the manuscript tradition is from the hand of Bar ʿAli himself' due to the evidence that later authors supplemented the work, as I will show in several places below significant overlap can often be found between the material in bar Bahlul's and bar ʿAli's lexicons as well as Ḥunayn's translations of the *Aphorisms*. As I will argue, these commonalities often should be considered strong evidence that the relevant material is derivative of Ḥunayn's lexicographical work.

45 G. Hoffmann (ed.), *Syrische-arabische Glossen: Autograph einer Gothaischen Handschrift enthaltend Bar ʿAli's Lexicon von Alif bis Mim* (Kiel 1874). The entries in this edition are numbered serially. For citations from this work, I therefore provide the page number followed by the entry number, thus: 10:1000.

46 R. Gottheil (ed.), *The Syriac-Arabic Glosses of Ishoʿ bar ʿAli* (Rome 1908–28).

hand and the Syriac and Arabic translations of the Hippocratic *Aphorisms* on the other. In making these comparisons I seek to determine two things. As mentioned above, bar Bahlul's *Lexicon* represents a compilation from several sources. Due to peculiarities in bar Bahlul's manner of citing his sources, which I detail below, the exact extent to which his *Lexicon* relied upon Ḥunayn's work is unclear. In the comparisons in the first chapter, then, I attempt to clarify this question. Following on from this, I shall assess the value of relevant Greek and Syriac lexicography for the study of Greek-to-Arabic translation.

In Chapter Two, I proceed to a more detailed treatment of Ḥunayn's translation techniques. I do this by focusing on his renditions of Greek words which in effect represent themselves in the Syriac *Aphorisms*. As I show, Syriac and Arabic adopted very different approaches to borrowing from the Greek. While such borrowing occurs relatively frequently in the Syriac version, it is extremely rare in the Arabic translation. The efforts made by Ḥunayn to avoid borrowing sometimes resulted in Arabic translations that explicate the sense of the Greek term in ways that can be creative and that shed light upon his translation praxis. Considering this category of terms also allows for the Greek lexicography contained in bar Bahlul's *Lexicon* to be more thoroughly considered.

In Chapters Three and Four I proceed to compare the four translations of the *Aphorisms* described above in the light of the ʿAbbāsid-era scholarly background as represented by the Syriac lexicons. Although these comparisons are organized around the more attenuated remains of the early Syriac and Arabic versions, by continuing to employ the methods of lexicographical comparison I regularly extend the discussions to consider the whole body of the *Aphorisms*. Although there is no strict division of subject-matter beyond this, Chapter Three tends to consider more strictly medical terminology, in particular disease-names, while Chapter Four tends more to treat theoretical and philosophical terminology. Finally, on the basis of these discussions, I consider the importance of Syriac sources for the main Arabic translations and the conclusions that may be drawn from them for the study of the broader Greek-to-Arabic translation movement.

Part One. The Syriac Lexicon of Bar Bahlul and the Syriac and Arabic Translations of the Hippocratic *Aphorisms*

Chapter 1

On the General Relationship Between Bar Bahlul's *Lexicon* and the Syriac and Arabic Translations of the *Aphorisms*

As discussed in the introduction, the lexicon of Ḥasan bar Bahlul is a very important source for the study of the history of Greek translation in the early ʿAbbāsid period. This work, compiled from several Syriac-Arabic lexicons, contains a large number of glosses written by some of the most important translators of philosophical and scientific works into Syriac and Arabic, including Ḥunayn ibn Isḥāq and Sergius of Reš ʿAynā among several others. Beyond Syriac, Arabic and Greek, many terms of Hebrew and Persian origin are defined in the *Lexicon.*[1] Religion, theology, philosophy, medicine and botany are only some of the subjects covered by the entries in the work.

Approaches to the Lexicographical Material

In his pathbreaking study *The Oriental Tradition of Paul of Aegina's* Pragmateia,[2] Peter E. Pormann developed techniques useful for the analysis of the entries of bar Bahlul's *Lexicon.* At the same time he clarified certain difficulties concerning the use of the *Lexicon* as a source for the translation movement.[3]

---

1 In the examples presented throughout, I have adopted the convention of referring to this work by the column and line of the entry presented, written in the text itself according to the following format: for 100:1, read column 100, line one. Citations from bar ʿAli's *Lexicon* will be given in the footnotes in the normal way.

2 P.E. Pormann, *The Oriental Tradition of Paul of Aegina's* Pragmateia (Leiden 2004).

3 Some of the conventions used in this work originate in Pormann's study, such as that of typing the translations of the Syriac elements of entries in plain face but the Arabic elements in italics. See Pormann, *Oriental Tradition*, 16 n. 20. Beyond these, I have introduced some new approaches. In Duval's edition, the first headword of every entry is set off in bold font from the rest of the entry's text. Because of this arrangement, at first glance it would appear that each entry defines solely the initial headword set off from the text in this manner, but this is not in fact the case. Although in general all of the headwords found under a given entry will be related to one another linguistically, strong and unpredictable variation in the authorship and subject matter of the entries is commonplace. In order to make this clear, I

Pormann's approach to the lexicographical material centred upon the identification of entries in the *Lexicon* defining terms derived from Greek and containing material attributed by bar Bahlul to Paul of Aegina, a seventh-century Alexandrian scholar of medicine whose work was important for the early Arabic medical tradition. Pauline material occurs with some frequency in the *Lexicon*, and furthermore the existence of Immanuel Löw's list of entries containing definitions attributed to Paul allowed Pormann to consider a significant number of terms.[4]

Despite sound beginnings, extension of Pormann's methods to the study of the material relevant to the broader translation movement has required some reconsideration of the editorial state of the *Lexicon*. In particular, an important oversight of the editor Duval's has made approaching the work somewhat difficult for succeeding generations of scholars. Duval made an impressive effort to locate and identify Greek terms in the lexicon. However, his index of Greek words remained arranged according to the place of the occurrence of the word in the lexicon, rather than being ordered alphabetically. This type of arrangement is not found in the following Syriac, Arabic and Persian indices, which are alphabetically ordered. For several reasons, including the character of Syriac transliteration of Greek words, often severe variations between conventions of transliteration, scribal errors and the relatively common placement of several Greek headwords within a single entry, systematic use of the Greek index in this state is impossible.

For this reason I have made an alphabetized list of the words represented in Duval's Greek index, which will be provided in an appendix to the present work. In the process I noticed that Duval's cross-referencing of his entries was not complete, so I have completed that task as a matter of course. Furthermore, alongside the Greek words for which Duval questioned his own attribution and those for which he did not hazard a guess, there is still ample room in my view to question and contest several of the attributions he

---

have placed all headwords in bold font regardless of their position in the entry. It is appropriate to mention here some further terminological distinctions concerning the *Lexicon*. In bar Bahlul's *Lexicon*, every entry consists of a headword or a series of headwords, each of which is given a definition. With only very rare exceptions, all of the headwords are written in Syriac characters, no matter the language of origin of the word in question.

4 I. Löw, 'Review of R. Payne Smith, *Thesaurus Syriacus*', *Zeitschrift der Deutschen Morgenländischen Gesellschaft* 47 (1893), 514–37.

made firmly. This is true especially when evidence from extant translations can be adduced, some examples of which I will give below.

Comparing the Lexicographical Material and the Translations

With Duval's Greek index now systematically accessible, I have proceeded to identify words which occur both in this index and in the Greek text of the Hippocratic *Aphorisms*. Although numerous Greek words identified by Duval in bar Bahlul's *Lexicon* are also present in the *Aphorisms*, these represent a definite minority of the words occurring in the latter work. Only about a third of the Greek words beginning with *alpha* in the Hippocratic work are also defined in the *Lexicon*. In systematically considering these entries, furthermore, this proportion suffers attrition due to various reasons. Some of these result from Duval's identifications, which at times are little more than guesses (as the editor regularly noted himself). Others may be proved incorrect with closer scrutiny, although this is relatively rare.

Studying the rendition of these words in the Syriac translation of the *Aphorisms*, I have separated out numerous terms represented in bar Bahlul's *Lexicon* that are in effect minimally Syriacized borrowings from Greek. These terms constitute the subject matter of Chapter Two below. Before proceeding to that material, however, in order to aid understanding of the relationship between the *Lexicon* and the translations in general, I wish to present entries for a range of Greek words that are rendered in the Syriac *Aphorisms* without recourse to the use of a borrowed Greek term. The material in the present chapter thus represents Greek words present in both the *Aphorisms* and bar Bahlul's *Syriac Lexicon* that begin with the letter *alpha*. Although this is something of an arbitrary selection, it has the advantage of providing a glimpse of the role of Greek scholarship in the translation of a range of concepts, including technical and non-technical words, and a variety of linguistic forms.

In considering this material I have focused particularly upon the relationships between the material in the lexicons and the translation equivalents given in the Syriac and Arabic versions of the *Aphorisms*. I have often supplemented these sources by reference to the translations cited in Manfred Ullmann's *Wörterbuch zu den griechisch-arabischen*

Übersetzungen des 9. Jahrhunderts.[5] These relationships can be used to provide firm answers to several outstanding questions regarding the role of Syriac in the Greek-to-Arabic translation movement.

Some of these questions are: How did Ḥunayn use Syriac in the production of his Arabic translations? How important was the Syriac scholarship undertaken prior to Ḥunayn, both for his Arabic and for his Syriac translations? Upon what methods did Ḥunayn's and other Syriac authors' lexicographical scholarship proceed? To what extent was this lexicography representative of or influential for the Arabic translations, and to what extent did the translators rely upon their glossaries in the production of the translations? Conversely, how well do the later compilations of bar Bahlul and bar ʿAli represent earlier stages of the translation movement? A fundamental question may be said to follow on the concern of Jourdain's quoted at the beginning of the Introduction: Was the Arabic translation of the *Aphorisms* performed on the basis of the original Greek text or rather on the basis of Ḥunayn's Syriac translation of the work?

Beyond the various characteristics that make it valuable for historical research into Greek-to-Arabic translation, bar Bahlul's *Lexicon* contains much material that well displays the independent reasoning and specific combinations of influence that gave ʿAbbāsid intellectual life its unique cast. For this reason, I have tended to give broad space to the entries rather than to restrict my treatments of them only to those elements which can positively be shown to relate directly to the translation movement. In doing so, I hope to demonstrate the value of this material beyond the confines of Graeco-Arabic studies, particularly for Syriac studies and ʿAbbāsid intellectual history more generally.

---

5 This lexicon provides extensive comparisons of the various techniques adopted by classical Arabic translators of Greek works. Ordered in the first instance according to the Greek alphabet, the terms to be treated are presented within their textual context along with the corresponding Arabic sentences in various translations. In what follows, I cite this work regularly for several different reasons. Perhaps most commonly, I use it to supplement the evidence from the early Arabic translation of the *Aphorisms*. Also, I refer to it in order to show the relationships obtaining between bar Bahlul's *Lexicon* and the broader translation literature. Where relevant, I discuss the characteristics of the various translations cited there.

The Authorship of the Entries of the Lexicon

Alongside these considerations, the fact that bar Bahlul included definitions written by several authors in his lexicon alongside his own material presents the student of the *Lexicon* with certain difficulties.[6] One goal of presenting the examples that follow is roughly to judge the frequency with which each author is referenced in the *Lexicon*, and to notice any patterns that the citations of individual authors follow. These tasks might seem straightforward at first, but they are complicated by the peculiar features of bar Bahlul's approach to referencing his authors. In particular, many of the definitions are not referred to any particular author. Yet these may not be assumed to have been written by bar Bahlul himself, for he writes in his prologue: 'For most of the terms contained in this lexicon whose author is not indicated, the text in them belongs to our teacher (*rabban*) Ḥunayn'.[7] For this reason I regularly refer to unattributed definitions as 'attributable to Ḥunayn', by which I intend to indicate the possibility that Ḥunayn did in fact write them. The degree of certainty with which any given unattributed definition may be attributed to Ḥunayn will be an important motif running through the entirety of this work.

Even for Henanišoʿ bar Serošway, an author whose name is more consistently referenced by bar Bahlul (although about whom little more is known), certain complications arise from bar Bahlul's account. Again in the prologue, bar Bahlul writes of this author: 'Henanišoʿ bar Serošway, the priest of Ḥirtā, whose lexicon is especially accurate, and fulfils Ḥunayn the physician'.[8] Following one possible interpretation of this statement, one might expect bar Serošway's material to overlap considerably with Ḥunayn's, thus providing further insight into the more-famous translator's glossographical activity. On the other hand, if bar Serošway's 'fulfilment' of Ḥunayn means primarily that the former writer tended to provide new information not mentioned by Ḥunayn, little insight into Ḥunayn's work will

---

6 For a full account of these authors, see the introduction to the edition of bar Bahlul's *Lexicon*, Duval, *Lexicon*, xiii–xxiv.

7 Duval, *Lexicon Syriacum*, xi. Ḥunayn's glossary at one time existed as an independent work, known as *Puššāq Šmāhē* 'The Interpretations of Names'. See U. Pietruschka, 'Puššāq šmāhē' und 'sullam': Mehrsprachige Wörterbücher bei Syrern und Kopten im arabischen Mittelalter', *Das Mittelalter* 2 (1997), 119–33.

8 Duval, *Lexicon Syriacum*, xi–xii.

be forthcoming from bar Serošway's glosses (although they will still provide interesting insight into tenth-century Syriac scholarship).

The situation regarding the material attributed by bar Bahlul to Paul of Aegina is perhaps even more confused. Pormann tentatively confirmed testimony in classical Arabic sources that Paul's *Pragmateia* was translated into Arabic by Ḥunayn by considering the extant texts of Paul's writing and certain entries attributed to Paul in bar Bahlul's *Lexicon*.[9] In the comparisons of the entries of Paul and Ḥunayn I make in the following chapters, two trends emerge that potentially complicate this narrative. In particular, in key instances the Arabic material attributed by bar Bahlul to Paul diverges significantly both from that attributed to Ḥunayn and from Ḥunayn's Arabic translations. Consideration of this material thus has the potential to extend our understanding of the Syriac-to-Arabic version of Paul's *Pragmateia.*

Despite all of these complexities, as I hope to show below, the Syriac lexicons produced by Ḥunayn's students and successors provide a wealth of interesting material that in general is highly relevant to the history of the Greek-to-Arabic translation movement. Continual reference to these entries provides valuable information regarding the scholarly background of these translations. At the same time it adds flesh to the otherwise spare remnants of the Syriac component of the process.

Greek Lexicography and Syriac Lexicography

By 'Greek lexicography', I intend the definitions of Greek words that either occur in the translations of the *Aphorisms* or that are related to them. By 'Syriac lexicography' I intend the entries in the lexicons for the Syriac equivalents of the Greek words as given in the Syriac *Aphorisms*. As a principle of organization, I have chosen to present the material according to the varying relationships observable between the Greek lexicography for a given word and Ḥunayn's translations of that word in his Arabic version of the *Aphorisms*.

In each section, I study several words in terms of the complex of lexicographical treatments and translation equivalents represented in the

9 This issue is discussed in several places in Pormann's book. For the traditional ascription of the authorship of the Pragmateia to Ḥunayn, see *Oriental Tradition*, 5. For summaries of the lexical and grammatical evidence, see ibid., 218–19 and 221, respectively.

Syriac and Arabic sources described in the Introduction. In the first section, I discuss words for which the relevant Greek-to-Arabic definitions in bar Bahlul's *Lexicon* agree better with Ḥunayn's Arabic translation equivalents in his Arabic version of the *Aphorisms* than do the Syriac-to-Arabic definitions in the *Lexicon* for the Syriac equivalents of those Greek words as given in the Syriac *Aphorisms*. In the second, I present words whose Syriac-to-Arabic definitions agree better with Ḥunayn's choices in his Arabic version of the *Aphorisms* than do the Greek-to-Arabic definitions in the *Lexicon*. In the third, I present words for which the Syriac and Greek definitions agree with Ḥunayn's Arabic choices to a more-or-less equal degree.

Syriac and Arabic Translations of Greek Words Beginning with *alpha* in the Hippocratic Aphorisms, with Reference to their Scholarly Background

Section One

As noted above, this first set of examples consists of Greek words whose entries in bar Bahlul's *Lexicon* agree more strongly with Ḥunayn's Arabic translations of these words in the *Aphorisms* than do the entries in the *Lexicon* for the words' Syriac equivalents as represented in the Syriac *Aphorisms*. This may be either because the Greek word is well-represented in the lexicons, or simply because the Syriac equivalent in the *Aphorisms* is absent from the lexicons entirely. In order to consider these complexes of definitions and translation equivalents, I begin by providing entries from bar Bahlul's *Lexicon* for the Greek word. I then proceed to discuss the various patterns observable in the renditions of that word in the several translations. Following this I consider the entries for the relevant Syriac words. These discussions will be supplemented by citations from other sources where appropriate.

1.1

ἁμαρτάνετε

181:18 ܐܡܪܛܐܢܗܛܗ ܚܛܘ اخطَوا ⁘

Amārṭānêṭê, they erred (*ḥṭaw*), *they erred* (akhṭaw).

Forms of the verb ἁμαρτάνω and the related noun ἁμάρτημα occur three times in the Hippocratic *Aphorisms*, all of them in aphorism i. 5. In each instance both al-Biṭrīq's and Ḥunayn's Arabic translations employ words derived from *khaṭi'a* 'to be mistaken' to translate these Greek words, while the Syriac translation gives words derived from *s<u>k</u>al* 'to make a mistake'. Regarding the second instance in the text there is some variation between the modern editions of the Greek original. Magdelaine includes this word, but Jones does not. Likewise in the translations under consideration here there is variation. Both Ḥunayn and the Arabic Palladius include this instance of the word, but the Syriac translation does not.

The Arabic and Syriac definitions given for ἁμαρτάνετε in the entry cited above from bar Bahlul's *Lexicon*, *ḥṭaw* and *ikhṭaw*, are etymologically related to one another and communicate broadly the same meaning, i. e. 'they erred'. While the Arabic gloss for ἁμαρτάνετε is related to the Arabic translations of ἁμαρτάνω in the *Aphorisms*, the Syriac gloss is not related to the equivalent found in the Syriac translation. Proceeding to consider the definitions in the lexicons for these two Syriac words, it is relatively clear that *ḥṭā* was more commonly associated with *khaṭi'a* than was *s<u>k</u>al* by the lexicographers. Here is an entry headed by the related word *sa<u>k</u>lā* 'fool':

1351:6 **ܣܟܠܐ** ܐܝܟ ܒܪ ܣܪܘ أحمق ܬܘܒ جاهل وأقول مايق غاوي سخيف. ܣܟ̈ܠܐ أقول سُخفاء. ܣܟܠܐ
ܡܢ ܝܘܠܦܢܗ. ܣܟܠܘܬܐ ܡܣܟܠܢܘܬܐ ܒܦܨ̈ܐ اساء. ܘܐܝܟ ܪܒܢ اساءة. ܡܣܟܠܢܘܬܐ ܕܒܥܠܘܒܝܘܬܐ ܗܝ
ܥܠܘܒܘܬܐ ܘܒܥܘܠܐ ܘܒܛܠܘܡܝܘܬܐ ܘܚܛܘܦܝܐ ܘܐܚܪ̈ܢܝܬܐ ܕܐܝܟ ܗܠܝܢ الجهالة الذنب الاساءة܀

Sa<u>k</u>lā according to bar Serošway, *a fool,* also *an ignoramus, and I say senseless, erroneous, a simpleton. Sa<u>k</u>lē I say, simpletons.* A fool for (all) his learning. Folly (*sa<u>k</u>lu<u>t</u>ā*), iniquity (*masklānu<u>t</u>ā*), in a manuscript *offence* (isā') and according to our teacher *offence* (isā'a). Iniquity (*masklānu<u>t</u>ā*) is through oppression and through injustice and rapine, and (according to) others the like of this, *ignorance, sin, offence.*

The following three entries define words related to the Syriac equivalent *ḥṭaw* given in bar Bahlul's entry at 181:18:

739:14 **ܚܛܐ** اخطأ. **ܚܛܐ** يخطي܀

Ḥṭā, he made a mistake (akhṭa'a). *Ḥṭē, he is making a mistake* (yukhṭī).

739:26 **ܚܛܗܐ** خطأ. **ܚܛܝܬܐ** خطيّة ܘܐܝܟ ܐܚܪܢܐ ذنب. **ܚܛܗ̈ܐ** ذنوب. ܒܪ ܣܪܘ **ܚܛܗ̈ܐ** ܕܡ ܒܥܘܡܗ
ܠܕܚܢܬܐ ܡܛܠ ܕܚܠܦ ܚܛܗܐ ܡܬܦܪܥ ܐܝܟ ܕܐܡܠ ܐܚܪܢܐ. **ܚܛܗܐ ܘܡܘܬܐ** خطيّة الزمان. **ܚܛܗܐ**

ܕܡܬܬܚܝܕܝܢ ܒܗܘܢ ܡ̈ܠܝܠܐ ܒܬܠܬܐ ܐ̈ܦܝܐ ܡܬܐܡܪܝܢ. ܐܘ ܒܡܠܬܐ ܚܛܝܢ. ܐܝܟ ܕܓܠܘܬܐ[10]
ܘܡܐܟܠܩܪ̈ܨܐ ܘܫܘܩ̈ܦܐ ܕܐܚܪ̈ܢܐ. ܐܘ ܒܣܘܥܪ̈ܢܐ. ܐܝܟ ܩܛܠܐ ܘܙܢܝܘܬܐ ܘܓܢܒܘܬܐ. ܐܘ
ܒܡܚܫܒ̈ܬܐ ܕܐܡܝܢ ܓܪܓ ܠܗ̇ ܠܪܡܘܬܐ. ܘܠܪܘܓܙܐ. ܘܪܚܡܬ ܟܣܦܐ. ܐܝܟ ܕܐܦ ܚܝ̈ܠܐ ܕܢܦܫܐ ܬܠܬܐ.
ܡܠܝܠܘܬܐ. ܘܨܒܝܢܐ. ܘܪܘܓܙܐ❖

*Ḥṭāhā, mistake (*khaṭa'*).* *Ḥṭiṯā, lapse* (khaṭī'a), and according to Zakariya, *sin* (dhanb). (According to) bar Serošway sacrifices are called *ḥṭāhā* because they are offered on account of sins, as if I had eaten [them]. *Ḥṭāhā yawmānā, faults of the time* (khaṭī'a al-zamān). Sins (*ḥṭāhē*) by which rational creatures are seized are expressed in three ways — for either they sin by means of words, such as lying, slander and other accusations, or by acts like murder, fornication and theft, or by thoughts which constantly excite pride, wrath and avarice — just as the powers of the soul are three: reason, will and appetite.

741:6 ܚܛܝܢܐ ذنوب. ܘܐܝܟ ܒܪ ܣܪܘܫܘܝ ܚܛܝܢܐ ܚܛ̈ܗܐ الخطايا. ܚܛܝܢܐ ܒܟܬܒ ܕܦܪܕ. ܚܛܝܬܐ ܕܒܪܐܝܬ
ܒܐܦܢ ܚܛ̈ܗܐ ܕܟܪܐ. ܚܛܝܬܐ ܐܝܬܝܗ̇ ܗܢܝܢܐ ܙܥܘܪܐ ܕܡܪܝܒ ܚܫܐ ܢܓܝܪܐ ܘܗܝ ܒܢܡܘܣܐ
ܡܬܚܝܒ الخطيّة. ܚܛܝܘܬܐ ܐܝܬܝܗ̇ ܣܘܓܐܐ ܕܨܒ̈ܘܬܐ ܕܥܒܪܝܢ ܦܘܩܕܢܐ. ܘܫܡܐ ܗܘ ܓܢܣܢܝܐ ܕܟܠ
ܐܝܟ ܓܢܣܐ ܠܟܠܗܘܢ ܙܢ̈ܝܐ ܕܚܛ̈ܗܐ ܠܘܬ ܐܠܗܐ ܘܠܘܬ ܒܢܝܢܫܐ الخطايا. ܚܛܝܬܐ ܗ̇
ܓܢܣܐ ܐܝܬܝܗ̇ ܕܟܠܗܘܢ ܣܥܘܪ̈ܢܐ ܡܬܚܝ̈ܒܢܐ ܘܐܝܬܝܗ̇ ܥܒܪ ܢܡܘܣܐ ܕܣܝܡ ܒܟܝܢܐ. ܘܒܟܬܒ ܕܦܪܕ.
الخطيّة. ܚܛܝܐ ܗܘ ܕܨܒܝܢܗ ܡܛܝܒ ܒܟܠܗ ܙܒܢ ܠܡܣܥܪܘ ܒܝܫܬܐ الخاطي❖

*Ḥṭyānā, sins (*dhunūb*)*, and according to bar Serošway, *heṭyānā*, sins, *errors*. *Ḥeṭyānā* in the *Book of Paradise*, sin (*ḥṭiṯā*), and less regularly as a masculine it is *ḥṭāhē*. *Ḥṭiṯā* is profit benefiting little (but) causing lengthy suffering, and is by the law condemned, *error*. Sinfulness (*ḥaṭāyuṯā*) is a multitude of things, (all of) which trangress a commandment. This name generally comprises as a class all types of transgressions, both those that relate to God and those that relate to mankind, *error*. Sin (*ḥṭiṯā*), this is a class that (includes) all blameworthy acts that transgress the law established in nature. In the *Book of Paradise*, *error*. The sinner (*ḥaṭāyā*) is one whose will is prepared at all times to accomplish evil, *sinner (*al-khāṭī*)*.

Both the Arabic translations and the evidence from bar Bahlul diverge significantly from the Syriac translation of the *Aphorisms*. However, the Syriac entries contain material that qualifies this discrepancy to a certain extent. Although the authors did not include any word related to *khaṭi'a* under the entry for *saḵlā*, it is relatively clear that the sense of that Arabic verb overlaps with those of both of these Syriac words (as does the Greek itself). This somewhat broader sense of *khaṭi'a* may be contrasted with the

10 Duval: ܕ. ܓܠܘܬܐ. The form used here in Duval's edition can only mean 'such as a cloak' (*ayk d-gulṯā*), so I have amended the text.

apparently narrower idiomatic sense of the related Syriac word *ḥṭā*, which according to the evidence in the *Lexicon* has a strongly legal connotation. Perhaps prompted by the close etymological relationship between *ḥṭā* and *khaṭi'a*, the Syriac lexicographers preferred to associate these two terms with one another, while tending less to associate the latter with *saklā*. When faced with a secular sense of ἁμαρτάνω such as those which occur in the *Aphorisms*, however, the broader sense of *khaṭi'a* allowed it to be employed in translation, while the narrower sense of *ḥṭā* could have suggested the choice of a different word.

It is nonetheless the case that the Greek entry relates more strongly to Ḥunayn's Arabic translation than does the entry for the equivalent given in the Syriac *Aphorisms*. Given that the definitions of the Greek word as well as many of the definitions of the Syriac word are left unattributed and are thus attributable to Ḥunayn, this discrepancy would seem to constitute evidence, albeit heavily qualified, against Ḥunayn's authorship of the Syriac version. Besides this, it should be noted that the entry for ἁμαρτάνετε clearly refers to the Greek language and not to a Syriac loan-word from Greek. However, while Duval did follow faithfully the transcription of the entry in his identification of the Greek term as the second-person plural imperfect, the Arabic and Syriac definitions are clearly third-person plural perfect forms. This would appear to indicate a weakness in the Greek lexicography, or at least in its transmission.

1.2

ἄνυδρος

209:12 ܐܢܝܘܕܪܘܣ ܒܪ ܣܪܘ̈ ܗ̄ ܡܚܣܪܬ ܡܢ ܡܝܐ عديمة الماء

Anyudros, bar Serošway, this is lacking water, lacking water.

In aphorism iii. 14, ἄνυδρος is used to characterize the season of autumn. Ḥunayn's Arabic translates it with *yābis* 'dry', while the Syriac gives *gliz men meṭrā* 'deprived of rain'. The previous three aphorisms also describe various seasons as dry, but employ the Greek word αὐχμηρός instead. The only occurrences of that word in the work are in those three aphorisms, and it is not represented in bar Bahlul's *Lexicon.* The Syriac version's translations of these three are identical to its translation of ἄνυδρος, i. e. *gliz men meṭrā* 'deprived of rain'. Ḥunayn's Arabic, however, differentiates between the two, translating αὐχμηρός with *qalīl min al-maṭar* 'having little rain' in each case. Ḥunayn's interpretation would seem to be that ἄνυδρος describes a more extreme condition than does αὐχμηρός. This distinction is absent from the Syriac version.

Bar Serošway's entry in bar Bahlul's *Lexicon* displays bi-lingual equivalence, but neither the Arabic nor the Syriac translations of the *Aphorisms* are reflected in it explicitly. However, none of the Syriac lexicography contains any material that could be considered relevant at all. Some of these entries run as follows:

494:23 ܓܳܠܶܙ يمنع⁘

Gālez, he obstructs.

496:2 ܓܠܝܙܘܬܐ عَدَم فقد. ܓܠܝܙܐ ܐܝܟ ܙܟܪܝܐ فقيد عديم. ܓܳܠܘܙܐ المانع وأقول السالب... ܓܠܝܙܐ معدوم ممنوع⁘

Glizuṯā, nonexistence, loss. Glizā, according to Zakariya *one lost, one wanting. Gālozā, preventing, and I say negative* (al-sālib)*... Glizā, nonexistent, forbidden.*

Although the definitions for these Syriac words have certain elements in common with the Greek entry, nothing in them gives any specific insight into Ḥunayn's Arabic translation of the term in the *Aphorisms.* Perhaps this is because the concision of the Greek negating prefix α- was only carried over into the Syriac translation by means of an extended phrase rather than a single word, thus making its representation in the lexicographical literature less straightforward. While none of the translations from the *Aphorisms* are represented in the entry for the Greek word, it does makes the sense clear in a general way, and so better relates to Ḥunayn's Arabic translation than do the Syriac entries. Thus it may be said that, for Greek words which as a rule were translated into Syriac by means of phrases rather than by single equivalents, it can sometimes be difficult to point to a clearly relevant correspondence in the Syriac lexicography.

Again in this case, we observe important discrepancies in interpretation between Ḥunayn's Arabic version and the Syriac translation. Thus, despite the above qualifications, it is entirely possible that the Syriac lexicography does not represent Ḥunayn's translation for the simple fact that Ḥunayn preferred a different word in his Syriac version. It also is possible that the discrepancy is due to the fact that Ḥunayn relied only upon the Greek text in his composition of his Arabic version of the *Aphorisms*.

1.3

αὐτόματον

57:18 ܐܘܛܘܡܘܛܘܢ ܒܨ̈ ܕܡܢ ܨܒܘܬ ܢܦܫܗ من ذاته من قبل نفسه ܐܚܪ̈ܢܐ ܐܘܛܘܡܘܛܘܣ من ذاته
من تلقا نفسه ܘܐܝܟ ܒܪ ܣܪܘ ܫܓܡܐ توليد لا أصل له܀

Awṭomoṭon in a manuscript, of its own accord, *by itself* (min dhātih), *of its own causing (*min qibal nafsih*)*. (In) others, *awṭomaṭos*, *by itself, of its own accord* (min tilqā nafsih). According to bar Serošway, chance, *born without any cause* (tawlīd lā aṣla lah).

58:1 ܐܘܛܘܡܐܛܘܢ من قبل نفسه܀

Awṭomāṭon, of its own causing (min qibal nafsih).

58:2 ܐܘܛܡܐܛܝܣܛܐ ܐܝܟ ܚܢܝܢ ܒܢ̈ܝ ܗܘ ܝܘܠܦܢܐ ܕܒܝܬ ܐܦܝܩܘܪܘܣ ܕܐܡܪܝܢ ܕܟܠܡܕܡ ܒܫܓܡܐ
ܘܕܠܐ ܒܛܝܠܘܬܐ ܪܕܐ ܘܡܢ ܐܘܛܘܡܐܛܘܢ ܫܪܐ ܗܘ ܡܢ ܨܒܘܬ ܢܦܫܗ يعني كل شيء لا يكون له أصل
بل يصدر من الإنسان إقتداء من ذاته܀

Awṭāmaṭisṭo,[11] according to Ḥunayn, those who held to the doctrine of the school of Epicurus, saying that everything occurs by chance, proceeds without forethought, and begins *awṭomaṭon*, that is, of its own accord. *It means everything that has no cause, but occurs in people spontaneously by itself* (iqtidā' min dhātih).

106:18 ܐܛܘܡܐܛܘܢ ܒܨ̈ ܫܓܡܐ ܐܘܟܝܬ ܡܕܡ ܕܗܘ ܡܢ ܨܒܘܬ ܢܦܫܗ ܗܘܐ ܘܐܝܟ ܣܪ ܠ ܠܐ
ܡܬܦܠܓܢܐ قائم بذاته غير منفصل شيء منهم يقوم من تلقاء نفسه ܐܚܪ̈ܢܐ ܕܡܢ ܢܦܫܗ ܩܐܡ ܠܥܠܡܐ ܐܘ
ܡܢ ܨܒܘܬ ܢܦܫܗ܀

Aṭomāṭon in a manuscript, chance (*šegmā*), that is, something that occurs of its own accord (*men ṣḇoṯ nefešeh*). According to Sergius, indivisible. *That which occurs by itself without being connected to anything else (*ghayr munfaṣil shay' minhum*), occurring of its own accord.* (According to) others, that which occurs by itself, is eternal, or is of its own accord.

The adjective αὐτόματος occurs six times in the *Aphorisms* in various forms. The Syriac version translates all of them according to the same general rule, using some form of *men ṣḇoṯ nefešeh* 'of its own accord' in each case. Ḥunayn's Arabic on the other hand shows marked variation. Thrice it gives a form of *min tilqā' nafsihi* 'of its own accord'. The other three cases are each translated uniquely according to the translator's understanding of the sense of the text. Thus in aphorism i. 2 *ṭaw'an* 'spontaneously' is found, in ii. 5 *alladhī lā yu'rafu lahu sabab* 'that which

11 Duval identifies this as a transcription of the Greek αὐτοματισταί. Discussion of the word αὐτόματος follows, but the entire entry is of interest.

has no known cause' is given, and in iv. 78 *'an ghayri shay' mutaqaddim* 'without anything preceding' is employed.

Two examples of translations of this word are found in the early Arabic version of the *Aphorisms*. Both instances translate with *ṭaw'an* 'spontaneously', including its version of aphorism i. 2. Here, Ḥunayn's version and the early Arabic version bear at least a superficial resemblance to one another. Ullmann notices other variations as well. In one example from Galen's *On Simple Drugs* Book 10, *min tilqā' nafsihī* 'of its own accord' is used. In another example from Galen's *On the Properties of Foodstuffs*, the phrase *min nafsihī* 'of itself' is employed.[12] Finally, the translation of Aristotle's *History of Animals* employs another different form, *min dhātihī* 'of itself', in the context of the description of a disease.[13]

Of these various translations, all except *ṭaw'an* 'spontaneously' and *min nafsihī* 'of itself' are represented in the Greek entries in the *Lexicon*. Several prominent definitions remain absent from the literature surveyed here, however, in particular the Arabic *min qibali nafsihī* 'of its own causing', which stands by itself in the entry at 58:1, and the Syriac *šegmā* 'chance'. A definition for *ṣḇoṯ nefešeh* also occurs in bar Bahlul's *Lexicon*:

1653:1 **ܨܒܘܬ ܢܦܫܗ** ܗ̄ ܡܢ ܨܒܘܬ ܢܦܫܗ ܒܨܚ̈ من تلقاء نفسه܀

Ṣḇoṯ nefešeh ('its own accord'), this is of its own accord (*men ṣḇoṯ nefešeh*). In a manuscript, *of its own accord* (min tilqā' nafsih).

An entry for the Syriac equivalent *šegmā* in bar Bahlul's *Lexicon* reads as follows:

1934:8 **ܫܓܡܐ** مُبهَم باطل. أقول كما يجي باتّفاق سهو܀

Šegmā, unintelligible, false. I say as it has been agreed upon, negligent.

Another in bar ʿAli's *Lexicon* gives some more relevant information:

ܫܓܡܐ ܕܠܐ ܦܘܪܫܢܐ. على الإطلاق من غير تفصيل. مُبهم. آخر باطل جزاف.[14]

Šegmā, without discrimination, *unrestrictedly, without measure. Unintelligible, also false, at random.*

12 For a detailed analysis of the various Syriac and Arabic translations of this work, see Pormann, 'The Development of Translation Techniques', *passim*.

13 Ullmann, *Wörterbuch zu den grechische-arabischen Übersetzungen*, 148.

14 Gottheil (ed.), *Syriac-Arabic Glosses*, II 411:3

The robust combination of lexicographical equivalents and theoretical discussion in the Greek entries may be contrasted with the slightness of the Syriac entries. The most common Arabic equivalent for αὐτόματος in the *Aphorisms* does appear in the Syriac entry for *ṣbo̱ṯ nefešeh*. However, both that equivalent and the translation given in Ullmann's citation of the Arabic *History of Animals* occur in the Greek entries. As well, several more detailed explanations of the term in the Greek entries are quite similar to Ḥunayn's explicating translations cited above, although they are not perfectly identical to them. As in the case of the translations of ἄνυδρος in the previous section, it may be that the most obvious explanation for these differences is that the standard Syriac equivalent for the Greek term αὐτόματος was a prepositional phrase as opposed to a single word. Whatever the reason for this, the strong variation between Ḥunayn's Arabic translation and the Syriac version constitutes evidence against the famous translator's authorship of the latter work.

Section Two

This section includes words for which the Syriac lexicography of bar Bahlul's *Lexicon* agrees better with Ḥunayn's Arabic translations than does the Greek lexicography.

2.1

ἀγαθός/ἀγαθά/ἀγαθοῦ

22:26 ܐ ܐܓܛܝܐ خير صالح خيرة صالحة⁘

Agaṯya, good (khayr), *good* (ṣāliḥ), *good* (khayra), *good* (ṣāliḥa).

22:27 ܐܓ ܐܓܐܛܐܘܣ صالح⁘

*Agaṯaus, good (*ṣāliḥ*)*.

24:8 ܐܓ ܐܓܗܘ ܐܝܟ ܒܪ ܣܪܘ ܛܒܐ خير⁘

Aghew according to bar Serošway good (*ṭāḇā*), *good* (khayr).

33:17 ܐܓ ܐܓܐܛܘܣ ܐܝܟ ܪܒܢ ܛܒܐ ܘܐܝܟ ܒܪ ܣܪܘ الخير التقى الصالح⁘

Agāṯos according to our teacher, good (*ṭāḇā*), and according to bar Serošway *good* (al-khayr), *piety* (al-tuqā*)*, *good* (al-ṣāliḥ).

Forms of this adjective occur numerous times in the *Aphorisms*. In general, Ḥunayn's Arabic translations of the word display a higher degree of variation than do the Syriac translations. The Syriac invariably translates with a form of either *ṭāḇ* 'good' or *šappir* 'fine'. Although the most common word used by Ḥunayn is *maḥmūd* 'praiseworthy' in its several forms, he employs other terms and phrases as well.

A certain division of technique occurs in some of Ḥunayn's Arabic translations of this word. For several instances of ἀγαθός that occur in the first four books of the *Aphorisms*, Ḥunayn added the word *'alāmatun* 'sign' to the translation without there being any corresponding Greek word in the source-text.[15] However, in several instances from the second half of the work, the synonomous term *dalīl* is found in a similar fashion.[16] The latter examples also display a strong tendency toward grammatical extension, especially in vi. 11, where five words are used to translate the single Greek adjective. While we do know from his *Risāla* that Ḥunayn translated Galen's *Commentary on the Aphorisms* into Arabic in multiple stages,[17] the variation between these translations of ἀγαθός in the first and second halves of the Hippocratic lemmas does not fit with the details of that account.[18]

The Greek lexicography does not extend very far beyond the listing of synonyms. While the Syriac definition *ṭāḇā* is also the most common translation in the *Aphorisms*, the Arabic definitions show very little overlap with Ḥunayn's Arabic translations of ἀγαθός. A form of the word *ṣāliḥ* 'sound' does translate ἀγαθός once, in aphorism ii. 2. Although the word

---

15 For example, in aphorism ii. 2, where he translated ἀγαθόν used as a predicate adjective with the phrase *fa-tilka 'alāmatun ṣāliḥa* 'then that is a good sign'.

16 For example, in aphorism vi. 11, where the bare predicate adjective ἀγαθόν is translated *kāna dhālika dalīlan maḥmūdan fīhim* 'that is a praiseworthy indication for them'.

17 Ḥunayn writes that he translated the first book of Galen's *Commentary on the Aphorisms* for one patron, and subsequently was asked to translate the rest for another. Bergsträsser (ed.), *Syrische und arabische Galen-Übersetzungen*, ٤٠.

18 The division defined by these translations of ἀγαθός occurs after the fourth book. The last occurrence of the word *'alāmatun* in translations of that Greek word is found in aphorism iv. 25, following occurrences of it in aphorisms ii. 2 and ii. 33. The first occurrence of the word *dalīl* in these translations is in aphorism vi. 11, following which it is also found in aphorisms vi. 37, vii. 5, vii. 41, and vii. 49. Ḥunayn's account of his Arabic translation of Galen's *Commentary on the Aphorisms* states that he translated the first section in one stage, then at a later stage translated the rest of the work. Since this account refers to Galen's *Commentary* and not necessarily to the lemmas themselves, it may not be of great relevance to this study in any respect. The pattern observed here clearly does not derive from the periodical translation mentioned in Ḥunayn's *Risāla*.

khayr 'good' does not translate ἀγαθός in the *Aphorisms*, the latter word is noted by Ullmann in quotations from the Arabic *Sentences of Menander*.[19]

A definition relevant to the Syriac equivalent *ṭāḇ* reads as follows:

785:7 ܛܳܒܳܐ خير صالح جواد. ܙܟ̈ܐ المختار من الشيء. ܛܳܒܽܘܬܳܐ جودة خيرورة صلاح. ܛܳܒ جيّد.
ܛܳܒ ما أحسن ويكون جيداً[20]...܀

Ṭāḇā, *good* (khayr), *good* (ṣāliḥ), *good* (jawād). (According to) Zakariya, *the choice part of something. Ṭāḇuṯā*, *goodness* (jūda), *goodness* (khayrūra), *a good condition* (ṣalāḥ). *Ṭāḇ*, *good* (jayyid). *Ṭāḇ*, *that which is very good* (mā aḥsanu wa-yakūnu jayyidan).

In these Syriac-to-Arabic definitions, Ḥunayn's translation choices in the *Aphorisms* are better represented. Although his preferred equivalent to ἀγαθός, *maḥmūd*, is noticeably still absent, the prominence of *jayyid* and related words make the Syriac lexicography more fully representative of Ḥunayn's translation technique than the Greek lexicography.

2.2

ἀγωγή

24:12 ܐܓܘܓܐ ܡܠܘܠܐ بربخ الماء ومجرى. ܐܓܘܓܐ ܐܝܟ ܒܪ ܣܪܘܫܘܝ ܢܗܪܘܪܐ نهير ܐܘܪܚܐ
ܕܡܝܐ[21] ܬܘܒ أنابيب قنى. ܐܓܘ̈ܓܐ ܐܝܟ ܚܢܝܢ ܒܝ̈ܒܐ ܘܡܬܟܬܒܐ ܒܘܒܝܐ أنواب مجرى وزاد
المروزي قناة الماء آخر ميزاب بربخ. ܐܓܘ̈ܓܐ قنى الماء مثاعب مجاري الماء. ܐܓܘܓܐ
ܘܩܕ̈ܝܢܐ ܐܝܟ ܒܪ ܣܪܘܫܘܝ مجارٍ ومخاريق في الارض܀

Agogā, drain, *drain of water, channel. Agogā*, according to bar Serošway a rivulet, *a rivulet*, path of water. Again, *pipes, ducts. Agogē* according to Ḥunayn channels (*biḇē*), also written *buḇyā, pipes, a channel. Al-Marwazī adds ducts of water, also a drain pipe, a channel. Agogē, ducts of water, drains, channels of water. Agogā wa-qāḏinā* (channels and watercourses) according to bar Serošway, *channels and cisterns*[22] *in the earth.*

A form of this Greek word occurs a single time in the *Aphorisms*. In aphorism v. 28, the phrase γυναικείων ἀγωγὸν 'the flow of women', in the sense of menstruation, was translated by Ḥunayn with *al-dam alladhī yajī'*

19 Ullmann, *Wörterbuch zu den griechisch-arabischen Übersetzungen*, 65.

20 Duval: جدا.

21 Duval writes here the single word ܐܘܪܚܐ (adding [*sic*]), following three manuscripts. Two other manuscripts give the reading I have employed, the sense of which is much easier.

22 Although Freytag gives definitions for this word, none of them fit the sense needed here. I proceed on the conjecture that this form *al-makhārīq* is a plural of the word *al-makhraq*, defined by Freytag *lapis in cisternae fundo e quo aqua emittur*, but for which he gives no plural form.

min al-nisā' 'the blood that comes forth from women', and by the Syriac translator with *dmā nešāyā* 'the blood of the woman'. Both of these translations make explicit the information implicit in the Greek phrase, although they are stylistically distinct.

An entry for the Syriac term *dmā* reads like this:

579:8 **ܕܡܐ** الدم ܟܝܡܘܣ ܪܛܝܒܐ ܘܫܚܝܢܐ ܕܐܝܬܘܗܝ ܨܘܪܬܗ ܡܢܐܝܬ ܡܢ ܐܣܛܘܟܣܐ ܕܐܐܪ

ܘܐܝܬܘܗܝ ܒܟܒܕܐ ܘܚܝܠܗ ܒܟܠܗ ܦܓܪܐ الدم܀

Dmā, blood, a wet and hot humour whose form derives properly from the element of air. It comes to be in the liver (*i̱taw b-ḵaḇdā*) and its power is in the entire body, *blood* (al-dam).

Although the relationships between the translations and the *Lexicon* are obscured by the fact that both the Greek original and the translations employ phrases to represent the concept in question, the supposedly Greek entry in fact refers to an etymologically-Greek Syriac term that has undergone significant modification in the latter tongue. This hints at a broader problem facing the study of the influence of Greek upon Syriac literature and philosophy. While a large number of borrowings from Greek into Syriac occurred, the conceptual ranges of these borrowings may differ significantly from those of their Greek antecedents. Although there is no specific entry for the equivalent Syriac phrase, the entry for *dmā* thus relates better to Ḥunayn's Arabic translation than does the entry for ἀγωγή.

2.3

αἰδοῖον

602:12 ܗܐܝܗܐܘܢ ܘܠܚܢܐ القضيب من الفحل܀

Hayêon, penises, *the penis of the male.*

Forms of this word occur twice in the *Aphorisms*. A distinct translation is used in each of these instances both in Ḥunayn's Arabic version and in the Syriac translation. In aphorism iii. 21, for the phrase σηπεδόνες αἰδοίων 'mortification of the genitals', Ḥunayn used *'afan fī al- furūj* 'putrification in the vulva' while the Syriac version gives *masyuṯā daḇ-maḥsānē* 'decay in the private parts'. For the second occurrence, in aphorism v. 22, Ḥunayn gives *al-farj* 'vulva' while the Syriac gives *qanyā* 'penis'.

The difference of interpretation between the Arabic and Syriac versions in aphorism v. 22 is striking. Whereas the Greek term may refer to the private parts of either gender, both the Arabic and Syriac terms employed here have etymological associations which clearly specify to which gender they refer:

al-farj literally means 'breach', while *qanyā* means 'rod'. This discrepancy thus is a further piece of evidence that the two translations were written by different authors.

The Greek entry in bar Bahlul's *Lexicon* does not correspond with the translations of the *Aphorisms*, especially given that Ḥunayn preferred to interpret αἰδοῖον with reference to female rather than male anatomy in both instances of the word in that work. An entry for the Syriac term *maḥsānē* is to be found in the *Lexicon* as follows:

1056:18 ܡܚܣܢܘܗܝ ܕܡܘܐܒ ܢܩܥܘܢ ܗ̄ عانة مواب تصيح تضجّ. ܡܚܣܢܐ ܘܐܙܒܐ ܐܝܟ ܒܪ ܣܪܘ̈ الحالبان الازبّ العانة الشعرة. ܣܦܘܬܐ ܕܡܚܣܢܐ ܒܟܬ̄ ܕܦܪܕ̈ ܐܡܪܝܢ ܕܬܚܬܝܬܗ ܗܝ ܕܟܪܣܐ العانة الفرج الحالبان܀

Maḥsānaw d-Mo'ab naq'un, this is *the loins of Moāb cry, shout.*[23] *Maḥsānē w-ezbē* ('the loins and the genitals') according to bar Serošway, *the hairy area around the loins,* (al-ḥālibān al-azabb),[24] *the hirsute loins. Sipwātē ḏ-maḥsānē* ('lips of the loins') *in the Book of Paradise*, they say the lower part of the abdomen, *pubes, vulva* (al-farj), *ureters.*

Although its attribution to Ḥunayn is somewhat difficult given its occurrence in close proximity to a Syriac definition from the *Book of Paradise*, the Arabic equivalent *al-farj* does occur in this entry. Thus the Syriac entry better corresponds with Ḥunayn's approach to translating αἰδοῖον in his version of the *Aphorisms*. Although the Greek entry is attributable to Ḥunayn, it clearly did not serve as his reference in the process of translating the *Aphorisms* into Arabic.

2.4

ἀκμή

276:13 ܐܩܡܐ ܡܫܘܚܬܐ. ܐܩܡ̈ܐ ܡܫܘ̈ܚܬܐ [*sic*][25] ܒܐ صنوف فنون أقران. ܘܐܝܟ ܒܪ ܣܪܘ̈ قامة: ܐܩܡܐ ܕܚܝܐ قامة لحياة ܒܐ السنّ܀

Aqmā, age. *Aqmē,* ages. In a manuscript, *types, varieties, peers.* According to bar Serošway, *stature. Aqmā ḏ-ḥayyē, stature of life.* In a manuscript *age* (al-sinn).

Forms of ἀκμή and the related verb ἀκμάζω occur six times in the *Aphorisms*. In all of these instances Ḥunayn's Arabic translation employs a

23 Isa. 15:4.

24 This word is somewhat obscure. The most obvious sense in the dictionaries would be 'umbilical veins'.

25 This is an abnormal plural. According to Payne-Smith the regular forms are ܡܫܘ̈ܚܬܐ and ܡܫܘ̈ܚܢ.

form of the word *al-muntahā*, while the Syriac gives a form of *'uzzā*, both meaning 'limit'. Al-Biṭrīq's translations of these words in aphorisms i. 8, i. 9, i. 10 and ii. 29 also exist. These exhibit greater variation than do Ḥunayn's. In the first two, the translator translated with a form of *al-ziyāda* 'increase'. For both of the instances of ἀκμή in i. 10, however, he translated with *muntahā marḍihim*, as did Ḥunayn. In aphorism ii. 29, which concerns the use of medicines at different stages of a disease, the early translator uses another different phrase. There, ἀκμάζω is found in the participial form ἀκμαζουσῶν 'at the apex' (of the disease). Al-Biṭrīq translated this with *in sa'idat al-'illa* 'if the disease rises', while Ḥunayn translated it with *iḏā ṣāra al-maraḍ ilā muntahāhu* 'when the disease comes to its utmost limit'.

Along with his citation of this example, Ullmann notes the use of *muntahā* for ἀκμή from both of these authors in their translations of Galen's *On Simple Drugs* Book Six.[26] Thus, while the early translator did know *al-muntahā* to be a possible equivalent to ἀκμή, he was also capable of using other, broadly synononomous translations. Ḥunayn's preference, however, appears to have been to use *al-muntahā* in a more standardized fashion, even when to do so required significant expansion relative to the source-text.

Nothing in the Greek entry in bar Bahlul's *Lexicon* relates to the translations given. An entry for the Syriac equivalent *'uzzā* runs as follows:

1413:17 ܥܘܙܐ ܒܟܝ شدة صعوبة منتهى. زاد المروزي سورة فورة عزّة. ܥܘܙܐ ܬܘܒ ܐܝܟ ܒܪ ܣܪܘ انتهاء الشيء الى الغاية ⁘

'Uzzā in a manuscript, *force, difficulty, utmost extreme* (muntahā). *Al-Marwazī adds vehemence* (sawra), *outburst, power*. *'Uzzā* again according to bar Serošway, *the extremity* (intihā') *of something unto the utmost.*

Muntahā appears in the first definition, which may be attributed to Ḥunayn by virtue of bar Bahlul's reference to 'a manuscript'. The entry shows a correspondence between the Syriac and Arabic equivalents as represented in the translations of the *Aphorisms*. Again, no such correspondence exists in the Greek entry given above.

2.5

ἀκρατῶς

145:6 ܐܩܪܛܘܣ ܒܪ ܣܪܘ ܐܬܪܐܬ ܡܫܡܫܬܐ ܕܢܦܫܐ أرآء النفس الضعيفة ⁘

---

26 Ullmann, *Wörterbuch zu den griechisch-arabischen Übersetzungen*, 86–7.

Ayqraṭos (according to) bar Serošway, weak consciousness of the soul (*terṯā nasisṯā ḏ-nepešā*), *weak conceptions of the soul* (arā' al-nafs al-ḍa'īfa).

Forms of the word ἀκρατής and related words occur three times in the *Aphorisms*. The available translations display no pattern of approaching these instances, but rather each is translated differently according to its context. In aphorism iii. 12, the word ἀκρατέα is used to describe the offspring of women who, having been with child in the course of a 'southerly, rainy, and calm' winter, give birth in a spring that is 'dry and northerly'. Ḥunayn in his Arabic translation rendered the adjective with the inner accusative *ḍa'īfa al-ḥaraka* 'weak of action', while the word *mḥilē* 'weak' is utilized in the Syriac version. Although the word *al-ḍa'īfa* does occur in bar Bahlul's entry for the Greek term above, its context is too specific for it to constitute an exact agreement. That is not the case in the following entry for the Syriac *mḥilā*:

1054:1 ܡܚܝܠܐ ضعيف. ܡܚܝܠܘܬܐ ضَعْف ⁘[27]

Mḥilā, *weak* (ḍa'īf), *mḥiluṯā* ('weakness'), *weakness* (ḍa'f).

The second instance, the word (νεύρων) ἀκράτειαν 'debility, impotence (of the nerves' in aphorism v. 16, occurs in the context of an enumeration of the potential negative influences of heat upon the body. The Syriac translates this with *tānuḇuṯā* (*ḏ-gyāḏē*) 'numbness (of the nerves)'. Although almost all manuscripts of Ḥunayn's Arabic read here *yaftaḥu* (*al-'aṣab*) (heat) conquers the nerves', there is a notable dissension which I discuss below. The early Arabic translation gives *yadhhabu bi-shidda al-'aṣab* 'destroys the strength of the nerves'.

An entry for the Syriac equivalent *tānubutā* reads as follows:

2074:21 ܬܢܘܒܘܬܐ خَدَر زوال الحِسّ. ܘܐܝܟ ܒܪ ܣܪܘ̈ ܬܢܘܒܘܬܐ ܕܗܘܝܐ ܒܨ̈ܒܥܬܐ ܡܢ ܩܘܪܐ ܣܓܝܐܐ ܡܘܬܐ خَدَر الأطراف ⁘

Tānuḇuṯā, *numbness (*khadar*), annihilation of sense.* And according to bar Serošway *tānuḇuṯā* is that which occurs in the fingers because of great cold, *numbness of the extremities.*

In the bilingual manuscript BnF 6734, there are found several alternatives to the dominant tradition *yaftaḥu* in aphorism v. 16. The text itself reads in

27 Duval: ضَعَف.

its place *khadar fī al-i'ṣāb* ‘numbness in the nerves’. A note in another hand, which in many places in the manuscript corrects variants toward more generally attested readings, reads *tafassukh wa-irkhā'* ‘dissolution and laxness’. The consonantal skeleton of the first word in the note (تفسّخ) is very similar in appearance to that of the dominant tradition (يفتح), so the two may readily have been confused. Furthermore, the second word is related to the reading found in Tytler’s edition, which adds *yarkhā* ‘relaxes (the nerves)’ to *yaftaḥu*. The correspondence between the Syriac entry for *tānuḇuṯā* and the translation found in the Paris manuscript is remarkable, but could be explained in different ways. It is possible for example that the scribe corrected Ḥunayn’s Arabic against the Syriac with the aid of Ḥunayn’s glossary.

For the third instance, the occurrence of ἀκρατής in aphorism vii. 40, Ḥunayn in his Arabic translation used yet another construction. In translating ἢν ἡ γλῶσσα ἐξαίφνης ἀκρατὴς γένηται, he wrote *matā 'adima al-lisānu baghtatan quwwatahu* ‘when the tongue loses its strength all at once’. The Syriac translation’s single manuscript is mostly effaced in this place; although the words *lan ḥayla* are discernible and may indicate a similar approach to that found in the translation of iii. 12, no systematic comparison is possible.

Although the Greek and Syriac entries are both representative of Ḥunayn’s translation of the *Aphorisms*, the specificity of the Greek entry makes it slightly less so than the Syriac. The entry for *mḥilā* at 1054:1 indicates a strong equivalence between the Arabic and Syriac translations of ἀκρατής in the *Aphorisms*. The source of bar Bahlul’s entry very well may have been Ḥunayn’s working glossary, or one of his Syriac-Arabic translations.

2.6

ἀνάγκη/ἀναγκαῖον

211:13 ܐܢܢܩܐ ܐܠܨܝܬܐ ضرورة⁘

Ananqe, necessity (*elṣiṯā*), *necessity* (ḍarūra).

211:14 ܐܢܢܩܘܣ ضروريّات⁘

Ananqos, *necessities* (ḍarūrīyāt).

Forms of this Greek word occur numerous times in the *Aphorisms*. The early Arabic translation, Ḥunayn’s Arabic translation, and the Syriac translation of the word all display some degree of regularity. The Syriac translation in particular is very regular in that it uses precisely the same word, *elṣā*, in all but one of these instances. The only exception is in aphorism vi. 58, where the Greek word is translated using the borrowed form *ananqē*.

Both of these translations and the transliteration are in consonance with the *Lexicon*'s entry at 211:13. In a majority of these cases Ḥunayn translated the word with a form of the phrase *wajiba ḍarūratan an* 'it is absolutely necessary that', which partially concords with the Greek entries in the *Lexicon*. In some places, he used the phrase *lā budda* 'it is inevitable', which was also the preferred phrase of al-Biṭrīq in his renditions of these instances.

As the single example of the borrowing *ananqē* indicates, ἀνάγκη was carried over into Syriac. This should colour somewhat any reading of the entries in bar Bahlul. That said, the definitions do not indicate a departure from the Greek word itself, and furthermore the headword given in the entry at 211:14 has a Greek grammatical form. The entry at 211:13 is an example of the tendency toward equivalent definitions in both target languages and perhaps shows that the borrowed Greek word was still somewhat obscure to Syriac speakers, or at least was not the usual standard. This corresponds to the evidence in the Syriac *Aphorisms*.

An entry relating to the Syriac equivalent *elṣā* in bar Bahlul's *Lexicon* reads as follows:

179:5 ܐܠܨܝܐ الواجب. ܐܠܨܝܬܐ ܒܨܚܚܐ ܗ̇ ܕܝܢ ܟܝܢܐܝܬ. ܐܠܨܝܬܐ ܒܪ ܣܪܘܫܘܝ ضروريّة.
ܐܠܨ اضطرّ ضايق آخر ضيّق اضطهد المروزي أجبَر وأقول لجّ لزّ. ܐܠܨܛܐ ܒܪ ܣܪܘܫܘܝ ضروريّات
المضايقات. ܐܠܝܨܘܬܐ أقول مشقّة اضطرار مضايقة اضطهاد مزاحم ازدحام. ܐܠܨܘܢ اضطهدوني
وأقول لجّوا عليّ لزّوني الجّوني❖

Ālṣāyā, necessity (al-wājib). *Ālṣāytā* in a manuscript, this is 'truly of nature'. *Ālṣāytā* (according to) bar Serošway, *necessity* (ḍarūriyya). *Elaṣ, to be damaged, narrow* (ḍāyiq), *also narrow* (ḍayyiq), *oppression, and (according to) al-Marwazī, to oppress. I say to torment, to bind. Ālāṣāṯā* (according to) bar Serošway *necessities, impediments. Aliṣuṯā, I say toil, damage, constriction, oppression, competition, crowdedness. Elṣun, they oppressed me, and I say they tormented me, they bound me.*

In this entry, another common element in Ḥunayn's translation of the *Aphorisms al-wājib* 'necessity' is present, thus making it slightly more representative of the translator's translation technique than the Greek entries.

The full phrase *yajibu min al-ḍarūra* still does not appear. It is found in an entry in in bar ʿAli's lexicon, however:

ܐܠܨܐ. ܗܘ ܡܢ ܐܢܢܩܐ يجب من الضرورة.[28]

Ālṣā, this is of necessity (*men ānānqē*), *absolutely necessary* (yajibu min al-ḍarūra).

Despite the broad correspondence between these various texts, and also the presence of ἀνάγκη in the Syriac language, the correspondence between Ḥunayn's translations and the Syriac entries in the lexicons is stronger than that obtaining between the translations and the Greek entries. The entry in bar ʿAli's *Lexicon* best reflects Ḥunayn's usage in the *Aphorisms*. Although this pattern strengthens the relationship between the Syriac lexicography and Ḥunayn's translations, the numerous cases in which Ḥunayn did not use any of these forms indicates that the translator did not work mechanically from the Syriac entries, but rather adapted his language to the context in which he worked.

2.7

ἀνάληψις

195:25 ܐܢܐܠܝܡܦܣܝܣ[29] التسلّق الصعود ܒ̈ ܐܢܐܠܝܘܢܦܣܝܣ ܣܘܠܩܐ السلّاق الصعود܀

Anālimpisis, ascent, rising. In a manuscript *anālionpisis*, the Ascension, *the Ascension, the rising.*

Forms of ἀνάληψις occur twice in the *Aphorisms*. In aphorism i. 3 ἀναλήψιες refers to restoration of the body by food. Ḥunayn rendered it with the phrase *kull taghdhiya* 'all feedings', the Syriac translator gave for it *mṯarsyānuṯā ḏ-mendriš* 'nourishment that is renewed', and the early Arabic translator translated it *malaʾ* 'repletion'. Although there is no entry in bar Bahlul's *Lexicon* exactly corresponding to the Syriac equivalent *mṯarsyānuṯā*, a related noun *tarsāyṯā* is represented in an entry that reads like this:

2089:5 ܬܪܣܝܬܐ حتي الغذاء القوت ܟܕ ܦܬܝܚܐ ܬ̄ ܘܙܩܝܦܐ ܣ̄. ܠܐ ܬܪܣܝܬܐ الهزال جاء به فولس في علل العين فقال إنّ الهزال ضيق العين وصغرها والسلّ ضيق صبى العين وحده܀

Tarsāyṯā, nourishment (al-ghidhā'), *nutriment,* when the *taw* has a short a-vowel and the *semkaṯ* has a long a-vowel. *Lā tarsāyṯā, emaciation* (al-huzāl). *Paul introduced it among*

28 Hoffmann (ed.), *Syrische-arabische Glossen*, 31:772.

29 According to Liddell-Scott, later Greek writers often wrote this word ἀναλήμψις, and it is clear that at least the head-word of the entry follows this convention.

the diseases of the eye. He said 'emaciation is weakness of the eye and its reduction, and consumption is the weakness of the pupil of the eye alone'.

The initial Arabic definition attributable to Ḥunayn shows strong agreement with the Arabic and Syriac terminology in the *Aphorisms*. Although not directly related to the translations considered here, the ophthalmological fragment of Paul is also of importance. This is in part due to its being represented in an entry with a Syriac headword.

In aphorism iv. 27, where ἀναλήψεσι signifies 'recovery, convalescence', Ḥunayn employed the hendiadys *yanqahu fa-yughdhā* 'he recovers and is fed'. The Syriac version translates here with *zabnā d-masyānuthon* 'the time of their being healed'. A short entry for a word related to the Syriac equivalent reads as follows:

991:7 ܡܐܣܝܢܐ الأساة الشفاة܀

Masyānā, healing (al-asā), *recovery* (al-shifā).

In this second case, Ḥunayn's interpretation differs from that of the Syriac translator. Interestingly, the Syriac lexicography for the first Syriac equivalent presented, *mṯarsyānuṯā*, in fact agrees to some extent with both of Ḥunayn's Arabic translations. This could indicate that Ḥunayn's Syriac translation likewise would have used a word related to *mṯarsyānuṯā* in both instances as well. Since the entry for ἀνάληψις in bar Bahlul's *Lexicon* defines a different and quite specific sense of the word, it does not overlap significantly with the Arabic translations. For its part, the Syriac lexicography does at least partially correspond with Ḥunayn's translations, despite the distinct interpretation adopted by the Syriac translator of the *Aphorisms*.

2.8

ἀνέλπιστος

215:11 ܐܢܛܝܠܝܦܛܝܐ ܐܝܟ ܣܪ ܓ̄ ܦܣܝܩܘܬ ܣܒܪܐ ܀

Antilipiṭyā according to Sergius, loss of hope.

A form of this word occurs once in the *Aphorisms*, in aphorism vii. 47. The Syriac version translates it *d-lā sabrā iṯaw* 'for whom there is no hope', while Ḥunayn's Arabic translation reads for it *laysa yurjā* 'he is not hoped for'. The Syriac translation is marginally related to Sergius' entry in the *Lexicon* presented above. The headword of the entry has a nativized form, indicating that it was taken over into Syriac. At the same time Duval's identification must be taken to be somewhat tentative, since the transcription does not very strongly match the expected Greek word. An entry for the substantial element of the Syriac translation, *sab̲rā*, reads as follows:

1298.5 **ܣܒܪܐ** ܐܝܟ ܒܪ ܣܪܘܫܘܝ ܣܘܟܝܐ ܕܐܝܠܝܢ ܕܥܬܝ̈ܕܢ ܕܢܐܬ̈ܝܢ ܘܡܫܬܡ̈ܥܢ. ܦܘܪܫܢܐ ܕܒܝܬ ܣܒܪܐ
ܠܣܘܟܝܐ ܗ̄ ܕܣܘܟܝܐ ܥܠ ܛ̈ܒܬܐ ܐܟܚܕ ܘܒܝ̈ܫܬܐ ܗܘܐ. ܣܒܪܐ ܕܝܢ ܥܠ ܛ̈ܒܬܐ ܒܠܚܘܕ. ܐܦܢ
ܡܚܠܛܐܝܬ ܡܬܪ̈ܓܫܝܢ ܒܗܘܢ ܡܛܠ ܦܫܝܛܘܬܐ ܘܥܝܕܐ وأقول الأمنيّة والأمل والرجاء للخير فقط...
ܣܒܪܐ ܐܝܟ ܚܢ ظنّ ويقال توهّم. ܣܒܪܢܐ ܐܝܟ ܒܪ ܣܪܘܫܘܝ أظنّ وأقول ܐܣܬܒܪܬ ܠܝ وقع لي.
ܣܒܪܬܐ بشرى. **ܡܣܒܪܢܘܬܐ** تبشير. **ܡܣܒܪܢܐ** ܐܝܟ ܙܟܪ المبشّر ✣

Sab̲rā according to bar Serošway, expectation of those things which are to come and that are renowned and proclaimed. The difference between hope and expectation is that expectation may be for good and evil together, but hope is solely for good, even if they may be felt in a mixed way, for the sake of simplicity and convention. *I say trust, hope, expectation* (rajā') *for good only*... *Sab̲rā* according to Ḥunayn, *opinion, and it is said supposition*. *Sābbar-nā* according to bar Serošway, *I suppose, and I say estabbrat̲ li, it occurs to me*. *Sb̲art̲ā, good tidings*. *Msabbrānut̲ā, giving good tidings*. *Msabbrānā* according to Zakariya, *a giver of good tidings*.

Some of this material is also present in an entry in bar ʿAli's *Lexicon*:

ܣܒܪܐ ܗ̄ ܣܘܟܝܐ ܕܐܝܠܝܢ ܕܥܬܝ̈ܕܢ ܕܢܐܬ̈ܘܢ ܐܘ ܡܫܬܡ̈ܥܢ. ܘܦܘܪܫܢܐ ܐܝܬ ܒܝܬ ܣܘܟܝܐ ܠܣܒܪܐ.
ܗ̄ ܕܣܘܟܝܐ ܥܠ ܛ̈ܒܬܐ ܐܟܚܕܐ ܘܣܒܪܐ ܕܝܢ ܥܠ ܛ̈ܒܬܐ ܒܠܚܘܕ [ܘܒܝ̈ܫܬܐ] ܗܘܐ.[30] ܐܦܢ
ܡܚܠܛܐܝܬ ܡܬܪ̈ܓܫܝܢ ܒܗܘܢ ܡܛܠ ܥܝܕܐ. أمل رجاء. والرجا للخير يفيض. ܒ̈ يقال **ܣܒܪ**
ܡܣܒܪܢܘܬܐ.[31]

Sab̲rā, this is expectation of those things which are to come that are renowned and proclaimed. The difference between hope (*sab̲rā*) and expectation is that expectation may be for good (and evil) together, but hope is solely for good, even if they be felt in a mixed way, for the sake of convention. *Hope, expectation. Expectation for good overflowing.* In a manuscript *it is said sb̲ar*, expectation.

Because bar ʿAli's *Lexicon* relied more exclusively on Ḥunayn's glossary than did bar Bahlul's, the latter's attribution of the material shared between the two entries to bar Serošway is somewhat problematic. On the one hand,

30 Gottheil: ܒܠܚܘܕ ܐ ܗܘܐ. Given the substantial similarity between these two definitions, Gottheil's reading appears to result from an omission. My reading follows Duval's text of Bar Bahlul's Lexicon as given above.

31 Gottheil (ed.), *Syriac-Arabic Glosses*, II 141:12.

it may merely be a mistake or a later interpolation. On the other, it may mean that bar Serošway reproduced Ḥunayn's definition of *sabrā* in his own work. This kind of reproduction would have significance for our understanding of the relationship between the glossographical works of Ḥunayn and bar Serošway.

2.9

ἀνταποδιδούς/ἀνταπόδοσις

206:26 ܐܢܛܦܘܕܝܕܘܣ ܒܪ ܗܘ̄ ܕܦܪܥ المكافي المجازي المقاوض܀

Anṭapudidus (according to) bar Serošway, that which recompenses (*d-pāreʿ*), *one who recompenses, one who apportions, one who exchanges.*

207:1 ܐܢܛܦܘܕܣܝܣ ܒܪ ܗܘ̄ جزاء مكافاة܀

Anṭapodsis (according to) bar Serošway, *reward, gratification.*

In aphorism 1. 12, the Hippocratic author refers to the ἀνταποδόσιες 'alternation' of cyclic periods of exacerbation as one of the phenomena which may be used to infer the specific characteristics of diseases. Ḥunayn's Arabic translation *tazayyud* 'increase' and the Syriac translation *tawseptā* 'increase' correspond in their interpretations, but the Arabic also explicates by adding *nāʾibatan* to give the sense of 'cyclic increase'. Al-Biṭrīq differed in his interpretation, giving *tadāwul* 'alternation'.

Some relevant entries in bar Bahlul's *Lexicon* for the Syriac equivalent run as follows:

2047:11 ܬܘܣܝ̈ܦܐ ܐܘܣܦܘܬ ܡܬܪܐ التفاضل والزيادات܀

Tawsipē, this means increases, *mutual striving, increases* (al-ziyādāt).

2047:12 ܬܘܣܦܬܐ ܐܝܟ ܒܪ ܣܪܘܫܘܝ ܬܘܬܪܬ ܡܫܘܚܬܐ ܕܪܘܫܡܐ ܕܐܝܬܝܗ̇ ܕܝ̈ ܒܨܒܘܬܐ
ܕܡܬܚܫܒܐ ܠܗ̇ ܡܢ ܠܒܪ ܕܠܐ ܗܘܐ ܡܢ ܟܝܢܗ̇ الزيادة. ܬܘܣܦܬܐ ܘܡܘܣܦܢܘܬܐ إعادة زيادة. ܒܝ̈
ܟܡܝܘܬܐ ܡܡܫܚܬܐ ܕܠܐ ܬܘܣܦ ܒܘܨܪ مقدار قصد܀

Tawseptā according to bar Serošway, an exceeding of the measure of the condition which characterizes a thing, occurring to it from without, that is not of its nature, *increase* (al-ziyāda). *Tawseptā w-mawspānutā, addition, increase*. In a manuscript, *kmāyutā mmaššaḥtā d-lā tawsep buṣār*, ('an amount measured without increase [or] deficit'), *an intended amount.*

Although the specific form used by Ḥunayn, *tazayyud*, is not present in these examples of relevant Greek and Syriac lexicography, the Syriac entries do contain the closely related form *al-ziyādāt* (increases). Thus, the Syriac lexicography better represents both the sense of this word in the *Aphorisms* and Ḥunayn's Arabic translation of the work than does the Greek lexicography.

2.10

ἀσθματικοί

227:13 ܐܣܛܡܛܝܩܘ ܗ̄ ܣܒܝܣܘܬ ܢܫܡܐ ضيق النفس܀

Asṭmṭiqo, this is closeness of breath (*sḇisuṯ nešmā*, lit. 'asthma'), *tightness of breath* (ḍīq al-nafas).

Forms of the Greek word ἄσθμα occur some four times in the *Aphorisms*. Both Ḥunayn's Arabic translation and the Syriac version are thoroughly consistent in their translations of these instances. The former gives *al-rabw* 'dyspnea, asthma' and the latter *lahāṯā* 'asthma, shortness of breath' for each occurrence. For the instance of the word in aphorism iii. 26 the early Arabic version is also extant, and in that place the word *buhr* 'laboured breathing' is employed. Besides this example, Ullmann notes others which show Ḥunayn's translation *al-rabw* to be a common choice beyond the *Aphorisms*.[32]

Although Duval's identification of its underlying Greek term must surely be correct, the entry at 227:13 does not echo the extant translations in any respect. However, in the definition of ἄσθμα/*al-rabw* found in Ḥunayn's translation of Galen's *Commentary on the Aphorisms*, there is some significant overlap in terminology. In particular, the word *ḍīq* 'tightness' both forms part of the definition in the *Lexicon* and figures prominently in Ḥunayn's translation of Galen's extended account of the meaning of the term in question.[33] If we turn to consider the entry for the Syriac equivalent *lahātā*, the significance of this can be clarified:

946:7 **ܠܗ̈ܬܐ** الربو صحّحه حنين. ܒܪ ܣܪܘ البهر اللهث܀

Lahāṯā, *asthma* (al-rabw). *Ḥunayn rectified it*. (According to) bar Serošway *laboured breathing* (al-buhr), *panting* (al-lahth).

In contrast to the entry for the Greek word at 227:13, the entry for the Syriac equivalent contains both Ḥunayn's preferred translation and the early

32 Ullmann, *Wörterbuch zu den griechisch-arabischen Übersetzungen*, 139–40.

33 Mimura (ed.), *Tafsīr Jālīnūs*, III, 72.

Arabic translator's as well. Furthermore, bar Bahlul appears to attribute to Ḥunayn the introduction of the term *al-rabw* as the equivalent of *lahāṯā*.

This example presents an opportunity for speculation regarding the varying roles played by Greek and Syriac lexicography in the production of Ḥunayn's Arabic translations. The centuries-old Greek-to-Syriac translation tradition allowed for very close translations of Greek texts into Syriac. In the case of ἄσθμα/*lahāṯā*/*al-rabw*, the Syriac terminology established in this process seems to have constituted the reference according to which Arabic terminology was established in its turn. To the extent that the Arabic translations used standardized terminology, such a lexicographical process would have preceded the translation of the texts themselves. If a strong Syriac role in this process may be inferred to have been present in the broader work of translation, this would mean that a Syriac exemplar read simultaneously with the Greek original would have been an important instrument for the careful Arabic translator.

Yet as the example from Galen's *Commentary on the Aphorisms* shows, the underlying Greek terminology was not effaced or forgotten in this process. Rather, precise etymological understanding of the Greek lexicon often was necessary for the accurate rendition of the more detailed works of Greek medicine and philosophy both into Syriac and into Arabic. Thus, bar Bahlul's entry for the term ἀσθματικοί seems to preserve notes used not for word-for-word translation, but rather for rendering detailed explanations of the term whenever it was encountered in the literature being translated. This suggests that Ḥunayn used a more complicated, tri-lingual Greek-Syriac-Arabic approach rather than relying solely upon either Greek or Syriac exemplars.

2.11

ἀφρώδης

268:26 **ܐܦܪܘܕܝܣܝܘܣ** ܐܝܬܘܗܝ ܪܥܘܬܢܐ ܡܬܬܬܐ ܡܢ ܗܝ ܕܪܥܘܬܐ ܀

Aprodisios is carrying foam, that from which foam (*ru'ṯā*) comes.

Forms of the noun ἀφρός and the related adjective ἀφρώδης occur three times in the *Aphorisms*. Ḥunayn's Arabic version translates all of these examples with a form related to the noun *zabad* 'foam', while the Syriac translation employs forms related to *ru'ṯā* 'foam'. The entry for *ru'ṯā* reads as follows:

1889:19 **ܪܘܥܬܐ** زبد رغوة. **ܪܘܥܬܐ ܕܢܝܛܪܘܢ** بورق. **ܡܪܥܬܢܘܬܐ** ܗܝ ܕܡܬܪܥܬܢ ܐܢܫ ܐܝܟ ܡܢ
ܕܝܘܐ ܐܝܟ ܐܢܫܝܢ. ܘܐܝܟ ܡܢ ܟܝܡܘܣ. ܐܚܪ̈ܢܐ. ܗܘܝܐ ܕܝܢ ܗܕܐ ܪܘܥܬܐ ܡܢ ܬܠܬ عِلل. ܐܘ ܡܢ
ܡܫܚܡܢܘܬܐ ܚܝܠܬܢܝܬܐ ܠܚܘܕ. ܐܝܟ ܩܕܪܐ. ܐܘ ܡܢ ܙܘܥܐ. ܐܝܟ ܕܒܝܡܐ. ܐܘ ܡܢ ܙܘܥܐ ܐܟܚܕ
ܘܡܘܙܓܐ ܕܡܫܚܡܢܘܬܐ. ܐܝܟ ܕܒ̈ܢܝ ܠܪ̈ܟܫܐ ܡܐ ܕܪܗܛܝܢ܀

Ru'ṯā, foam (zabad), *froth* (raghwa). *Ru'ṯā ḏ-niṭrun, borax. Mar'tānuṯā*, this is when a man foams at the mouth, whether due to a devil as the people say (*ayk nāšin*), or because of humours. (According to) others, this foam occurs due to three causes, either solely because of intense heat, as for example a pot, or because of motion, as for example in the sea, or because of a combination of motion and heat, as for example horses when they run.

This entry, attributable to Ḥunayn, presents an interesting contrast between folk medicine and learned medicine. These contradictory perspectives are allowed to stand side-by-side. Since the entry for the Greek word contains only a Syriac definition while the Syriac entry contains Ḥunayn's Arabic equivalent *al-zabad*, the latter is better representative of the translator's approach.

Section Three

Finally, for these words, both the Greek and the Syriac lexicography represent Ḥunayn's Arabic translations of the *Aphorisms* equally well.

3.1

αἷμα

132:10 **ܐܝܐܝܡܐ** ܗܘ ܕܡܐ ذكر جبريل بن بختيشوع أن الدم اسمه باليونانية ܐܝ, ܐܝܡܐ܀

Ayaymā, this is blood (*dmā*). *Jibrīl ibn Bukhtīshū' said that the name of blood in Greek is* ay aymā.

135:14 **ܐܝܡܐ** ܒܪ ܣܪܘ̄ ܕܡܐ الدم܀

Aymā (according to) bar Serošway, blood (*dmā*), *blood (*al-dam*)*.

636:27 **ܗܡܐܛܘܣ** ܘܐܝܟ ܪܒܢ ܗܡܐ الدم܀

Hemāṭos, and according to our teacher *hemā*, *blood* (*al-dam*).

This word is translated consistently in both Ḥunayn's Arabic translation and the Syriac translation, the former giving *al-dam* and the latter giving *dmā*, both of which mean 'blood'. The only exception in either work occurs in aphorism v. 33, where Ḥunayn's Arabic compresses the Greek phrase αἷμα ἐκ τῶν ῥινῶν ῥυέν 'blood flowing from the nostrils' into the single word *al-ru'āf* 'nosebleed'. The straightforward definitions of the Greek word are equivalent to the translations of the term in our texts.

The entry for the Syriac term *dmā* reads like this:

579:8 **ܕܡܐ** الدم ܟܘܡܘܣ ܪܛܝܒܐ ܘܫܚܝܢܐ ܕܐܝܬܘܗܝ ܐܕܫܗ ܕܝܠܢܐܝܬ ܡܢ ܐܣܛܘܟܣܐ ܕܐܐܪ ܘܐܝܬܘܗܝ ܒܟܒܕܐ ܘܫܘܠܛܢܗ ܒܟܠܗ ܦܓܪܐ الدم❖

Dmā, *blood*, a wet and hot humour whose form derives properly from the element of air. It comes to be in the liver (*iṯaw b-ḵaḇdā*) and its power is in the entire body, *blood* (*al-dam*).[34]

In this entry, also attributable to Ḥunayn, the traditional humoural view of the physicians concerning blood is stated. Notably, this more extended definition is present in the entry for the Syriac word, but absent from the entries for the Greek equivalent. Because the words in all three languages are strongly synonomous, there is a general concord amongst the entries and the translations.

3.2

ἀκριβῶν (ἀκριβής)

277:25 **ܐܩܪܒܝܐ**[35] ܘܐܩܪܝܒܘܢ ܐܝܟ ܒܪ ܣܪܘܫܘܝ ܬܪܝܨܐ ܚܬܝܬܐ. **ܐܩܪܒܝܐ** حقّ واضح❖

Aqrbya and *aqribon* according to bar Serošway, correct, true (*ḥattiṯā*). *Aqrabeya*, *true*, *evident*.

278:19 **ܐܩܪܒܝܐ** ܒܟܬܒ ܕܦܪܕܝܣܐ ܗ ܬܪܝܨܘܬܐ ܐܘ ܝܬܝܪܘܬܐ❖

Aqrabeya in the *Book of Paradise*, this is rightness or excess.

Forms of ἀκριβής occur five times in the *Aphorisms*. In three cases found in aphorisms i. 4 and i. 5 that reference diet, both Ḥunayn's version and the Syriac translation employ consistent translations. For these instances the former gives *al-bāligh* 'extreme', while the latter employs the word *ḥattiṯā* 'truly'. For the occurrence of the adverbial form of the word in the phrase ἀκριβείην κράτισται 'are truly best' in aphorism i. 6, Ḥunayn's version translates with the single word *ajwad* 'best', while the Syriac version gives *ḥattiṯuṯā ṭāḇ miṯrān* 'are truly and entirely good'. Finally, in aphorism iv. 59 the adjective occurs in a description of fevers. Both the Arabic and Syriac versions here adopt different approaches from those given above. The Syriac

34 Although I have already provided this entry in the discussion of ἀγωγή above (unit 2.2), I repeat here for ease of reference.

35 Duval: ܐܩܪܒܝܐ.

gives *kad saggi arikā* 'when it (the tertian fever) is very long', while the Arabic gives *aṭwal mā takūn* 'the longest (tertian fevers) that occur.

The Syriac translations on the whole are more literal than the Arabic translations due to the latter's omitting to translate the specific adverb in aphorism 1. 6. The entries in bar Bahlul's *Lexicon* agree somewhat with these Syriac translations, but less so with the Arabic texts. Nor does the entry for the Syriac equivalent *ḥattiṯā* contain much more of direct relevance for them:

782:13 ܚܬܝܬܐ الصحيح الخالص الصرف المحض ܙܟܪ. زاد المروزي راسخ تامّ. ܚܬܝܬܘܬܐ صحّة خلاص صرف حقيقة يقين. ܚܬܝܬܐܝܬ الحقيقة. ܚܬܝܬܐ ثابت راسخ محض صحيح يقين܀

Ḥattiṯā, correct, sincere, pure (al-khāliṣ), *uncut, pure* (al-maḥḍ), (according to) Zakariya. *Al-Marwazī adds firm, complete. Ḥattiṯuṯā, sound, integral, pure, true, certain. Ḥattiṯā'iṯ, true. Ḥattiṯā, established, firm, pure, correct, certain.*

Neither the Greek nor the Syriac entries relate to Ḥunayn's translation. Furthermore, the rather severe differences between the two translations' renditions of ἀκριβής constitute evidence against Ḥunayn's authorship of the Syriac *Aphorisms*. This is also the most probable reason for the discrepancy between the Arabic translations and the Syriac lexicography.

3.3

ἀλφοί

178:17 ܐܠܦܘ ܗ̄ ܒܗܩܝܬܐ البهق܀

Alpo, this is tetter (*behqiṯā*), *tetter* (al-bahaq).

This term occurs in the *Aphorisms* a single time, in aphorism iii. 20. The main Syriac and Arabic versions both translate it using the same terms that are found in the entry above, *behqiṯā* and *al-bahaq*. The early Syriac translation for this aphorism also exists, and for this term it appears to give *ḥḵāḵā* 'itch, mange'.[36] There is thus a clear correspondence between Ḥunayn's entry in bar Bahlul and the translations in both the Arabic and Syriac versions. This stands in contrast to the earlier Syriac translation, which appears to give evidence for a development toward greater lexicographical precision in the Syriac translation tradition.

36 Although some text of the aphorism has dropped out, it is likely that *ḥḵāḵā* does translate ἀλφοί.

Although the translation for this aphorism does not exist in any of the fragments of the early Arabic version, according to Ullmann the translator al-Biṭrīq's preferred translation of the term ἀλφός was also *al-bahaq*, as shown by several examples from his translation of Galen's *On Simple Drugs* Book Six.[37] Therefore, while the available Syriac examples evince terminological development, in contrast the Arabic examples show terminological stability.

The entry for the Syriac term *behqiṯā* in the *Lexicon* reads like this:

361:28 **ܒܗܩܝܬܐ** بهق ܘܐܡܪܝܢ ܦܘܠܘܣ ܘܒܪ ܣܪܘܫܘܝ **ܒܗܩܝܬܐ** ܕܡܒܗܩܐ ܐܝܟ ܢܘܪܐ ܘܡܨܡܚܐ الوضح وهو البهق البرص والبهق أصحّ ⁘

Behqiṯā, tetter (bahaq). Paul and bar Serošway say, tetter that glows like fire and shines. *Spotting* (al-waḍaḥ), *which is tetter, leprosy* (al-baraṣ), *but tetter is more correct.*

The Arabic *al-bahaq* and Syriac *behqiṯā* are derivable from the same Semitic root and would appear to be related. The Syriac word's clear etymology from the sense 'to shine', which has no analogue in Arabic, makes it more likely that it originates in the former language. Furthermore, the Syriac word occurs several times in the *Peshitta*, demonstrating its use from an early date.[38] The early Arabic translator al-Biṭrīq's use of the word in his translations of Galen means that, if an adaptation from Syriac did occur, it was prior to Ḥunayn's career.

3.4

ἅμα

181:17 **ܐ̈ܡܐ** ܐܡܪ ܒܪ ܣܪܘܫܘܝ معاً ⁘

Āmā according to bar Serošway *accompanying* (maʿan).

This Greek adverb occurs once in the *Aphorisms*, in aphorism ii. 46. Ḥunayn translated it *ma'an* 'accompanying', while the Syriac translates *aḵḥḏā nehwon* 'at once'. Bar Serošway's Arabic definition in the *Lexicon* agrees exactly with the text of Ḥunayn's translation. Bar Bahlul's entry for the Syriac equivalent *aḵḥḏā* likewise agrees while giving some further relevant information:

37 Ullmann, *Wörterbuch zu den griechisch-arabischen Übersetzungen*, 97.

38 For example, in Lev. 13:4.

155:22 ܐܟܚܕܐ مَعاً والذي جاء به حنين في موضع بالجملة❖

Akḥdā, accompanying (maʿan), *and that which Ḥunayn introduced in one place,* (*namely*) *'altogether'* (bil-jumla).

3.5

ἀμόργη

184:1 ܐܡܘܪܓܐ ܠܗ ܛܛܪܐ ܕܥܨܪܐ ܕܙܝܬܐ عكر الزيت ܒܦܢ ܥ. ܐܡܘܪܓܐ ܠܗ ܡܝ̈ܐ ܕܙܝܬܐ. ܪܒܢ. ܡܕܡ
ܕܫܟܒ ܡܢ ܡܫܚܐ ܕܙܝܬܐ ما يرسب تحت الزيت اذا عصر من الزيتون❖

Amorgē, the lees of the oil of the olive (*teṭrā ḏa-'ṣārā ḏ-zaytā*), *the lees of oil* (ʿakar al-zayt), in an old manuscript. *Amorgē*, the lees of oil (*mayyē ḏ-zaytā*). (According to) our teacher, the part of olive oil that settles, *that which settles at the bottom of oil when it is pressed from olives.*

A form of this Greek term appears in aphorism vii. 45, where it used figuratively to describe a flow of pus that is a sign of death in one suffering from a disease of the liver. Both Ḥunayn's Arabic translation and the Syriac translation differ slightly from the entry in bar Bahlul's *Lexicon* given above. The Arabic gives *thufl al-zayt* 'lees of oil', while the Syriac translation gives *teṭrā ḏ-mešḥā*, again meaning 'lees of oil'.

The Greek entry at 184:1 contains a descriptive definition of ἀμοργή directly attributed to Ḥunayn, which allows us to compare the translator's Syriac writing to the text of the Syriac *Aphorisms.* Ḥunayn in the entry employs the phrase *'ṣārā ḏ-zaytā* for 'olive oil', while the Syriac translation uses a different word, *mešḥā*, which strictly speaking simply means 'oil'. Although minor, this discrepancy reinforces the sense that Ḥunayn was not the author of the Syriac *Aphorisms*.

Two entries related to the Syriac equivalent *teṭrā* in bar Bahlul's *Lexicon* read as follows:

2057:13 ܛܛܝܪܐ ܒܦܢ ثخين خاثر كدر. ܘܐܝܟ ܒܪ ܣܪܘ عكر. ܘܒܦܪܕ ܘܛܐܛܪ ܠܗ ܗ̄ ܥܟܪ ܠܗ ܠܛܛܪܗ❖

Tṭirā in a manuscript, *thick, turbid, impure*. And according to bar Serošway, *dregs* (ʿakar). And (according to) the *Book of Paradise w-ṯāṭar leh*, this is 'he stirred up its dregs'.

2057:18 ܛܛܪܐ كدر. ܛܛܪܗ ܢܡܨܘܢ ܐܝܟ ܒܪ ܣܪܘ كدره يمصّون❖

Teṭrā, impure. Teṭreh nemṣun according to bar Serošway, *they drank from the dregs.*[39]

39 Although *al-kadar* is not defined in this way in the dictionaries, the sense is clear from the context.

Although these do not reflect Ḥunayn's Arabic translation of the Greek term, an entry in bar ʿAli's *Lexicon* does:

ܛܛܝܪܐ الخاثر والثقل والعكر والكدر والدردي.[40]

Tṭirā, concentrates, lees, dregs, impurities, sediments.

None of the Greek or Syriac entries in bar Bahlul agree exactly with Ḥunayn's Arabic translation. Since my way of proceeding relies on bar Bahlul's *Lexicon* and not bar ʿAli's, the agreement between the latter's entry for *tṭirā* and Ḥunayn's translation of ἀμόργη in the *Aphorisms* does not bear upon the placement of this example in the organization of the chapter.

3.6

ἀνήρ

199:6 ܐܢܕܪܐ ܝܘܢܐܝܬ ܠܓܒܪܐ ܒܝ ܐܢܕܪܢܐ رجل ܀

Andrā, in Greek, a man. In a manuscript *andrānā, man.*

210:8 ܐܢܐܝܪ ܒܪ ܣܪܘܫܘܝ ܠܓܒܪܐ رجل ܒܝ ܐܢܐܝܕ ܀

Anayr, bar Serošway, man, *man.* In a manuscript *anayd.*

In aphorism v. 69, the word ἀνδράσι occurs. The Syriac translates it *b-gaḇrê*, and Ḥunayn's Arabic gives for it *fī al-rijāl*. In this case, all three words are synonomous with one another in a strong sense, and so it is not very surprising to see the translations in agreement with the definitions in the *Lexicon*. A brief entry in bar Bahlul's *Lexicon* for the Syriac equivalent further confirms it:

447:4 ܓܒܪܐ رجل ܀

Gaḇrā, a man (rajul).

3.7

ἄνθρακας (ἄνθραξ)

216:15 ܐܢܬܪܐܩܣ ܒܪ ܣܪܘܫܘܝ ܠܓܘܡܪܐ جمر ܀

Anṯrāqês, bar Serošway embers (*gumrē*), *embers* (jamr).

This word is found in aphorism v. 11, where the odour given off when the sputa of consumptive patients is poured over embers is mentioned as a sign of death. The Syriac translates it with *gumrē*, while the Arabic gives the

40 Gottheil (ed.), *Syriac-Arabic Glosses*, II, 475:12.

etymologically-related *jamr*, both of which mean ‘embers’. These translations agree precisely with bar Serošway’s definition at 216:15.

Ullmann notices several contexts wherein ἄνθραξ signifies ‘carbuncle’, a disease of the eye, including one citation from Galen’s *On Simple Drugs* Book Six and four from Dioscorides’ *Materia Medica*.[41] The Arabic translations for these occurrences of the term vary noticeably from one another. Although three of them give *jamr* or *jamra*, in one case the word is transliterated, and in another a different name is given to it, *al-nār al-fārisī* ‘Persian fire’. Although the single Syriac translation of ἄνθραξ in the *Aphorisms* has nothing to do with this sense of the word, it allows us to refer to the entry for the Syriac term found in bar Bahlul, which does relate to it:

466:20 ܓܘܡܪܐ جمر. ܓܘܡܪ̈ܐ الجدري وقد سمّى فولوس جنساً من الخراجات بهذا الاسم.
ܓܡܘܪܬܐ جمرة وذكرها ايضاً فيما يخرج في العين. ܘܐܝܟ ܒܪ ܣܪܘܫܘܝ ܫܘܚܢܐ ܒܝܫܐ ܥܝܕ̈ܐ ܕܗܘܐ
ܒܝܩܕܢܐ نار فارسيّة وكذلك قال مسيح أي الجمرة وهي النار الفارسيّة܀

Gumrā, ember (jamr). *Gumrē, smallpox* (al-jadrī). *Paul has named a type of swelling by this name. Gmurṯā, ember. He also mentioned it among those things that come forth in the eye.* And according to bar Serošway the common cancer (*šuḥnē bišê ʿyāḏē*) which occurs due to burning, *Persian fire* (nār fārsīya). *And likewise Masīḥ said this is* al-jamra, *which is Persian fire.*

This entry provides evidence that allows for the implications of preceding scholarship to be clarified. Pormann’s account of this term in his work on Paul of Aegina notes two of the senses found here. Specifically, in Ḥunayn’s *Ten Treatises on the Eye*, ἄνθραξ is found defined as *al-jadrī* ‘smallpox’.[42] Pormann calls this text ‘corrupt’, evidently on the reasonable grounds that smallpox is not an eye disease. Bar Bahlul’s entry for the Syriac equivalent *gumrā* cited here makes these two senses of ἄνθραξ homonymous on the authority of Paul, and is thus the likely source for the confusion noted by Pormann. It may be hoped, furthermore, that detailed consideration of the translations of the Greek term in Dioscorides’ work on the basis of this entry would reveal the rationale behind their variations as well.

This example serves to emphasize the importance of the Syriac tradition for studies of Arabic medicine. Howsoever it may be acquired, awareness of the proper Syriac equivalents for Greek terminology is a prerequisite for

41 Ullmann, *Wörterbuch zu den griechisch-arabischen Übersetzungen*, 112.

42 Pormann, *Oriental Tradition*, 189.

consulting the Syriac-to-Arabic lexicographical tradition. Since the extant traces of this tradition contain significant portions of the infrastructure upon which the Greek-to-Arabic translations and independent Arabic works of medicine were performed, they hold the potential of clarifying otherwise anomalous characteristics of the Greek-to-Arabic translation movement.

It is notable that this entry is absent from Löw's catalogue of entries in Bar Bahlul's *Lexicon* containing definitions attributed to Paul of Aegina. Löw's material largely, if not entirely, consists of etymologically Greek terms, so it is perhaps not surprising that this example of a definition of Paul's given for an etymologically-Syriac word does not figure there. This is an indication that more, perhaps many more, examples of Paul's glossographical work await discovery in bar Bahlul's *Lexicon*.

3.8

ἀπόστημα/ἀποστήματα

251:23 ܐܦܘܣܛܝܡܐ خراج܀

*Aposṭimā, abscess (*khurāj*).*

251:24 ܐܦܘܣܛܝܡܛܐ الأورام الحادّة ܒ̈ ܐܘܟܝܬ ܩܘܒܝܢܐ الدمّلة ܕܗܘܝܢ ܒܒܪܝܘܬܗ ܕܦܓܪܐ ܦܘ̄
الأورام الحادّة التي لم تنضج ܒܪ ܣܪܘ̄ الخراجات التي فيها مدّة الدبابل[43] والدمامل܀

Aposṭimāṭā, sharp inflammations (al-awrām al-ḥādda). In a manuscript, its meaning is inflammations (*qubyānā*), *boils* (al-dummala) that occur on the outside of the body. (According to) Paul, *sharp inflammations that have not suppurated*. (According to) bar Serošway, *abscesses that have pus inside of them, ulcers (*al-dabābil*), boils.*

253:21 ܐܦܘܣܛܝܡܐ ܙܥܘܪܐ ܕܗܘܝܐ ܒܩܪܢܐ ܪܒܬܐ ܕܥܝܢܐ ܕܠܘܬ ܢܚܝܪܐ الناصور الحادث
في الماق الأكبر. ܘܡܐ ܕܦܩܥ ܡܬܩܪܐ ܐܝܓܝܠܘܦܣ܀

Aposṭimā z'urā ('small abscess'), this occurs in the great corner of the eye which is (near) to the nose. *Fistulas* (al-nāṣūr) *that occur in the great corner of the eye*. When it bursts it is called *aêgilops*.

264:26 ܐܦܣܛܡܐ علة الرحم دبيلة تكون في الرحم܀

Apsṭmā, a disease of the womb, an ulcer that occurs in the womb.

Forms of ἀπόστημα and closely related words occur some seven times in the *Aphorisms*. In most cases, Ḥunayn's Arabic and the Syriac translate regularly, the former giving a form of *khurāj* 'abscess' and the latter a form

43 *Dabābil*, a plural of *dabla*, a word that Freytag glosses '*vomica, apostema; morbus in ventre*'. He does not include this particular plural form.

of *qubyānā* 'inflammation'. There are two exceptions to this in these two translations. In aphorism vii. 36 forms of ἀπόστημα occur twice, first in reference to swellings on the outside of the body and second in reference to those that are inside of the body. The Syriac uses *qubyānā* to refer to both, but for the second instance Ḥunayn breaks his habit, translating the word with *al-dabīla* 'ulcer'. The second exception is in aphorism vii. 78, where the Syriac alters its pattern to translate with *mapaqtā* 'inflammation, eruption of the skin'. This translation is similar to the Arabic *khurāj* in its metaphorical logic of derivation, both being derived from verbs meaning 'to go out'.

None of the lemmas containing this term survive in the fragments of the early Arabic translation. Ullmann notices several translations of this term, however, and the renderings taken from Galen's *On Simple Drugs* Book Six allow for the development of the Arabic tradition to be considered in the light of the entries in bar Bahlul's *Lexicon*. In these three examples, the early translator prefers in each case *al-awrām* 'inflammations', while Ḥunayn used equivalents like *al-kharājāt* and *al-dubayla* that tack closely with the examples from the *Aphorisms* given above.[44] Thus the citations of Ḥunayn and Paul in the entry at 251:24 relate more closely to the early Arabic translation, while bar Serošway's definitions there are closer to Ḥunayn's translation.

The entries found in the *Lexicon* reflect several senses of this Greek word. The single-word definition at 251:23 would fit well in a working translator's glossary and matches Ḥunayn's preference in the *Aphorisms* exactly. The entry at 251:24 introduces significantly more symptomatological detail. Although Arabic predominates, the most common Syriac equivalent of ἀπόστημα found in the *Aphorisms*, *qubyānā*, is found near the beginning in a definition attributable to Ḥunayn. It may be noted that the specification in the entry that ἀποστήματα/*qubyānē* occur 'on the outside of the body' does not agree with the usage found in the Greek original of the *Aphorisms* or in the Syriac translation, if it is to be taken as a general characterization.

44 Ullmann, *Wörterbuch zu den griechische-arabischen Übersetzungen*, 125–6.

The opthalmological entry at 253:21 is strongly related to an entry of bar Bahlul's on ἀγχίλωψ/αἰγίλωψ 'lachrymal abscess' discussed by Pormann in his work on Paul of Aegina, which reads as follows:

606:8 ܗ ܓܠܘܦܘܣ ثؤلول[45] ܘܐܝܟ ܦܘ ܐܦܘܣܛܝܡܐ ܙܥܘܪܐ ܕܩܪܢܬܐ ܪܒܬܐ ܕܥܝܢܐ ܗܝ ܕܠܘܬ ܢܚܝܪܐ ܕܡܬܦܬܚܐ
ܘܡܛܝܐ ܠܓܪܡܐ ܘܐܝܓܝܠܘܦܐ ܦܫܘܦܬܐ ܕܥܝܢܐ ܘܕܢܚܝܪܐ خُراج يكون ما بين ماق العين العظم والأنف وينفجر وإن
ضيع صار ناسوراً. ܘܐܝܟ ܒܪ ܣܪܘ ܩܪܢܬܐ ܕܥܝܢܐ ܕܡܫܓܠܐ ܘܐܬܡܬܚܐ الناسور في العين ܒ الغرب وريح
الغرب.

Heglopos, a wart. According to Paul a small abscess (*aposṭimā z'urā*) of the great corner of the eye (near) to the nose, when it breaks and reaches the bone. And *aykilopā, an abscess occurring between the great corner of the eye and the nose when it has broken. If it is neglected it becomes a fistula* (*nāsūr*). According to bar Serošway, a corner of the eye that abscesses and swells, *fistulas in the eye*. In a manuscript, *the West and the West Wind.*[46]

The phraseology of Paul's definition in this entry strongly resembles that of the unattributed definition of *aposṭimā minora* at 253:21. The Syriac descriptions of the affliction in the two entries are especially close, while the Arabic versions differ in some very slight details. It probably must be admitted, following Pormann, that in the entry at 606:8 there is some confusion of the two Greek terms which refer to this type of abscess before and after it has burst (ἀγχίλωψ and αἰγίλωψ, respectively).[47] However, if the transcription of the former term is to be recognized by the use of a *kāp* and that of the latter by the use of a *gāmal*, it would appear that the entry at 253:21 more accurately reflects the distinctions in the Greek terminology.

Given that the entry at 253:21 is unattributed, it is possible that it was written by Ḥunayn. Comparison with Pormann's example shows, however, that the entry at 606:8 overlaps significantly with the extant Arabic translation of Paul's *Pragmateia*. There are some slight differences between the two entries that correspond to readings in the Arabic translation of Paul's work. However, when comparing these, no clear pattern emerges. For example, the entry at 253:21 corresponds with the Arabic *Pragmateia* in calling fistulas *nāṣūr* against 606:8's *nāsūr*, yet 606:8 and the *Pragmateia* call the corner of the eye *al-'aẓm* while 253:21 calls it *al-akbar*.[48] Thus it

45 Duval: تولول. The reading given is Pormann's.

46 For Pormann's treatment of this entry, see *Oriental Tradition*, 156.

47 Ibid.

48 Ibid., 157.

appears that fragments which rely upon Paul may be found to exist in the *Lexicon* without identification. It bears repeating here that the attribution to Ḥunayn of any particular unidentified entry in the *Lexicon* requires some external corroboration in order to be considered certain.

The entries for the two Syriac equivalents of ἀπόστημα given in the *Aphorisms* read as follows:

1133:28 **ܡܦܩܬܐ** ܫܟܝܪܬܐ ܕܢܦܩܢ ܒܦܓܪܐ البثور السمجة الظاهر في الجسد. ܘܬܘܒ ܕܐܬܝܗܘܢ ܫܟܝܪܬܐ ܕܗܘܝܢ ܒܥܠܝܫܘܬܐ ܕܡܫܟܐ ܕܪܝܫܐ قروح الخراج. **ܡܦܩܬܐ** ܒܢ̈ إخراج خراجات وكلّ شيء يخرج من البدن يكون به البُحران قال المروزي عن حنين أنّ بقراط يستعمل ذلك على كلّ شيء يخرج من البدن فيه البحران؛

Mapqāṯā, pustules (*šaḵirṯā*) that appear on the body, *ugly pustules that appear on the body*. Again, sores (*al-buthūr*) on the surface of the skin of the head, *sores* (al-qurūḥ), *abscesses* (al-khurāj). *Mapaqṯā* in a manuscript, *breaking out of abscesses* (ikhrāj kharājāt). *Crises occur by virtue of anything that comes out from the body. Al-Marwazī said on the authority of Ḥunayn that Hippocrates used this (word) for anything that comes out from the body in which are crises.*

1721:6 **ܩܘܒܝܢܐ** ܐܝܟ ܚܢܝܢ احتقان. ܘܒܪ ܣܪܘܫܘܝ ܟܠ ܪܛܝܒܘܬܐ ܕܡܬܟܢܫܐ ܒܝܬ ܬܪܝܢ ܩܠܦܐ أورام حارّة جراحات. المروزي الخراجات وآخرون نزلات دُبلات؛

Quḇyānā, according to Ḥunayn *congestion* (iḥtiqān). And (according to) bar Serošway, any moisture that gathers together between two layers (of skin). *Hot swellings, lesions.* (*According to*) *al-Marwazī abscesses* (al-kharājāt). (*According to*) *others catarrhs* (nazalāt), *ulcers* (dubalāt).

While these Syriac entries refer to words whose scope of meaning is somewhat narrower than that of ἀπόστημα, they display a greater variety of terminology, more direct explanation of medical phenomena, and a strong tendency to branch out into discussions of broader medical theory. In the entry for *quḇyānā*, bar Serošway's description of the term is simple and direct and does not resort either to exotic terminology or to the listing of synonyms. On the other hand, al-Marwazī's account of Ḥunayn's teaching on Hippocrates' doctrine of the crisis in the entry for *mapaqṯā* extends the discussion beyond the everyday treatment of nagging sores into the significance of such sores for the prognosis of disease. This entry again shows the extent to which Syriac medical discourse had been nativized. Rather than referring Ḥunayn's account of Hippocrates' teaching to the Greek word, bar Bahlul records it for the Syriac equivalent instead. Despite the inherent interest of the Syriac entries, both the Greek and the Syriac lexicography represent Ḥunayn's translations of ἀπόστημα in the *Aphorisms* equally well.

3.9

ἀρθρῖτις

98:25 ܐܘܛܪܝܛܝܣ ܐܝܟ ܒܪ ܣܪܘ̄ ܟܐܒ ܫܪ̈ܝܬܐ وجع المفاصل ❖

Awtriṭis, according to bar Serošway pain of the joints (*keḇ šaryāṯā*), *pain of the joints* (wajʿ al-mafāṣil).

Forms of ἀρθρῖτις occur twice in the *Aphorisms*. Both the Syriac and Arabic translations agree with bar Serošway's entry in the *Lexicon*. Ḥunayn's Arabic translation does introduce a slight variation of style by using the singular in the phrase *waj ' al-mafāṣil* 'pain of the joints' to translate ἀρθρίτιδες in aphorism iii. 16, but the plural *awjā' al-mafāṣil* 'pains of the joints' to translate ἀρθριτικά in iii. 20. The Syriac uses the same form *keḇ šāryāṯā* 'pain of the joints' in each case, as does the fragment of the early Syriac translation of iii. 20.

A definition of the Syriac equivalent reads as follows:

857:9 … ܟܐܒ ܫܪ̈ܝܬܐ وجع المفاصل ❖

Keḇ šāryāṯā, pain of the joints (wajʿ al-mafāṣil).

Thus in this straightforward example, the Greek and Syriac lexicography represent Ḥunayn's Arabic translation equally well.

3.10

ἀριστερά

299:22 ܐܪܣܝܛܪܐ ܣܡ̈ܠܐ ܐܝܟ ܒܪ ܣܪܘ̄ الشمال اليسار ❖

Arsiṭrā, the left. According to bar Serošway *the left, the left side*.

Forms of ἀριστερά occur twice in the *Aphorisms*. Both instances refer to the sympathetic relationship between the thinning of one of the breasts of a woman pregnant with twins and the miscarriage of one of her children. Ḥunayn's Arabic and the Syriac translate in similar ways, the former with *al-aysar* and the latter with *semālā*, both meaning 'the left'. These translations are fully reflected in the entry in the *Lexicon*. A short entry for the Syriac equivalent reads like this:

1359:16 ܣܡ̈ܠܐ أقول اليسار الشمال ❖

Semālā, I say the left side (al-yasār), *the left.*

3.11

ἄρρην

303:12 ܐܪܪܘܢ ܐܝܟ ܪܒܢ ܕܟܪܐ ذكر ܀

Arron according to our teacher, male (*deḵrā*), *male* (dhakar).

This word is translated consistently in both the Syriac and Arabic *Aphorisms*. Ḥunayn's Arabic employs *al-dhakar* 'male' in various forms and the Syriac uses the related word *dḵar* 'male'. These translations concord almost exactly with Ḥunayn's definition of the Greek word in the *Lexicon*. An entry related to the Syriac equivalent likewise agrees with Ḥunayn's translation:

574:24 ܕܟܪܐ ܫܡܐ ܡܫܘܕܥܢܐ ܕܓܢܣܐ ܒܓܢܣܐ ܕܡܬܦܪܫ ܒܐܙܕܘܘܓܘܬܐ ܦܪܝܫܐ ܒܗܘ ܙܪܥܐ ܣܓܝܐܐ. ܡܛܠ ܐܐ
ܢܬܚܠܦܘܢ ܠܡܡܘܢܘܬܐ ܕܐܓܢܣܐ الذكر الإحليل. ܕܟܪܐ كبش ذكر. ܒܢܝ̈ ܕܟܪ̈ܐ أولاد الكباش وهي الحملان.
ܕܟܪܐ ܒܢܝ̈ ܕܝ̈ܨܐ كباش الثياتل ܀

Deḵrā, a name that indicates the sex in a species that is distinguished in marriage (by) abundant seed for the continuation of the species, *male* (al-dhakar), *urethra* (al-iḥlīl). *Deḵrā, a male sheep. Banay deḵrē, the children of the ram, which are lambs. Deḵrē*, children of the ibex (*banay dayṣē*), *a ram, wild goats* (al-thayātil).

3.12

ἀρχή

293:5 ܐܪܟܐ ܫܘܪܝܐ ܐܘ ܪܫܝܬܐ ܗܘ ܕܝܘܢܝܐ ܐܪܟܐ ܐܡܝܪ ابتداء رئيس الامم الصحيح ܘܐܝܟ ܒܪ ܣܪܘ
ܗܘ ܕܝܘܢܝܐ ܐܪܟܢܐ ܐܡܝܪ ܠܗ ܀

Arkā, in the Greek *arkā* means beginning (*šurāyā*) or heading, *beginning* (ibtidā'), *the rightful leader of the nations.* According to bar Serošway, in Greek it is '*arkānā*'.

293:19 ܐܪܐܟܝ ܥܒܪܝܐ ܐܘܟܝܬ ܪܫ ܥܡܐ ܢܬܩܪܐ ܀

Arāḵay 'Eḇrāyā, that is, he was called leader of the Hebrews.

304:1 ܐܪܫܝ ܗܘ ܫܘܪܝܐ ܪܫܝܬܐ ابتداء رأس ܀

Arši, this is beginning (*šurāyā*), heading, *beginning* (ibtidā'), *heading*.

Forms of ἀρχή occur several times in the *Aphorisms*. The Syriac translates with forms of *šurāyā* 'beginning', while Ḥunayn's Arabic gives forms of *al-awwal* 'beginning'. Al-Biṭrīq's usual equivalent for these instances was *bad'* 'beginning'. The only exception in the latter is found in the translation of aphorism i. 12, where the phrase *min awwal al-maraḍ* 'from the beginning of the disease' is employed.

The entries taken from the *Lexicon* converge somewhat with the examples found in the *Aphorisms*. Both *šurāyā* and *al-ibtidā'* are represented in the entries at 293:5 and 304:1, each of which is attributable to Ḥunayn. However, Ḥunayn's usual equivalent for ἀρχή *al-awwal* is not represented in either of them. The entry in bar Bahlul's *Lexicon* for the usual Syriac equivalent for ἀρχή *šurāyā* reads as follows:

1957:11 **ܫܘܪܝܐ** ܐܝܟ ܒܪ ܣܪܘ ܐܝܬܘܗ̄ ܡܢܬܐ ܡܫܘܚܬܐ ܕܙܒܢܐ. ܕܢܩܦ ܠܐܝܠܝܢ ܕܡܫܬܪܝܢ. ܘܡܬܚܡܢܐ
ܕܥܒܕܐ ܘܕܙܒܢܐ. ܕܙܒܢܐ ܓܝܪ ܡܬܝܕܥ ܗܘ ܕܥܒܕܐ ܕܣܘܥܪܢܐ ܐܝܟܢܐ ܕܗܘ ܥܕܡܐ ܠܥܒܕܐ ܕܣܘܥܪܢܐ
ܐܚܪܢܐ ܐܘ ܕܐܝܬ ܠܗ ܕܡܬܚܡܐ ܕܙܒܢܐ ܡܦܣܩܐ. ܘܠܬܘܡܬܗܘܢ܁ ܡܠܝܢ ܠܥܒܕܐ ܐܡܪ ܐܢܐ ܘܠܙܒܢܐ ܫܘܪܝܐ
ܡܬܬܩܝܡ. ܡܛܠ ܕܠܝܬ ܥܒܕܐ ܕܠܐ ܡܫܬܪܐ. ܘܠܐ ܙܒܢܐ ܕܠܐ ܫܘܪܝܐ الابتداء. **ܕܠܐ ܫܘܪܝ**، ܐܝܟ ܙܟܪ
ابديّ܀

Šurāyā according to bar Serošway, it has the meaning of the beginning of (some) time which accompanies those (things) that begin, defining both the action and the time. For the meaning of time is that of the action of an affair of some sort up until the action of some other affair, or (the action of an affair) which has a beginning at a definite time. And I say that beginning refers both to action and to time. For there is no action that does not begin, and no time without a beginning. *Beginning* (al-ibtidā'). *D-lā šurāy* according to Zakariya, *eternal (*abadī*)*.

Bar Serošway introduces questions of the nature of time in this somewhat extended discussion of the sense of this Syriac word. However, the Greek and the Syriac lexicography are equally unrepresentative of Ḥunayn's Arabic translations of ἀρχή in the *Aphorisms*. Assuming that Ḥunayn was not in fact the author of the extant Syriac *Aphorisms*, this could be due to the fact that Ḥunayn preferred a different word in his own Syriac translation.

3.13

ἀσθενής

245:20 **ܐܣܬܗܢܝܣ** ܐܝܟ ܒܪ ܣܪܘ ܡܚܝܠܐ ضعيف܀

Astênis according to bar Serošway, weak (*mḥilā*), *weak* (ḍaʿīf).

Forms of ἀσθενής occur several times in the *Aphorisms*. Ḥunayn's Arabic translation employs words related to the verb *ḍaʿufa* 'to be weak' in all instances. The Syriac version for its part uses the adjective *mḥilā* 'weak' in all instances. Despite the fact that both display a relatively similar degree of regularity, Ḥunayn's version tends slightly more toward expanding the texts than does the Syriac translation. In aphorism ii. 49, for example, Ḥunayn translated the phrase κῆν ὦσιν ἀσθενέες ἢ γέροντες with *wa-in kāna ḍa'īfata al-badan aw shaykha* 'and if they are weak or old', using the inner accusative *ḍa'īfata al-badan* which literally means 'weak in the body'. The Syriac translation of this phrase is *ap sāḇā iṯayhon aw mḥilē* 'though they are old or weak'. The Syriac text is also perhaps notable in that the two adjectives are in reverse order from the Greek and Arabic versions.

Ullmann also notes a text from Book Six of Galen's *On Simple Drugs* that contains a form of ἀσθενής. There, the early translator al-Biṭrīq and Ḥunayn both translated the phrase ἀσθενεστέρα τὴν δύναμιν in the same way, giving *ḍa'īf al-quwwa* 'weak in strength' for it.[49] The entry at 1054:1 bar Bahlul's *Lexicon* for the Syriac equivalent *mḥilā* further confirms these terms' synonymity:

1054:1 ܡܚܝܠܐ ضعيف. ܡܚܝܠܘܬܐ ضَعْف⁛[50]

Mḥilā, weak (ḍa'īf). *Mḥiluṯā, weakness* (ḍa'f).

3.14

ἀχλύς

157:16 ܐܟܠܘܣ ܘܐܟܘܠܘܣ ܬܘܒ ܐܝܟ ܒܪ ܣܪܘܫܘܝ ܥܡܛܢܐ الظلمة. ܘܬܘܒ ܐܟܠܘܣ ܥܡܛܢܐ ܘܥܢܢܐ الغمام القتام الضباب⁛

Aklus or again *akulus* according to bar Serošway, darkness (*'amṭānā*) , *darkness* (al-ẓulma). Again *aklus*, darkness, clouds, *clouds, gloom, mist.*

In aphorism iii. 5, the word ἀχλυώδεες appears in a list of disorders that occur due to south winds. Ḥunayn translated this word with the phrase *ghishāwatun fī al-baṣar* 'a veil in the vision', while the Syriac version employs the phrase *'amṭānā ḇa-ḥzāṯā* 'darkness in the vision'. Although the definition in bar Bahlul overaps generally with the Syriac translation, there is no specific reference to an ophthalmological condition. Furthermore, Ḥunayn's equivalent *ghishāwa* is lacking. Neither is the latter found in the entry for the Syriac equivalent *'amṭānā*:

1441:22 ܥܡܛܢܐ ܒܨܚ̈ ظلمة شديدة تحدث نهاراً من غيم أسود. ܕܗܐ ܐܬ̇ܐ ܐܢܐ ܠܘܬܟ ܒܥܡܛܢܐ ܕܥܢܢܐ ܗ̄ ܕܝܢ ܒܥܡܘܕܐ ܕܥܢܢܐ آتيك في ظلمة الغيم. ܥܡܛܢܐ ܬܘܒ ܚܫܘܟܐ ܕܠܐ ܡܬܚܫܝܢ ܗܘ ܒܗ ܒܥܝܢܐ ظلام⁛

'Amṭānā in a manuscript, *severe darkness occurring during the day because of a black cloud. D-hā āṯē enā lwaṯaḵ b-'amṭānā ḏa-'nānā*, this is in the pillar of the cloud, *I come to*

49 Ullmann, *Wörterbuch zu den griechisch-arabischen Übersetzungen*, 139.

50 Duval: ضَعْف. This entry is also cited in unit (2.5) above.

you in the darkness of the cloud.[51] *'Amṭānā* again, darkness in which the stars cannot be seen, *darkness*.

Nor again is it found in the entry for *'amṭānā* in bar ʿAli's *Lexicon*:

ܥܡܛܢܐ الظلام. والظللمة ضباب. ܘܗܘ ܚܫܘܟܐ.[52]

'Amṭānā, gloom, darkness, mist. It is darkness (*ḥešoḵā*).

As in the discussions of ἀκριβής and ἀρχή above (units 3.2 and 3.12, respectively), Ḥunayn's preferred Arabic translation in the *Aphorisms* is present neither in the Greek lexicography nor that of the relevant Syriac equivalent. Furthermore, as in the cases of ἄνυδρος and αὐτόματον (units 1.2 and 1.3, respectively, the Syriac version employs a phrase rather than a single word in translating ἀχλυώδεες. This may be the reason it escaped representation in the lexicons. On the other hand it is impossible to rule out that Ḥunayn preferred a different Syriac word from *'amṭānā* to translate ἀχλυώδεες in his Syriac version of the *Aphorisms*. The word *ḥešoḵā* 'darkness' mentioned in the entry of bar ʿAli's above is be a natural place to begin searching for a potential alternative. A relatively long, unattributed entry for that word runs as follows:

779:3 **ܚܫܘܟܐ** ܗ̄ ܚܝܠܐ ܐܝܬܝܐ ܘܬܠܝܦܐ ܕܢܬܝܐ ܕܡܬܢܝܬܐ ܡܥܒܕܢܘܬܗ ܘܡܪܓܫ ܒܚܣܝܪܘܬܗ
ܒܚܣܝܪܘܬܐ ܕܢܘܗܪܐ. الظلمة. **ܡܚܫܟ** ܡܚܫܟܠ. ܐܝܟ ܗܘ ܕܠܡܚܫܟܘ ܥܝܢܝܟ ܘܠܡܦܪܬܘ ܢܦܫܟ يظلم
عينيك ويذيب نفسك. **ܡܚܫܟ** ܚܫܘܟܐ ܕܥܝܢܬ ܡܚܫܟܢ ܥܝܢܝܟ. ܐܝܟ ܗܘ ܕܐܡܪ ܦܠܘܛܐ ܡܦܫܪ ܘܡܚܫܟ
المساء يروح ممسى. **ܚܫܘܟܐ** ܐܬܘܬܐ ܠܛܠܠܐ ܕܒܥܡܛܢܐ ܚܦܝܐ. ܕܒܠܝܠܘܬܐ ܢܘܗܪܐ ܡܬܚܦܝܢ.
ܡܬܬܚܝܬ [illegible] ܡܛܠ ܕܠܐ [illegible] ܚܫܘ̈ܟܐ. ܡܛܠ ܕܠܐ ܒܥܝܢܐ ܠܥܡܛܢܐ
ܚܕܝܡ ܚܫܘܟܐ. ܐܠܐ ܐܝܠܝܢ ܕܥܝܢ ܠܚܘܕ ܘܠܝܬ ܒܗܘܢ ܦܫܝܛܘܬܐ. ܗܘ ܕܒܠܝܠܘܬܐ ܢܘܗܪܐ
ܡܬܚܦܝܢ. ܕܐܠܐ ܐܢ ܒܕ ܡܛܠ ܒܠܝ ܢܘܗܪܐ ܒܡܒܪܝܢܘܬ ܠܐ ܗܘܐ ܚܫܘܟܐ. ܕܠܐ ܗܘܐ ܒܪ ܚܝܠܐ
ܐܝܬܘܗܝ ܚܫܘܟܐ. ܡܬܚܫܒܐ ܡܢ ܗܕܐ ܕܐܢ ܢܦܩ ܐܝܟ ܦܥܠܢܐ ܒܢܘܗܪܐ ܘܡܬܦܫܪܐ ܠܗ ܡܫܬܟܚܬ
ܕܐܝܟ ܕܠܡܦܪܫ ܢܘܗܪܐ ܠܐ ܢܦܠ ܒܗ. ܒܪ ܥܒܕܬܗ ܗܘܐ ܒܗ ܚܫܘܟܐ. ܘܗܘܐ ܐܢ ܚܝܠܐ ܐܝܬܘܗܝ
ܗܘܐ ܠܗ ܥܠ ܐܝܟܢܐ، ܕܚܙܝܐ ܐܝܬ ܒܪ ܗܘܐ ܠܗ الظلمة. ܘܬܘܒ **ܚܫܘܟܐ** ܐܝܟ ܕܐܢܫ ܐܡܪܘ
ܠܒܝܬܐ ܗܘ ܕܡܢ ܛܠܠܐ ܕܒܥܡܛܢܐ ܐܬܦܫܪ. ܘܡܫܚܠܦܐ ܡܦܪܫܢܐ ܚܝܠܐ ܐܡܪ ܕܐܝܬܘܗܝ ܚܕ ܡܢ ܥܡܚܠܐ
ܚܝܠܐ ܡܕ̈ܡܝܐ ܕܐܝܬܘܗܝ ܦܝܫܢ̈ܝܐ ܠܓܘܫܡܐ ܕܐܝܬܝܗܘܢ. ܥܦܪܐ. ܘܐܪܥܐ. ܢܘܪܐ. ܘܡܝ̈ܐ. ܘܐܐܪ.
ܡܠܐܟܐ. ܚܫܘܟܐ.❖

Ḥešoḵā, this is a fluid substance that hinders vision, whose action and sensibility are known through the absence of light. *Darkness* (al-ẓulma). *Maḥšeḵ*, to darken, as in 'it darkens your

51 Exod. 19:9.

52 Gottheil (ed.), *Syriac-Arabic Glosses*, II, 220:13.

eyes and consumes your soul', *it darkens your eyes and consumes your soul. Mḥaššeḵ*, the darkness of the place of the setting of the sun, as in 'he approached Palestine early and late'. *The evening, he went in the evening. Ḥešoḵā* is the shadow of a dense body, which consists of the absence of light. It is defined as a shadow because it has no substance, and it is of dense bodies because not all bodies bring about darkness, but only those that are dense and which have no transparency in them. Its consisting in the absence of light means that, but for the complete absence of light, there would be no darkness. For darkness is that which does not have substance. It is ascertained from this (example): If someone pitches a tent at mid-day, and it mostly covers him, such that light entirely does not reach him, simultaneously there is darkness in it. But if it had substance, whensoever someone sought to do so, he might bring it into being.[53] *Darkness.* Again, *ḥešoḵā* according to the people, they say it is an accident that occurs on account of the shadow of a body. But the blessed commentator[54] said that it is a substance, one of the seven primary substances that come to be in the sixth, which are heaven, earth, fire, water, air, angels and darkness.

In this very interesting entry, two contradictory accounts of the nature of darkness are presented side-by-side. One of these may easily be linked with the Peripatetic conception of darkness, while the other is presented within a theological context. In my opinion it is likely that Ḥunayn wrote the Peripatetic-leaning material in the entry, while bar Bahlul himself appears to prefer the theological account.

Another, shorter entry contains a word closely related to Ḥunayn's equivalent for ἀχλύς in the *Aphorisms*, *ghishāwa*:

780:15 **ܚܫܟܐ** الظُلمة. **ܚܫ̈ܟܢܐ** الدوار والسدر. ܘܐܝܟ ܙܟܪܝܐ الظلمة الغشوة. ܒ̈ ܠܠܝܐ ܕܠܐ ܣܗܪܐ
ظلمة ليل بلا قمر ❖

Ḥeškā, darkness. Ḥeškānē, dizziness, vertigo. According to Zakariya, *darkness, covering* (ghishwa). In a manuscript, a night with no moon, *the darkness of a night without a moon.*

Whatever the case may be, neither the Greek lexicography nor that for the Syriac equivalent found in the *Aphorisms* accords with Ḥunayn's Arabic translation of this word.

---

53 See Aristotle's account of darkness as a privation, given in his definition of light in *On the Soul*, Book II.7, 418b9. See also J. de Groot, *Aristotle and Philoponus on Light* (London 1991), *passim*.

54 This would seem to be a reference to Theodore of Mopsuestia, an influential theologian of the Church of the East. See A. Mingana (ed.), *Commentary of Theodore of Mopsuestia on the Nicene Creed* (Cambridge 1932), 16.

Conclusion

The Composition of the Lexicon's *Entries*

Before proceeding to consider the relative importance of the Greek and Syriac lexicography for Ḥunayn's Arabic translation, some analysis of the composition of the entries of bar Bahlul's *Lexicon* may prove instructive. For this reason I shall consider here the quantities of definitions contained in the Greek and Syriac entries and the frequency with which the various authors cited by bar Bahlul appear in them. Although these counts are approximate, rely significantly on my subjective judgment, and in a few places in the examples of Syriac lexicography are taken from abridged entries, they still should provide a general idea concerning the varying patterns of Greek and Syriac scholarship discoverable in bar Bahlul's *Lexicon*.

In the selections above, I presented 41 entries containing definitions of Greek words. These 41 entries contain 65 headwords. Of these 65 headwords, 27 were left unattributed by the compiler, 10 are referred to 'a manuscript', and four are attributed expressly to Ḥunayn. Thus, following bar Bahlul's own statement regarding unattributed definitions discussed in the opening section of this chapter, 41 of the 65 definitions of these Greek entries are attributable to Ḥunayn.[55] Of the remaining, 18 are attributed to bar Serošway, two to Sergius, two to Paul of Aegina, two to 'others' and one to Jibrīl ibn Bukhtīshūʿ.

38 entries for Syriac words occur above, containing 134 definitions. Of these 134, 65 were left unattributed, 10 are referred to 'a manuscript', and six are attributed expressly to Ḥunayn. All told, then, 81 are attributable to Ḥunayn. Of the remainder, 20 are referred to bar Serošway, ten were provided by bar Bahlul himself with the phrase 'I say' (*aqūl*), seven are referred to Zakariya, five to al-Marwazī, four to the *Book of Paradise* and three to 'others'.

A little less than two-thirds of the entries in both categories are attributable to Ḥunayn, so bar Bahlul's level of reliance upon the famous translator may be said to be comparable in both Greek and Syriac. The two

55 Although the attribution to Ḥunayn of unattributed entries may of course be challenged in any specific case, I see no reason to dispute the general validity of bar Bahlul's statement.

categories naturally differ in the lists of authors to whom bar Bahlul attributed definitions. Five authors are mentioned as sources for the definitions of Greek words: Ḥunayn, bar Serošway, Sergius, Paul and Jibrīl ibn Bukhtīshūʿ. For the definitions of Syriac words, however, seven authors are cited: Ḥunayn, bar Serošway, bar Bahlul himself, Zakariya, al-Marwazī, Paul and the *Book of Paradise*. This points to a readily-intuitable fact, namely that the number of Syriac-speaking authors working in Greek was less than that of such authors working in Syriac during this period.

Several patterns emerge in comparing these two sets of figures. Most obviously, the Syriac entries tend to include more headwords than do the Greek entries, or, to put it another way, the Greek entries tend to define very specific senses of the words in question. Furthermore, the definitions for Syriac headwords are more likely to be extended beyond the simple listing of synonyms. In general, there tends to be a reasonably clear distinction between the glosses attributed to the various authors. In particular, regarding the problem of the relationship between the lexicography of Ḥunayn and that of bar Serošway mentioned at the beginning of the chapter, it appears that the two authors usually offer independent interpretations. However, there are examples of significant overlap between the two, as in the discussion of ἀνέλπιστος in unit (2.8).

Greek Lexicography, Syriac Lexicography and the Arabic Translations

While numerous Greek words identified by Duval in bar Bahlul's *Lexicon* are also present in the *Aphorisms*, they represent a definite minority of all the words found in the Hippocratic work. Only about a third of the words beginning with *alpha* are also present in the *Lexicon*. In considering these entries systematically, furthermore, this proportion suffers attrition from various causes. Some of these result from Duval's identifications, which at times are or appear to be little more than guesses. Others may be proved incorrect with closer scrutiny, although this is relatively rare. Also significant are Duval's identifications which declare etymologically-Greek Syriac words to be Greek without qualification, as for example regarding the entry for ἀγωγή treated above in unit (2.2).

Despite all of these qualifications, it is clear that relevant examples of Greek-to-Arabic lexicography are discoverable in the *Lexicon*. That said, it is also clear that a significantly larger number of Syriac-to-Arabic entries of the *Lexicon* of bar Bahlul (and that of bar ʿAli as well, where I have cited it) are representative of Ḥunayn's Arabic translation of the *Aphorisms*. When the Greek-centred approach I have followed in this chapter is taken into account, the latter point is only made sharper. Since the *Lexicon* is much more broadly representative of the Syriac language than it is of the Greek, an approach to Ḥunayn's translation that took the words of the Syriac *Aphorisms* as its starting point would very likely display a similar pattern of agreement between the lexicography and the Arabic translations.

Perhaps the easiest explanation for this would be that the lexicographers often worked by reading together copies of Ḥunayn's Syriac and Arabic translations and extracting the equivalents found therein. This evidence also may indicate that Ḥunayn's Arabic translation of the *Aphorisms* was made with some sort of reference to a Syriac exemplar. However, this does not necessarily mean that the work was translated solely from Ḥunayn's Syriac version. It is here that the Greek entries of bar Bahlul's *Lexicon* can really contribute to the argument. This may be seen in the discussion of the translations of the word ἀσθματικοί (unit 2.10 of this chapter), perhaps the strongest example given above. There, the Arabic equivalent in the *Aphorisms* is found in the entry for the Syriac equivalent, and bar Bahlul adds that Ḥunayn had 'rectified' the relationship between the two languages. While the Greek entry contains neither the Syriac or Arabic equivalents, it does reflect quite well Ḥunayn's rendition of Galen's explanation of the sense of ἄσθμα in his commentary on the aphorism. Even with the caveat that Ḥunayn composed his Syriac translation of the Hippocratic lemmas separately from his Syriac version of Galen's *Commentary*, this example still gives evidence that a certain division of labour between Greek and Syriac lexicography was a part of Ḥunayn's translation praxis.

Here too, however, the continuing uncertainty regarding the authorship of the Syriac translation is keenly felt. If it were certain that Ḥunayn did in fact compose the work, comparisons amongst the Greek original and the several translations could be expected to determine quite clearly whether he relied more on the Greek original or the Syriac in producing his Arabic version. As it is, however, if we are to assume that Ḥunayn was the author of the Syriac *Aphorisms*, there begins to appear a certain inconsistency in the evidence. Despite some exceptions, a strong relationship exists between bar

Bahlul's Syriac-Arabic lexicography and Ḥunayn's Arabic version of the *Aphorisms*. However, there also exist at times very severe differences between the textual interpretations of the Syriac and Arabic versions of the Hippocratic work, as well as important differences in style. Thus, although we may be reasonably sure that a Syriac version played some role in the production of Ḥunayn's Arabic translation, it seems just as unlikely, if not more so, that the extant Syriac *Aphorisms* was the text he actually used.

With that said, the examples presented above demonstrate clearly that the Syriac lexicons contain an abundance of material relevant to Ḥunayn's Greek-to-Arabic translation. Despite often strong variations between Ḥunayn's Arabic translation and the Syriac version, the equivalents found in the latter often provide a reasonably good guide for uncovering Ḥunayn's Syriac-Arabic equivalencies. Even when it seems clear that an equivalent given in the Syriac *Aphorisms* was not preferred by Ḥunayn in his own Syriac translation, the content of bar Bahlul's entries may be used to trace possible alternatives. With the general relationship between these translations and the Syriac lexicons thus clarified, it should be possible to make informed use of the latter in order to make reference to any significant Syriac influence upon Ḥunayn's Arabic translation praxis.

Chapter 2

Greek Loan-words in the Syriac *Aphorisms* and Ḥunayn's Arabic Translation Techniques

In the previous chapter, I examined the relationships between the Syriac and Arabic translations of the Hippocratic *Aphorisms* and the *Syriac Lexicon* of Ḥasan bar Bahlul with the primary aim of gaining an understanding of the part played by Greek and Syriac sources in the production of Ḥunayn ibn Isḥāq's Arabic translations. Building on that material, in this second chapter I seek to elucidate further the relationship between the lexicographical scholarship of Ḥunayn and his school and the translator's approach to medical translation.

In a number of important contributions, Sebastian Brock has traced the development of Syriac receptivity to Greek style and vocabulary.[1] A spirit of admiration for the cultural achievements and intellectual expertise of classical Greek writers found its expression in the changes Syriac writers made to their language over the course of several centuries. Grammatical constructions and idioms borrowed from Greek came to be more and more prominent in the usage of Syriac writers and thinkers. As part of this process, Greek loan-words came to be relied upon ever more greatly in place or in absence of native Syriac equivalents.

As will be demonstrated below, there is strong evidence to suggest that this receptivity to Greek vocabulary was not shared by the Arabic literary audience. In fact, in his Arabic translation of the *Aphorisms*, Ḥunayn very often made extensive efforts to avoid using vocabulary derived from the Greek. This is one of the most salient differences between the Syriac and Arabic approaches to the translation of the *Aphorisms*.

---

1 Most recently, in S. Brock, 'Charting the Hellenization of a Literary Culture: The Case of Syriac', *Intellectual History of the Islamicate World* 3:1–2 (2015). See also idem., 'From Antagonism to Assimilation: Syriac Attitudes to Greek Learning', in N. Garsoïan et al. (eds), *East of Byzantium: Syria and Armenia in the Formative Period* (Washington, D.C. 1980), 17–34; as well as papers collected in *Syriac Perspectives on Late Antiquity* (London 1984). Also of importance for this subject is A.M. Butts' recently published monograph *Language Change in the Wake of Empire: Syriac in its Greco-Roman Context* (Winona Lake, IN 2016).

Duval's Greek index to bar Bahlul's *Lexicon* regularly includes what are in effect etymologically Greek Syriac words. Because of this, one of the more obvious uses of this index is to trace the effects of the contrasting Syriac and Arabic approaches to Greek loan-words. In order to do this I have identified numerous examples of translations in the Syriac *Aphorisms* wherein the Greek word is in effect left untranslated in the Syriac version. In these cases, that is, a Greek loan-word in Syriac stands for the very Greek word from which it was derived. I have proceeded to analyse the translations and lexicographical treatments of these words along similar lines to those adopted in the previous chapter. Rather than focusing primarily upon the part played by the lexicography in these relationships, however, here I categorize the material according to the character of Ḥunayn's Arabic translations of these words.

In the first part, I present studies of Greek words whose Arabic translations in Ḥunayn's version of the *Aphorisms* display a high degree of instability, usually owing to the translator's use of clause-length explicating translations. In the second part, I treat Greek words whose Arabic translations by Ḥunayn in the *Aphorisms* are relatively stable, but which show evidence for the translator's having worked to establish new terminological equivalents. In the third part, I present Greek words for which both the Arabic and the Syriac translations either deploy nativized equivalents derived from that self-same Greek word, or for which there is no reason not to assume continuity between Ḥunayn's Arabic translation techniques and the earlier stages of the translation movement.

In adopting this method of organization, I hope first and foremost to point out potential consequences of Syriac's Hellenizing tendency for Ḥunayn's Arabic translations. In a broader context, these consequences could be shown to represent a kind of negative Syriac influence upon the translations. These studies would then constitute test cases which could be used to answer certain questions. Firstly, how deep was the influence of the trend toward adoption of Greek vocabulary in Syriac medicine? In other words, did the Syriac glossographers treat these Greek words as fully native, or were etymologically Syriac equivalents resorted to in order to explain them? If not, to what extent did the absence of a significant effort in developing native vocabulary on the part of Syriac translators influence or limit Ḥunayn's Arabic translation technique?

Many of the Greek words that Syriac medical writers adopted were relatively central to the art of medicine. For this reason, detailed consideration of these words allows for a closer approach to the history of medicine strictly speaking than was afforded by the words treated in the first chapter. This approach thus will regularly display the value of bar Bahlul's *Lexicon* for the history of Syriac and Arabic medicine and medical translation.

Section One

In this section, I compare the translations and lexicographical background of Greek words in the *Aphorisms* for which the Syriac version of that work employs the self-same borrowed from the Greek, and for which Ḥunayn's Arabic translations display a high degree of instability.

1.1

αἱμορροΐδες

67:21 **ܐܘܡܘܕܪܐܣܝܣ** التوت وهو جنس من البواسير ❖

Awmudrasis, al-tūt,[2] *which is a type of haemorrhoids* (al-bawāsīr).

616:7 **ܗܡܘܪܘܐܝܕܝܣ** ܗ̄ ܥܪܩܐ ܕܚܕܪ، ܠܒܝܬ ܡܦܩܬܐ. ܟܕ ܡܬܦܣܩ ܢܦܩ ܡܢܗ ܕܡܐ ܣܓܝܐܐ العرق الدقيق الذي حول المقعدة وينقطع ويخرج منه دم كثير ❖

Hēmuruidēs, this is the vein that surrounds the anus, when it is cut and there flows forth from it much blood. *The fine vein that surrounds the anus, when it is cut and there flows forth from it much blood.*

637:5 **ܗܡܘܪܪܐܝܕܝܣ** بواسير ܒܝ ܗ̄ ܡܡܘܪܕܘܐܝܕܝܣ ❖

Hēmurraidēs, *haemorrhoids* (al-bawāsīr). In a manuscript, it is *mmurduaidēs*.

Forms of the word αἱμορροΐς occur four times in the *Aphorisms*. For all of these examples, the Syriac translation gives a form of the self-same word borrowed from Greek. For three occurrences of the word clustered together in book six of the *Aphorisms*, Ḥunayn gives *al-bawāsīr* as a translation. However, for the other instance, found in aphorism iii. 30, Ḥunayn gives a five-word exegetical translation, *infitāḥ afwāh al-'urūq min asfal* ('the opening of the mouths of the veins from below'). As will be seen in other places below, this aphorism in particular contains several exegetical

2 *Al-tūt* means 'mulberry', but it appears that a different sense is intended here.

translations. It may be that Ḥunayn consciously preferred to explicate here in response to the context of Galen's commentary on the text.

This explicating translation appears all the more exceptional when the broader translation tradition as treated by Ullmann is taken into account. Along with the citation of one of the aphorisms from book six mentioned above, the translations of forms of αἱμορροΐς from three other works are cited in his *Wörterbuch*. All of these likewise employ a form of *al-bawāsīr*.[3]

Turning to the entries in bar Bahlul's *Lexicon*, the definition found at 616:7 explains the symptoms of the disease without providing a single-word equivalent. The Syriac and Arabic glosses correspond to one another almost exactly. The only significant variation is the addition of the word 'fine' (*al-daqīq*) to the Arabic definition. The definition provides a technical explanation of the phenomenon which, while detailed, does not overlap significantly with the exegetical translation in Ḥunayn's version of aphorism iii. 30. In contrast, the definition given at 637:5 simply provides *al-bawāsīr* as a synonym for the Greek word, and thus could easily have been drawn from a translation or from a translator's working glossary.

1.2

εἰλεός

128:17 **ܐܝܠܐܘܣ** ܒܢܝ̈ ܡܦܩܢܐ ܐܠܗܐ ܚܘܣ نوع من أنواع القولنج يقذف فيه الإنسان الثفل معنى اسمه يا رب أرحم وجع ألمعا ܘܐܝܟ ܒܪ ܣܪܘ **ܐܠܝܐܘܣ** ܕܐܝܬܘܗ̇ ܟܐܒܐ ܕܗܘܐ ܒܡܥ̈ܝܐ ܘܐܝܬܘܗ̇ ܕܡܣܬܟܢܘܬܐ. ܘܐܝܠܝܢ ܕܡܝܬܝܢ ܒܗܢܐ ܡܘܬܐ ܫܘܐ ܠܡܬܪܚܡܘ ܗܘܐ ܠܗܘܢ ورم المعا القتّال܀

Ailāos in a manuscript, it is glossed 'God have pity'. *One of the types of colic in which people discharge sediment. The meaning of its name is 'Oh my Lord have mercy'. Pain of the bowels.* According to bar Serošway *alêaws*, which is a disease that occurs in the bowels and is perilous. Those that die this death deserve to have pity shown to them. *A deadly inflammation of the bowels.*

27-167:25 **ܐܠܝܐܘܣ** ܗܘ ܕܐܝܬܘܗ̇ ܟܐܒܐ ܘܡܥܨܪܢܘܬܐ ܘܗܦܘܟܝܐ ܕܡܥ̈ܝܐ. ܘܟܘܪܗܢܐ ܕܗܘܐ ܒܡܥ̈ܝܐ ܡܚܝ̈ܠܬܐ. ܠܗ ܠܟܘܪܗܢܐ ܩܪܐ ܟܘܪܕܘܦܘܣ ܗܪܐ. ܘܠܐ ܡܬܐܣܝܢܐ. ܗܘ ܗܢܐ ܟܐܒܐ يا رب أرحم܀

Alêaos, this is pain, contortion and recession (*hpuḵyā*) of the bowels. A disease that occurs in the small intestine. He called this disease *krodopos* (χορδαψός)[4]. It cannot be treated. This pain is *'Oh my Lord have mercy'*.

---

3 Ullmann, *Wörterbuch zu den griechisch-arabischen Übersetzungen*, 82–3.

4 According to Duval's identification. The word is defined in Liddell-Scott as '*a disease in the great guts*, identical to εἰλεός in the small ones'.

Forms of εἰλεός occur three times in the *Aphorisms*, and the Syriac translation gives the borrowed Greek word for all of them. Ḥunayn's Arabic version of the work, for its part, shows what appears to be a definite process of development. His translations run as follows:

iii. 22 القولنج الشديد الذي يسمّيه اليونانيون إيلاوس

The severe colic that the Greeks call *īlā'ūs*

vi. 44 القولنج المعروف بإيلاوس وتفسيره المستعاذ منه

The colic known as *īlā'ūs* and whose explanation is 'that from which refuge is sought' (*al-musta'ādh minhu*)

vii. 10 القولنج المستعاذ منه

The colic from which refuge is sought (*al-musta'āḏ minhu*)

In the first example, Ḥunayn gives a description and a transliteration of the Greek term without giving the disease a native Arabic name. In the second, he both gives the transliteration and provides an Arabic name for the disease. In the third, he writes only the Arabic name given in the second example. This could be explained by saying that, when Ḥunayn began his translation of the *Aphorisms*, no accepted Arabic equivalent for εἰλεός existed. Being discontent with the transliteration of the Greek, he endeavoured to introduce a new Arabic name for the term.

A definition attributable to Ḥunayn is found in each of the two relevant entries from bar Bahlul. Arabic predominates in the first, while Syriac predominates in the second. Both describe symptoms of the disease, but the two descriptions do not overlap significantly. The Syriac definition is somewhat more detailed than the Arabic. Neither provides a single native name for the disease, but both suggest calques that are roughly equivalent to one another.[5]

There is some evidence that the thirteenth-century commentator al-Kīlānī had recourse either to bar Bahlul's *Lexicon* or to work that drew upon it. Al-Kīlānī begins his discussion of εἰλεός in his commentary on aphorism iii. 22 by repeating again Ḥunayn's translation, 'The severe colic that the Greeks call *īlā'ūs*'. He then writes, 'its meaning is "My Lord, have mercy"'

5 Pormann, *Oriental Tradition*, 57–8.

(*ma'nāhu rabb arḥam*), which is almost identical to the definitions given in the entries from bar Bahlul.[6]

1.3

ἐπίπλοος

647:6 ܗܦܝܦܠܘܣ ܐܝܟ ܒܪ ܣܪܘ̄ ܗ̄ ܠܒܘ̈ܫܐ الثرب ؞

Hêpiplos according to bar Serošway, this is adipose membranes, *adipose membranes* (al-tharb).

Forms of this Greek word occur three times in the *Aphorisms*. The Syriac translation gives the borrowed Greek word in each case. Ḥunayn in his Arabic version translated each of these instances slightly differently. For the occurrence of the word in aphorism v. 46, he employed the long explicating translation *al-ghishā' al-bāṭin min ghishā'ī al-baṭn alladhī yusammā al-tharb* 'the innermost membrane of the membranes of the belly which is called *al-tharb*'. For the occurrence in aphorism vi. 58, he gave simply *al-tharb* 'the adipose membrane'. Finally, in aphorism vii. 55, he preferred the usage *al-ghishā' al-bāṭin* 'the interior membrane'.

The entry in bar Bahlul's *Lexicon* attributed to bar Serošway conforms reasonably well with Ḥunayn's Arabic translations. Ullmann notes some variation in the approaches to translating this word found in other Arabic sources. Whereas in the Arabic version of Aristotle's *History of Animals al-tharb* serves in place of forms of ἐπίπλοος, the word *al-marāqq* 'diaphragm' is employed in the Arabic version of the same author's *Parts of Animals.*[7]

1.4

κίνδυνος

1737:17 ܩܘܢܕܝܢܘܣ ضيق شدة خطر جهد ؞

Qundinus, narrowness, severity, danger (khaṭar), *struggle.*

1769:11 ܩܝܘܢܕܝܢܘܣ ܒܟܬ̈ ضيق أو شدة. ܐܝܟ ܦܘ̄ هلاك ܘܐܝܟ ܒܪ ܣܪܘ̄ الضرورة ؞

Qyundinus in a manuscript, *narrowness or violence*. According to Paul, *destruction* (halāk), and according to bar Serošway, *harm.*

1775:7 ܩܢܕܘܢܘܣ الجهد الخطر الضيق الشدة ؞

Qindunus, struggle, danger (khaṭar), *narrowness, severity.*

6 N. Carpentieri et al. (eds), *Sharḥ al-Kitāb al-Fuṣūl li-Aḥmad ibn Muḥammad Al-Kīlānī* (ARABCOMMAPH/editions/al-Kīlānī/al-Kīlānī bk. i.- iv. 72), 58.

7 Ullmann, *Wörterbuch zu den griechisch-arabischen Übersetzungen*, 259.

In the Syriac version of the *Aphorisms*, the various forms of κίνδυνος occurring in the *Aphorisms* are all translated with the self-same word borrowed from the Greek. This approach extends to the compounds ἐπικίνδυνος and ἀκίνδυνος as well. In his Arabic translation, Ḥunayn adopted varying approach. He used the equivalent *al-khaṭar* 'danger' most frequently, but at times preferred instead phrases like *lā yu'min 'alayh* '(the patient) is not safe from'.

Translations of forms of ἐπικίνδυνος and ἀκίνδυνος survive in the early Arabic version of aphorism iv. 43. The former is rendered there with the phrase *aqrab ilā halāk* 'closer to destruction' while the latter is translated *ab'ad ilā halāk* 'further from destruction'. Importantly, the use of *halāk* here places al-Biṭrīq's approach to translating κίνδυνος in close agreement with the definition of the word attributed to Paul of Aegina in bar Bahlul's entry at 1769:11. In contrast, Ḥunayn's usage in the *Aphorisms*, *al-khaṭar*, occurs in the unattributed entries from the *Lexicon* cited above.

1.5

κιρσός

1781:9 **ܩܝܪܣܘ** ܐܝܟ ܪܒܢ الخلط الأسود الذي يحدث في عروق الساقين. يسمّيه أهل الشام الدالية وهو العرق المدينيّ. ويقال له أيضاً ܩܢܘ܀

Qirsu according to our teacher, *black humours that occur in the veins of the legs. The folk of Syria call it* 'al-dāliya', *which is varicose veins* ('irq al-madīnī, *lit. veins of the city-dweller'*). *It is also called qnaw.*

1848:18 **ܩܪܣܘ** ܐܝܟ ܒܪ ܣܪܘ̄ العرق المدينيّ܀

Qrsu according to bar Serošway, *varicose veins.*

Forms of the word κιρσός occur three times in the *Aphorisms*. The Syriac version gives a form of the borrowed Greek word in each case. Ḥunayn's Arabic translation adopts a different approach for each instance. In aphorism vi. 21, Ḥunayn employed the translation *ittisā' al-'urūq allatī tu'raf bil-dawālī* 'the expansion of the veins that is known as varicose veins (*al-dawālī*)'. Forms of κιρσός occur twice in aphorism vi. 34, and for the first of these, the translator used a different explicative translation, *al-'urūq allatī tattasi' allatī tu'raf bil-dawālī* 'veins which have expanded that are known as varicose veins (*al-dawālī*)'. For the second, the single word *al-dawālī* serves.

In the entry for κιρσός at 1781:9 in bar Bahlul's *Lexicon*, Ḥunayn gives an aetiology for the disease and then mentions two different names for it. One of these is *al-dāliya*, the singular of *al-dawālī*, which he links to the 'folk of Syria'. He explains this word with the phrase *'irq al-madīnī* 'veins of the city-dweller'. Another entry for κιρσός in Duval's Greek index to bar Bahlul's *Lexicon* begins with a native Syriac name for the disease, *dalāyṯā*, and reads as follows:

> 577:2 **ܕܠܝܬܐ** العريش والعروق التي تنبع في الساقين المعروفة بالدوالي وباليونانيّة **ܩܝܪܣܘܣ** قورسوس الاغصان الطويلة التي في الكرمة الممتدّة. ܒܼ **ܕܠܝܬܗ ܐܪܡܝܬ ܒܐܪܥܐ** قضبانها. ܐܝܟ ܙܟܪܝܐ ܘܐܝܟ ܒܪ ܣܪܘܫܘܝ **ܕܠܝܬܐ** ܫܒܘܩܐ ܕܓܘܦܢܐ ܕܣܠܩܝܢ ܥܠ ܐܝܠܢܐ ܘܡܫܬܒܩܝܢ ܕܠܐ ܟܣܚܐ. ܠܘܬ ܐܚܪ̈ܢܐ ܕܝܢ **ܬܐܡܢܘܣ** ܐܝܬܘܗ̄ اغصان الكرمة التي تتعرّش.

> *Dalāyṯā, bowers, and the veins which emerge in the legs known as* al-dawālī (al-ʿurūq allatī tanbaʿ fī al-sāqayn al-maʿrūf bil-dawālī), *and in Greek qirsus,* qūrsūs. *Branches in the vine that are outstretched.* In a manuscript, *dalāyṯāh armyaṯ b-ar'ā* (its branches extended in the earth), *its branches.* According to Zakariya and according to bar Serošway *dalāyṯā*, the shoots of the vine which arise upon the tree and are left without pruning. According to others, *tamnos* (θάμνος) is *the branches of the vine that are trellised.*

The initial description of varicose veins in this entry agrees with Ḥunayn's translations of κιρσός in the *Aphorisms* in important respects. In this case, the Syriac word *dalāyṯā* serves as a locus for the establishment of the Arabic equivalent *al-dāliya*.[8] The following definitions suggest the metaphorical extension of the sense of 'vine-shoots' or 'trellised vines' to the veins on the legs of those suffering from the disease. It could be argued that the entry at 1781:9 indicates that Ḥunayn established *al-dāliya* in literary Arabic medical terminology. His attribution of the usage to *ahl al-shām* 'the folk of Syria' may refer to speakers of Syriac, or alternatively to Arabic speakers in Syria who had taken the Syriac word over into their vernacular.

1.6

λήθαργος

> 969:18 **ܠܝܬܪܓܘ ܛܥ̈ܝܐ** ضلال. **ܠܝܬܐܪܓܘܣ** ܐܝܬܘܗ̄ ܡܬܛܥܝܢܘܬܐ. **ܠܝܬܪܓܝܩܐܝܬ** ܡܬܛܥܝܢܐܝܬ بالنسيان.

> *Liṯargo, wanderers* (ḍullāl). *Liṯārgos*, this is forgetfulness. *Liṯargiqā'iṯ*, forgetfully, *forgetfully* (bil-nisyān).

---

8 *Al-dāliya* is derived from *dalāyṯā*, according to Brockelmann.

Λήθαργος occurs in the *Aphorisms* once, in aphorism iii. 30, in the form of the plural substantive λήθαργοι. Its context is a list of diseases that occur in middle age. The Syriac gives the borrowed Greek word, while Ḥunayn's Arabic gives a five-word explicative translation, *al-ḥummā allatī yakūnu ma'ahā al-sahar* (the fever with which insomnia occurs). This example again seems to emphasize the lengths to which Ḥunayn went in avoiding the inclusion of transliterated Greek terms in his version of the *Aphorisms*.

Ullmann notes translations of this word and the related form ληθαργικός.[9] One of these is an occurrence of the word in Galen's *Commentary on the Aphorisms*, the context of which is given as a fragment taken from al-Rāzī's *Ḥāwī.* Although Mimura's edition of Galen's work gives a substantially different text from that found in the *Wörterbuch*, they do agree that in this context Ḥunayn gave a transliteration of the Greek word rather than providing a native equivalent.[10] Several citations from the Arabic version of Dioscorides' *Materia Medica* likewise transliterate this Greek word. One example from Book 11 of Galen's *On Simple Drugs* gives a native equivalent. There, the phrase τὰ ληθαργικὰ καὶ καταφορικὰ πάντα πάθη is translated *fī jamī' 'ilal al-nisyān aw fī subāt* 'in all the diseases of forgetfulness or in sleeping sickness'.

Of all the available translations, this last is the closest to any of the definitions of the term collected by bar Bahlul, whereas Ḥunayn's explicating translation in aphorism iii. 30 is not reflected in any substantial way in that entry from the *Lexicon*. The final headword in the entry *litargiqā'it* is a nativized adverb, and the Arabic equivalent is etymologically related to the Syriac equivalent *metnašyānutā.* A short entry for the Syriac equivalent mentioned in the *Lexicon* reads as follows:

1197:11 **ܡܬܢܫܝܢܘܬܐ** ܐܝܟ ܒܪ ܣܪܘ̈ النسيان ❖

Meṯnašyānuṯā according to bar Serošway, *forgetfulness* (al-nisyān).

1.7

μελαγχολία/μελαγχολικά

990:14 **ܡܐܢܩܘܠܝܩܝܐ** ܐܝܟ ܒܪ ܣܪܘ̈ ܚܘܠܛ ܚܫ̈ܒܐ. ܘܐܒܕܢܘܬ ܦ̇ܘܪܫܢܐ ܕܗܘܐ ܡܢ ܝܬ̈ܝܪܘܬܐ فساد الفكر ❖

Mānkoliqyā according to bar Serošway, disorder of the mind and annihilation of the

9 Ullmann, *Wörterbuch zu den griechisch-arabischen Übersetzungen*, 391.

10 Taro Mimura (ed.), *Tafsīr Jālīnūs*, II, 7.

intelligence occurring without fever, *disorder of the mind.*

1017:10 ܡܐܢܩܘܠܝܩܝܐ ܐܝܟ ܒܪ ܣܪܘ ܫܘܚܠܦ ܚܘܫܒܐ ܘܐܒܕܢܘܬ ܗܘܢܐ فساد الفكر ❖

Mānkoliqyā according to bar Serošway, disorder of the mind and annihilation of the intelligence occurring with fever, *disorder of the mind.*

1021:15 ܡܐܠܢܩܘܠܝܐ سوداء ❖

Mêlankolyā, melancholy (sawdā').

1021:20 ܡܐܠܢܩܘܠܝܐ الوسواس الاحتراق السوداويّ ❖

Mêlankolyā, burning melancholy madness.

1021:16 ܡܐܠܢܩܘܠܝܩܝܐ سوداويّ. حنين الوسواس. وكذلك قال المروزي ܘܐܝܟ ܒܪ ܣܪܘ ܐܕܫܐ ܐܝܬܘܗܝ ܕܫܢܝܘܬܐ ܡܢ ܡܪܬܐ ܐܘܟܡܬܐ الصرع من المرّة السودوي ❖

Mêlankoliqya, melancholy. (*According to*) *Ḥunayn, delusion* (waswās), *and likewise said al-Marwazī.* And according to bar Serošway it is a type of madness (occurring) due to black bile, *epilepsy due to black bile.*

1085:3 ܡܠܐ ܐܝܟ ܒܪ ܣܪܘ الحُزن الكره ܒܣܝܪܘܬܐ ❖

Mlē according to bar Serošway, *dejection, abhorrence*, abhorrence.

Forms of the word μελαγχολία and related words occur several times in the *Aphorisms*. The Syriac *Aphorisms* consistently utilizes a form of the borrowed Greek word. Ḥunayn's Arabic translations develop relatively consistently from the word *al-sawdā'* 'melancholy', but in several cases expand the text. For example, in aphorism iv. 9, the Greek phrase τοὺς… μελαγχολικοὺς is translated *man al-ghālibu 'alayhi al-mirra al-sawdā'*, 'those in whom black bile predominates', while the Syriac gives simply *l-mêlankoliqāyē* 'for (those who are) melancholic'. For instances that refer more particularly to the disease 'melancholy', the phrase *al-waswās al-sawdāwī* 'melancholy delusion' is usually given in Ḥunayn's translation. In aphorism iii. 14, these two approaches are combined, producing the phrase *al-waswās al-'āriḍu min al-sawdā'* 'delusion produced by melancholy'. The numerous texts wherein Ḥunayn varied his approach to translating this Greek word display on the one hand the translator's reader-oriented style, but on the other hand indicate that the Arabic medical lexicon had not fully adopted a single, catch-all equivalent word that referred both to the disease and to its underlying humoural aetiology.

Examples of translations of μελαγχολικά survive in both the earlier Syriac and the early Arabic versions. The early Syriac version in particular utilizes significantly different terminology when compared with the later Syriac version. For the occurrence of the term in aphorism iii. 20, the fragment of the *Aphorisms* taken from the *Syriac Epidemics* translates with the phrase *bnay merṯā ukkāmṯā*[11] 'diseases (literally 'sons') of black bile'. This is a good example of the historical trend towards lexical Graecization in Syriac between the sixth and ninth centuries.

The early Arabic version of aphorism vi. 23 is also extant. The aphorism reads as follows:

Ἢν φόβος ἢ δυσθυμίη πολὺν χρόνον ἔχουσα διατελῇ, μελαγχολικὸν τὸ τοιοῦτον.

If fear or despondency continue for a long time, the affliction is melancholic.

Ḥunayn in his Arabic version translated the final phrase μελαγχολικὸν τὸ τοιοῦτον with the words *fa-'illatuhu sawdawiyatun* 'then his illness is melancholic', while al-Biṭrīq employed the phrase *fa-dhālika yaṣīr ilā al-mirra al-sawdā'* 'then that results in black bile'. The clear difference in interpretation extends beyond the varying approaches to the grammatical force of the nominal predicate to the terminological treatment of μελαγχολικόν. Whereas Ḥunayn employed an adjective derived from the standardizing term for melancholy illness *sawdawiya*, the early Arabic translator preferred to make reference to the humoural sense of the Greek term.[12]

The entries in bar Bahlul's *Lexicon* given above display a relatively strong relationship with the translations of μελαγχολία in the *Aphorisms*. An entry for the equivalent of μελαγχολικά in the *Syriac Epidemics* occurs under the headword *merṯā* in bar Bahlul's *Lexicon*:

1163:7 **ܡܪ̈ܬܐ** ܒܢ̈ܝ مرّة. **ܡܪܬܐ ܣܘܡܩܬܐ** ܐܝܟ ܒܪ ܗܘܪ ܐܬܝܬܝܗ̇ ܒܡܘܡܘܣ ܕܚܡܝܡܐ ܘܝܒܝܫܐ
ܘܡܬܩܪܝܐ ܡܪܬܐ ܡܢ ܐܘܣܛܘܟܣܐ ܕܢܘܪܐ ܘܐܝܬܝܗ̇ ܦܠܛܘܬܗ ܕܡܪܬܐ ܘܫܘܠܛܢܗ ܒܐܘܣܛܘܟܣܐ المرّة
الصفراء. **ܡܪܬܐ ܐܘܟܡܬܐ** ܐܝܟ ܒܪ ܗܘܪ ܐܬܝܬܝܗ̇ ܒܡܘܡܘܣ ܩܪܝܪܐ ܘܝܒܝܫܐ. ܘܡܬܩܪܝܐ ܡܪܬܐ ܡܢ
ܐܘܣܛܘܟܣܐ ܕܐܪܥܐ. ܘܐܝܬܝܗ̇ ܦܠܛܘܬܗ ܕܟܠܝܬܐ. ܘܫܘܠܛܢܗ ܣܓܝ ܒܛܚܠܐ المرّة السوداء. **ܡܪ̈ܬܐ**

11 Kessel: ܒܢ̈ܝ ܡܪܬܐ ܐܘܟܡܬܐ.

12 For a discussion of the treatment of this aphorism in the later Arabic tradition, see N.P. Joose and P.E. Pormann, 'Commentaries on the Hippocratic *Aphorisms* in the Arabic Tradition: The Example of Melancholy' in P.E. Pormann (ed.), *Epidemics in Context* (Berlin 2012), 211–50.

ܢܨܘܦܬܐ ܐܝܟ ܒܪ ܣܪܘܫܘܝ المرّة الناصعة. ܡܪܬܐ ܚܪܘܥܬܐ ܐܝܟ ܒܪ ܣܪܘܫܘܝ المرة الغبراء. ܡܪ̈ܬܐ
ܡܥܝܕܐܝܬ ܒܙܩܦ ܪܫܐ܀

Merṯā in a manuscript, *bile*. *Merṯā sumāqṯā* ('red bile') according to bar Serošway, it is a hot and dry humour that is constituted properly of the element of fire. Its dwelling is in the gall, and its power is in the stomach, *yellow bile*. *Merṯā ukkāmṯā* according to bar Serošway, it is a cold and dry humour whose constitution is properly of the element of earth. Its dwelling is in the spleen, and its power is around the kidneys, *black bile*. *Merṯā naṣopṯā* according to bar Serošway, *clear bile*. *Merṯā ḥaru'ṯā* ('yellow bile') according to bar Serošway, *dust-coloured bile*. *Merāṯā*, usually with the long-a vowel, the head.

1.8

φρενῖτις

1497:16 ܦܪܢܝܛܝܣ ܒܟ̈ ܝ ܫܢ̈ܝܐ ܐܡܝܢܐ ܕܥܡ ܐܫ̈ܬܐ سرسام جاء به برسام܀

Pêrniṭis in a manuscript, chronic ravings occurring with fevers, *phrenitis* (sarsām), *he introduced phrenitis* (birsām).

1607:3 ܦܪܢܝܛܝܣ ܒܟ̈ ܝ ܫܢ̈ܝܐ ܐܡܝܢܐ ܕܥܡ ܐܫ̈ܬܐ سرسام وهو البرسام ويقال ورم الدماغ. ܦܘ
برسام ܘܠܡ ܙܟܪܝܐ ܘܒܪ ܣܪܘܫܘܝ ܠܡܘܡ̈ܐ ܚܡܝ̈ܡܐ ܕܒܪܫܐ الأورام الحارّة التي تعرض في الرأس البرسام
الجنون. ܠܡܘܡܐ ܚܡܝܡܐ ܕܓܕܫ ܒܡܘܚܐ ܕܪܫܐ الورم الحارّ الحادث في الدماغ܀

Prêniṭis in a manuscript, chronic ravings that (occur) with fevers, *phrenitis* (sarsām), *which is phrenitis* (birsām). *It is said* (*to be*) *swelling of the brain.* (According to) Paul, *phrenitis* (birsām), and according to Zakariya and bar Serošway, hot swellings that are in the head, *hot swellings that happen in the head, phrenitis* (birsām), *madness.* A hot swelling that occurs in the brain, *hot swellings that occur in the brain.*

Forms of words related to φρενῖτις occur three times in the modern editions of the *Aphorisms*.[13] As discussed below, an additional occurrence is attested as a secondary reading for the word νεφριτικοῖσιν 'kidney disease' in Magdelaine's edition of aphorism vi. 11, based in part on the Arabic and Syriac translations of the work considered here. In translating three of these four occurrences, the Syriac translator employed the etymologically-Greek borrowing *prêniṭis*. For the occurrence in aphorism vi. 11, however, the word *ṣāḇrā* 'raving' is given instead.

Ḥunayn's Arabic translations of φρενῖτις in the Hippocratic lemmas display a high degree of instability. For the instance of the word in aphorism

13 A fourth occurrence is found in aphorism vii. 83, but since this aphorism was not included in any of the translations under consideration, it is outside the scope of the present work.

iii. 30, the long explicating translation *al-hummā allatī yakūn ma'hā ikhtilāṭ al-'aql* 'the fever with which disorder of the mind occurs' is given. In that found in aphorism iv. 72, a different explicating translation reads *al-hummā allatī ma'a waram al-dimāgh* 'the fever that occurs with swelling of the brain'. The Arabic translations of the occurrences of words related to φρενῖτις in aphorisms vi. 11 and vii. 12 both give the word *al-birsām* 'phrenitis'. In several manuscripts of the various Arabic commentaries on the *Aphorisms*, the alternate form *al-sarsām*, also meaning 'phrenitis', occurs in place of *al-birsām.*[14]

This equivalence between *al-sarsām* and *al-birsām* is somewhat controversial in the Arabic tradition. For example, in the text of the Hippocratic lemma given in Amīn al-Dawla ibn al-Quff's commentary on aphorism vi. 11, the form *al-sarsām* is employed rather than *al-birsām*. In his commentary, ibn al-Quff writes, 'In some manuscripts *al-birsām* appears for *al-sarsām*, but this is a mistake. Hippocrates' saying concerns diseases, and *al-birsām* is one of the diseases of the chest'.[15] Ibn al-Quff seems to have relied upon the Persian etymology of these two words in making this judgment: in that language, *sar* means 'head', *bir* means 'chest', and *sām* in combination with these signifies 'disease'.[16]

However reasonable this argument may be, the entries which Duval identified as relating to φρενῖτις in bar Bahlul's *Lexicon* provide clear evidence that Ḥunayn and other translators considered the two words to be equivalent and to refer to a disease of the brain. While these entries also do refer obliquely to the origin of this equivalence, the evidence they give is somewhat contradictory. In the entry at 1497:16, which bar Bahlul refers to 'a manuscript' and so is therefore relatively strongly attributable to Ḥunayn, *sarsām* is given as the first Arabic equivalent for φρενῖτις. This is followed

14 Mimura lists some of these variations in the apparatus to his edition of the Arabic version of Galen's *Commentary on the Aphorisms*. Mimura, *Tafsīr Jālīnūs*, VI, 24 n. 253.

15 Nicola Carpentieri et al. (eds), *Al-Uṣūl fī Sharḥ al-Fuṣūl li-Abī al-Faraj ibn al-Quff* (ARABCOMMAPH/editions/QUF book 6), 17.

16 The particular distinction between these two disease-names appears to have been lost in the centuries intervening between the translation movement and ibn al-Quff's lifetime. For an earlier explanation of these terms written by the medical theorist Ya'qūb al-Kaskarī, see P.E. Pormann, 'Theory and Practice in the Early Hospitals in Baghdad: Al-Kaškarī on Rabies and Melancholy', *Zeitschrift für Geschichte der arabisch-islamischen Wissenschaften* 15 (2003), 242.

by the phrase *jā'a bih birsām* 'he introduced for it *birsām*'. This would seem to be reasonable grounds for attributing its introduction to Ḥunayn. However, in the entry at 1607:3 *birsām* is again made synonymous with φρενῖτις in a definition attributed to Paul. Although traditionally the authorship of the Arabic translation of Paul's *Pragmateia* has been ascribed to Ḥunayn, in that case it would still be unclear what exactly bar Bahlul intended in citing Paul as a distinct source.

Most of the elements of the various translations of the *Aphorisms* are found in the Greek entries cited above. The one missing phrase, *ikhtilāṭ al-'aql* in Ḥunayn's translation of iii. 30, does occur in an entry for the etymologically Syriac equivalent of φρενῖτις, *ṣaḇrā*:

1654:7 **ܨܒ̈ܪܐ** ܡܢ ܨܒܘܪܘܬܐ ܒܨ̈ܚܚܐ وسواس ܘܐܝܟ ܒܪ ܣܪܘܫܘܝ اختلاط العقل الهذيان ذهاب العقل. وآخرون اختلاط الذهن܀

Ṣaḇārā, from *ṣāḇoruṯā*, in a manuscript *delusion* (waswās), and according to bar Serošway *disorder of the mind* (ikhtilāṭ al-ʿaql), *raving, loss of reason.* (*According to*) *others, disorder of the mind* (ikhtilāṭ al-dhihn).

Section Two

In this section, I compare the translations and lexicographical background of Greek words in the *Aphorisms* for which the Syriac version gives the self-same word borrowed from the Greek as an equivalent, and for which Ḥunayn's Arabic translations display a high degree of stability.

2.1

ἀθληταί

330:22 **ܐܬܠܝܛܘܬܐ** ܐܬܠܝܛܐ مصارع مناضل مكادح. ܐܝܟ ܒܪ ܣܪܘܫܘܝ الشجاع البطل. ܐܝܟ ܚܢܝܢ صريع. ܒܨ̈ܚܚܐ **ܐܬܠܝܛܘܬܐ** الابلاء بين يدي السلطان.[17] ܒܟܬܒܐ ܕܦܪܕܝܣܐ ܟܠ ܪ̈ܘܪܒܢܐ ܘܚܝܠܬܢܐ ܕܢܨܝܚܝܢ ܒܩܪܒܐ ܦܪ̈ܝܫܐ ܡܫܒܚܢܐ܀

Aṯlayṭuṯa, an athlete (*aṯlayṭā*), *a wrestler* (muṣāriʿ), *a fighter* (munāḍil), *a striver* (mukādiḥ). According to bar Serošway, *courageous, brave*. According to Ḥunayn, *a wrestler* (ṣirrīʿ). In a manuscript *aṯlayṭuṯā, the good things present with the sultan.* In the *Book of Paradise*, all of the great nobles who are mighty and glorious in battle.

This word occurs a single time in the *Aphorisms*, in aphorism i. 15. The Syriac version gives the borrowed Greek word, while Ḥunayn's Arabic

---

17 Duval: السلبطان.

translates it with *al-ṣirrī'ūn* 'wrestlers'. Ullmann notes examples of Arabic translations for ὁ ἀθλητής and the related word ἀθλητικός from a variety of works. A text from the Hippocratic *On Regimen* uses the same form as that found in the *Aphorisms,* but the usual word employed there is the related *al-muṣāri'*, also meaning 'wrestler'.[18]

These translations roughly correspond to the definition attributed explicitly to Ḥunayn in bar Bahlul's *Lexicon*, *ṣirrī'*. The series of synonyms given at the beginning of the entry indicate a certain instability in the reception of the term in Arabic, contrasting with the regularity of the attested translations. The word seems to have been thoroughly integrated into the Syriac language, such that no single native synonym needed to be cited to clarify its meaning.

2.2

ἀποπληξία

251:6 **ܐܦܘܠܘܟܣܝܐ** ܫܘܬܩܐ سكتة ܐܝܟ ܙܟܪܝܐ ܒܨܚܚܐ ܐܦܘܦܠܝܟܣܝܐ ܘܐܝܟ ܣܪܓܝܣ ܡܫܬܠܚܢܐ.
ܘܗܟܢ ܒܪ ܣܪܘ܀

Apolo<u>k</u>sia, stroke (*šuttāqā*), *stroke* (sakta), according to Zakariya in (one) manuscript, *apopli<u>k</u>sia*, and according to Sergius 'being deprived' (*meštalḥānā*), and likewise bar Serošway.

253:25 **ܐܦܘܦܘܠܝܩܝܐ** ܦܘܠܘܣ ابولقسيا بطلان الحسّ والحركة في الاعضاء الرئسية ܘܐܡܪ
ܐܦܘܩܪܐܛܝܣ ܕܪܓܠܗ ܥܒܕ ܐܦܘܦܠܝܟܛܐ܆ معناه إنّ هذا الراقد عرض في الساق وحدها. ܟܘܪܗܢܐ
ܗܘ ܕܐܒܕܢܐ ܕܚܠܐ ܘܡܬܬܙܝܥܢܘܬܐ. وقال مرّة فالج ܘܬܘܒ **ܐܦܘܦܠܟܣܝܐ** ܫܘܬܩܐ سكتة܀

Apopoli<u>k</u>ia (according to) Paul, abūliqsīya, *nullity of sense and action in the governing parts.* Hippocrates says that his leg became apoplectic; *its meaning is that this sleeping occurred in one leg only.* This disease consists of the loss of sense and action. *He said another time, hemiplegia* (fālij). Again, *apople<u>k</u>sia,* stroke, *stroke.*[19]

263:8 **ܐܦܠܦܐܣܝܐ** ܒܪ ܣܪܘ ܫܘܬܩܐ السكتة܀

Aplpāsia (according to) bar Serošway, stroke (*šuttāqā*), *stroke* (sakta)

265:12 **ܐܦܣܠܣܝܐ** ܐܝܟ ܒܪ ܣܪܘ ܡܘܬܐ ܕܡܢܫܠ موت الفجأة܀

Apslsia, according to bar Serošway sudden death (*mawtā <u>d</u>-menšel*), *sudden death* (mawt al-faj'a).

---

18 Ullmann, *Wörterbuch zu den griechisch-arabischen Übersetzungen*, 75.

19 I have followed Pormann in the reading of this passage and in much of the translation. Pormann, *Oriental Tradition*, 19.

Forms of ἀποπληξία, ἀπόπληξις, and the related adjective ἀπόπληκτος occur seven times in the *Aphorisms*. Both the Syriac translation and Ḥunayn's Arabic version use generally well-established equivalents for these instances, the former giving a form of the borrowed Greek word, the latter giving a form of *al-sakta* 'stroke'. There are exceptions in both versions; although they are relatively minor, their description will bring up a few points of interest.

In aphorism vi. 56, Ḥunayn's Arabic version employs the hendiadys *al-sakta wal-fālij* 'stroke and hemiplegia' to translate the phrase ἀποπλεξίην τοῦ σώματος.[20] The Syriac too departs from its normal course in rendering this phrase. Instead of using the borrowed Greek term, it translates with *mrašlutā* 'paralysis'. It may be that both Ḥunayn and the translator of the Syriac *Aphorisms* were motivated to modify their usual approach to translating ἀποπληξία in this aphorism by the context of the aphorism, which mentions several other diseases of the head, or by Galen's commentary, which discusses the generality of the effects of phlegm and melancholy in such cases.[21] Another exception occurs in the Arabic translation of aphorism vii. 40. There, Ḥunayn rendered the phrase ἢ ἀπόπληκτόν τι τοῦ σώματος with *aw istarkhā 'uḍwun min al-a'ḍā* 'or if one of the parts slackens'. The Syriac in this case only slightly departs from the other examples discussed, giving *aw medem men pagrā apoplêṭiqiya nehwā*, 'or a part of the body is apoplectic'.

One relevant text from the early Arabic version also survives. In aphorism iii. 16, the term ἀπόπληκτοι occurs in the context of a list of diseases. While Ḥunayn's Arabic and the Syriac follow their usual approach as described above, al-Biṭrīq's version translates the word with *al-fālij* 'hemiplegia'. This equivalent overlaps with the exceptional hendiadys used by Ḥunayn in aphorism vi. 56, but as an isolated example little can be concluded solely on the basis of it.

If we turn to the entries in bar Bahlul's *Lexicon*, however, it is possible to descry a certain division between the various authors' approaches to the Greek term in question which may broaden the implications of the single early Arabic example. In the definitions attributed to Paul of Aegina in the

20 Mimura's edition differs slightly from Tytler's text, which reads simply *al-fālij* 'hemiplegia'.

21 Mimura (ed.), *Tafsīr Jālīnūs*, VI, 129–30.

entry at 253:25, the extended descriptions of the symptoms of the disease do not include Ḥunayn's preferred equivalent *al-sakta*. Instead, this word occurs alongside the strongly synonomous Syriac word *šuttāqā* after a restated headword. If the verb *qāla* 'he said' may be taken to refer to Paul, however, bar Bahlul does attribute the equivalent *al-fālij* to the translation of the work of Paul.

The repeated pairing of *al-sakta* and *šuttāqā* is also notable. Even though they are not clearly related in a formal etymological sense, these two words do share a common sense-development from roots meaning 'to be silent', and bear a certain phonetic resemblance to one another as well. The prominence of that native Syriac equivalent in these entries combined with the presence of several relatively extensive and complimentary definitions gives the impression that the borrowed Greek word was somewhat obscure in Syriac. Yet at the same time *šuttāqā* is not very well represented in the lexicons considered here. Only a single-word entry pairing it with *al-sakta* in bar ʿAli's *Lexicon* occurs in them.[22]

The other equivalent given in the Syriac *Aphorisms* is better represented in the lexicons. Bar Bahlul's entry for *mrašluṯā* runs as follows:

1162:27 **ܡܪܫܠܘܬܐ** ܒܨܚ خَدَر[23] ܗܘ ܕ ܕܙܘܥܐ ܒܠܚܘܕ ܒܠܥܕ ܪ ܠܚܒܠܐ ܢܚܒܪ ܐܘ ܢܬܒܨܪ ܣܓܝ ويقال له
الاسترخاء. ܘܐܝܟ ܒܪ ܣܪܘ **ܡܪܫܠܘܬܐ** ܡܢ ܪܘܫܠܐ الاسترخاء من العصب. **ܡܪܫܠܘܬܐ ܕܦܪܨܘܦܐ**
ܕܡܢ ܚܕ ܓܒܐ ܐܝܟ ܒܪ ܣܪܘ ܗܘ ܕܩܪܝܢ ܠܗ ܩܘܢܝܩܘܣ ܘܐܦ ܡܘܣ ܘܐܦ ܩܦܣܐ ܟܠܒܢܐ اللقوة.܀

Mrašluṯā in a manuscript, *numbness* (khadar). That is, that movement (considered) by itself is lost or greatly diminished, without sensation.[24] *Slackening* (al-istikhrā) *is said for it.* According to bar Serošway *mrašluṯā* is from *rušālā* (paralysis), *slackening* (al-istikhrā) *of the nerves. Mrašluṯā ḏ-parṣupā* (paralysis of the face) is of one side, according to bar Serošway, they read this for several types of canine convulsions (*haw da-qrin leh quniqus w-ap mus w-ap qpāsā ḵalbānā*),[25] *paralysis of one side of the face* (al-laqwa).

That a word related to the exceptional usage found in Ḥunayn's Arabic version of vii. 40, *al-istikhrā,* would appear so prominently in the entry for the exceptional usage *mrašluṯā* found in the Syriac version of vi. 56 is

22 Gottheil (ed.), *Syriac-Arabic Glosses*, II 425:16.

23 Duval: خَذَر.

24 Literally, 'that movement by itself without sensation is lost or greatly diminished'.

25 Both *quniqus* and *qpāsā ḵalbānā* are defined as 'canine convulsions'. Although *mus* is obscure, it is clearly related to these by the force of the definition.

interesting. Given the evidence already presented that the Syriac and Arabic *Aphorisms* were authored by different people, this may be due to Ḥunayn's having used this Syriac equivalent in his Syriac version of the work rather than the borrowed Greek word.

2.3

ἄρωμα

657:15 **ܗܪ̈ܘܡܐ** أفاويه ܘܐܝܟ ܒܪ ܣܪܘܫܘܝ العطر الطيب. ܒܟܬܒܐ ܕܦܪܕܝܣܐ ܒܣܡ̈ܐ ܓܒܝ̈ܐ ܕܡܕܟܝܢ. **ܗܪ̈ܘܡܐ** طيب܀

Êrumē, *aromatics* (afāwīh), and according to bar Serošway, *perfume, scent* (al-ṭīb). In the Book of Paradise, choice perfumes that purify. *Êrumē*, *scent*.

This word occurs once in the *Aphorisms*, in the phrase ἢ ἐν ἀρώμασι πυρίῃ 'fomentations containing aromatics' in aphorism v. 28. The Syriac gives the slightly modified borrowing *êrumē* in the phrase *šuḥānā ḏa-ḇ-êrumē* 'fomentations with aromatics'. Ḥunayn's Arabic version gives for this phrase *al-takmīd bil-afāwīh* 'fomentations with aromatics'. The early Arabic translation of this aphorism also exists, and for this phrase employs *al-bakhūr bil-ṭīb* 'fumigation with scent'.

Ullmann notes some examples of the related adjective ἀρωματικός and verb ἀρωματίζω. One of these is taken from Galen's *On Simple Drugs* Book Six, where both the early Arabic version and Ḥunayn's version give the same basic form *aṭyabu rīḥan* 'strongest in scent' for the superlative ἀρωματικώτερον. The other two examples are taken from Dioscorides' *Materia Medica.* In the first of these the translator employs the verb *yuṭayyibu* 'he makes scented' to translate the verb ἀρωματίσαντες, while in the second he uses the phrase *(fī) adwiyatin mimmā yaqa'u fīhi al-afāwīh* '(as for) a drug that has in it aromatics' to translate the substantive ἀρωματικάς.[26]

Although *êromē* is for our purposes here both a Greek and a Syriac word, we can compare entries for the native Syriac equivalent *besmē* 'perfumes', given in the entry at 657:15, to get a better sense of the possible distinctions to be made between the Greek and Syriac lexicography:

26 Ullmann, *Wörterbuch zu den griechisch-arabischen Übersetzungen*, 137–8.

408:25 ܒܣܡܐ العطّار. ܒܝܬ ܒܣܡܐ المجمرة. ܒܣܡܐ ܒܙ ܐܣܡܟܬ ܗ̄ التلذّذ التنعّم. ܒܣܡܐ ܪܝܫܝܐ ܐܝܟ ܒܪ ܣܪܘܫܘܝ الطيب من العود والمسك والعنبر وما يشبهه. ܒܣܡܐ بخور عطر. ܒܣܡܢܐ الطيب. ܒܣܡܐ ܡܬܩܢ ܒܣܡܐ عطّار ❖

Basāmā, perfumer (al-ʿaṭṭār). *Bat̲ besmē, censer. Besāmē* with a long a-vowel on the *semkat̲, pleasure, enjoyment. Besmā rišāyā* ('choice perfumes') according to bar Serošway, *scent of incense, musk, amber, and the like. Besmā, frankincense, perfume. Besmānā*, scent. *Besāmā mt̲aqen*, perfumers, *perfumers.*

Much of the material in these entries overlaps with that found in the entry at 657:13 for *êromē*. However, Ḥunayn's translation in the *Aphorisms, al-afāwīh*, is notably found only in the latter. This constitutes evidence that in Ḥunayn's Syriac translations of the word ἄρωμα and related terms would have themselves tended in general to employ *êromē* rather than *besmē*.

2.4

ἐπιληψία

143:11 ܐܝܦܝܠܡܐܣܝܐ ܒܢ̄ الصرع ܗ̄ ܦܝܠܝܦܣܝܐ ❖

Aipilmasia, in a manuscript *epilepsy* (al-ṣarʿ), that is *pilipsia.*

144:20 ܐܝܦܝܠܝܦܝܣܝܐ ܒܢ̄ ܢܦܘܠܬܐ ܕܡܢ ܫܠܝ سقوط الفجأة البغتة ❖

Aipilipisia, in a manuscript falling suddenly, *sudden, unexpected falling.*

646:22 ܗܦܝܠܝܡܣܝܐ ܐܝܟ ܦܘ̄ ܗܢܘ ܡܬܚܐ ܕܦܓܪܐ ܟܠܗ. ܥܡ ܢܟܝܢܐ
ܕܡܕܒܪܢܘܬܐ ܐܝܟ ܡܕܒܪܢܝܬܐ امتداد الجسد مع مضرة تنال الأفعال الرئيسة ❖

Êpilimsia according to Paul, this is rigour of the entire body, with injury of the governing power. *Rigour of the body with harm befalling the governing powers.*

647:21 ܗܦܝܠܝܡܣܝܐ ܐܘܚܕܢܐ ܐܣܬܘܪ ܪ̈ܓܫܐ الصرع ܘܡܦܘܠܬܐ ܘܡܫܪܝܘܬܐ ܕܟܠܗ ܦܓܪܐ ❖

Êpilimsia, its meaning is the seizure of the senses, *epilepsy* (al-ṣarʿ), falling and paralysis of the entire body.

Ἐπιληψία and related words occur six times in the *Aphorisms*. Both Ḥunayn's Arabic and the Syriac translation are almost entirely consistent in their renditions of them, the former translating with forms of *al-ṣarʿ*, the latter with the borrowed Greek word. There are no important exceptions. Ullmann's citations from works attributable to Ḥunayn likewise give *al-ṣarʿ* or related words, while those from works attributed to al-Biṭrīq usually give transliterations.[27] In the early Arabic version of the *Aphorisms*, the word is

27 Ullmann, *Wörterbuch zu den griechisch-arabischen Übersetzungen*, 256–7.

translated *junūn* 'madness'. In the fragments of the *Aphorisms* found in the Syriac *Epidemics*, the word is also transliterated.

Of the four entries for the term found in bar Bahlul, one is attributed to Paul of Aegina, while three are attributable to Ḥunayn. The text attributed to Paul at 646:22 contains equivalent Arabic and Syriac translations of his definition of the term, but does not include Ḥunayn's standard translation *al-ṣar'*.[28] The entry for the word at 144:20 again displays strong parallelism between the Syriac and Arabic definitions, but does not contain *al-ṣar'* either. The entry at 143:11, strongly attributable to Ḥunayn by virtue of the citation of 'a manuscript', merely lists *al-ṣar'* without explanation, accompanied by a variant Syriac transliteration. The entry at 647:21 gives a more detailed explanation in Syriac, with *al-ṣar'* inserted in the middle. None of the entries contain a single-word native Syriac equivalent. This pattern may indicate that Ḥunayn was responsible for the introduction of *al-ṣar'* as an equivalent for ἐπιληψία, or at least that it was established in the period intervening between al-Biṭrīq's translations and his own.[29]

2.5

καῦσος

1688:10 **ܩܐܘܣܘ ܘܩܐܘܣܘܣ** تشنج. ܘܐܡܪ ܒܪ ܣܪܘܫܘܝ ܐܘܩܕܢܐ ܡܘܩܕܢܝܬܐ الحمى المحرقة. ܘܐܡܪ ܚܘܢܝܢ ܐܫܬܐ ܕܡܢ ܡܣܪܝܘܬܐ ܕܗܝܘܠܐ ܚܡܝܡܬܐ ܕܠܓܘ ܥܪ̈ܩܐ ܀

Qāwso and *qāwsus, a spasm.* According to bar Serošway, it is burning (*mawqdānitā*), *burning fever* (al-ḥummā al-muḥraqa). According to Ḥunayn, a fever occurring due to the rotting of the hot matter that is inside the veins.

Forms of this and related Greek words occur some five times in the *Aphorisms*. In all but one case, the Syriac version gives the self-same word borrowed from the Greek, while Ḥunayn's Arabic version translates with a form of *al-ḥummā al-muḥraqa* 'burning fevers' without exception. The one exception in the Syriac version is found in aphorism iv. 54, where the phrase ἐν πυρετοῖσι καυσώδεσιν 'in burning fevers' occurs. This adjectival usage contrasts with the usual use in other contexts of καῦσος as a substantive

28 Pormann, *Oriental Tradition*, 17–18. His comparison of this text with the relevant passage from the Arabic translation of Paul's Pragmateia displays important differences between the two.

29 See the discussion of colocynth in Pormann, *Oriental Tradition*, 217–18.

standing alone, as in aphorism iii. 30. For this phrase, the Syriac translation gives *eštāwāṯā mawqḏāniṯā* 'burning fevers'.

Ullmann notes an occurrence of the related verbal form καυσόομαι in Galen's *On Simple Drugs* Book Six. In that place, the early Arabic translation of the work employs the transliterated Greek word as an equivalent in the phrase *al-ḥummā allatī tud'ā qawsūs* 'the fever that is called *qawsūs*'. The later version attributed to Ḥunayn also adopts a different approach from that attested in the translator's version of the *Aphorisms*, employing a hendiadys in the phrase *li-man yajid lahīban wa-tawaqqudan* 'for the one he finds blazing and burning'.

By virtue of the presence of strong Syriac material in the entry in bar Bahlul's *Lexicon*, we may infer that the borrowed Greek word was relatively unfamiliar to Syriac speakers. The definitions match both Ḥunayn's translations in the *Aphorisms* and the exceptional Syriac translation in aphorism iv. 54. The Syriac definition attributed to Ḥunayn is a good example of a likely citation from his glossary.

2.6

τέτανος

788:23 ܛܝܛܐܢܘܣ ܗ̄ ܡܩܝܣܘܬܐ التشنّج؞

Ṭêṭānus, that is rigors (*mqaysuṯa*), *spasms* (al-tashannuj).

789:8 ܛܝܛܐܢܘܣ[30] ܐܚ̇ܕܬܐ ܙܩܬܐ قال مفسّر كناش فولس أنّه الكزاز ويعني به التشّنج ويسمّيه التمدّد وأقول أنّه تحدّب؞

Ṭêṭānus, this is tetanus (*zqāṯā*). *The interpreter of the* Compendium *of Paul says that it is tetanus* (al-kuzāz), *meaning by it spasms* (al-tashannuj). *He named it* tamaddud, *and I say that it is* taḥaddub.

789:11 ܛܝܛܐܢܝܩܐܝܬ ܡܬܩܦܦܣܝܢ الذين يعرض لهم الامتداد الكزازيّ؞[31]

Ṭêṭāniqā'iṯ meṯqappsin (they were afflicted with tetanus), *those to whom rigours* (al-imtidād) *occur, those with tetanus (*al-kuzāzī*).*

802:13 ܛܝܛܐܢܘܣ ܡܩܝܣܘܬܐ التشنّج ܛܝܛܐܢܘܣ ܐܡܪ؞

Ṭiṭānus, rigours (*mqaysuṯa*), *spasms* (al-tashannuj). He says *ṭêṭānus.*

Forms of the word τέτανος occur nine times in the *Aphorisms*. Both Ḥunayn's Arabic translation and the Syriac version translate the word

30 Duval: ܛܝܛܐܢܘܣ.

31 This entry goes unlisted in Duval's Greek index.

consistently, the former with forms of *al-tamaddud* 'rigours', the latter with forms of the borrowed Greek word. Three translations of the Greek word survive in the fragments of the early Arabic translation, where they are consistently translated with forms of *al-kuzāz* 'spasms'. Furthermore, Ullmann notes an example from Aristotle's *History of Animals*, which gives *al-kuzāz* as a disease of horses.[32]

The precise sense of the term τέτανος was unstable even in the later Greek tradition, and this instability was carried over into the Arabic medical tradition as well.[33] This is quite clear in the entries from bar Bahlul's *Lexicon*. Some of the discussions of the equivalents of this term bear on important questions regarding the relationship between the Syriac and Arabic medical traditions. In particular, the relationship between those glosses attributed to Paul and the rest of the lexicographical material needs to be addressed.

The Syriac equivalent *zqātā* at the beginning of the entry at 789:8 is attributable to Ḥunayn. A definition attributed to the commentator on the *Compendium* of Paul follows, which gives the equivalent *al-kuzāz*. However, this definition is heavily mediated by the writer of the entry, who glosses *al-kuzāz* with *al-tashannuj* 'spasms'. The writer then refers back to the commentator for the equivalent *al-tamaddud* before giving his own equivalent *al-taḥaddub*.

When we consider the entry in bar Bahlul's *Lexicon* for the Syriac equivalent *zqātā*, the picture is clarified somewhat:

> 698:12 ܙܩܛܐ كزاز ويقال على الحدبة والنقلة والقدماء يسمّونه التمدّد وحُنين يخصّه بالتشنّج والتحدّب ولا
> يسمّيه الكزاز. ܙܩܛܐ ܕܡܢ ܒܣܬܪܐ ܐܝܟ ܦܘ كزاز من خلف. ܐܙܕܩܛܘ ܐܝܟ ܒܪ ܣܪܘ تشنّجوا. ܙܩܛܐ
> ܡܩܝܣܘܬܐ التخبيل التشنيج ❖
>
> *Zqāṯā, tetanus (*kuzāz*), which is said of humps. The translators and the ancients called it* al-tamaddud, *and Ḥunayn specified it with spasms and hunching* (al-tashannuj wal-taḥaddub) *but did not call it* al-kuzāz. *Zqāṯā ḏ-men bestrā* according to Paul, *tetanus* (kuzāz) *in the back. Ezdqeṯ* according to bar Serošway, *they had spasms* (tashannajū). *Zqāṯā mqaysuṯa, nullification of the senses* (al-takhbīl), *effectation of spasms* (al-tashnīj).

An apparently related entry occurs in bar ʿAli's *Lexicon*:

32 Ullmann, *Wörterbuch zu den griechisch-arabischen Übersetzungen*, 671.

33 Pormann, *Oriental Tradition*, 265.

ܙܩܛܐ ܟܐܒܐ ܐܝܬܘܗ̇. ܕܗܘܐ ܡܢ ܩܘܕܡܐ ܘܡܢ ܒܣܬܪܐ ܐܟܚܕܐ. ܐܘ ܡܢ ܩܘܕܡܐ ܐܟܚܕܐ ܘܒܣܬܪܐ. ܝܘ̈. ܛܝܛܐܢܘܣ: الكزاز والتقلّص ويقال على الحدبة وحنين يخصّه بالتشنّج والتحدّب ولا يسمّيه الكزاز:[34]

Zqāṯā is a disease that occurs from the front and from the back simultaneously, or from the front at once and the back.[35] The Greeks called it *ṭêṭanus*, *spasms and contraction* (al-kuzāz wal-taqalluṣ), *which is said of humps. Ḥunayn specified it with spasms and hunching* (al-tashannuj wal-taḥaddub) *but did not call it* al-kuzāz.

The material in both these definitions for *zqātā* strongly agrees with that found in the entry at 789:8. There, again, *al-kuzāz* and *al-tamaddud* are attributed to the commentator on Paul, while the writer of the entry provides *al-tashannuj* and *al-taḥaddub* himself. In his entry for *zqātā*, bar Bahlul attributes *al-tamaddud* to the ancients and the translators (*al-qudamā' w-al-naqala*) as an equivalent for *zqātā*, credits Ḥunayn with the specification of the disease by *al-tashannuj* and *al-taḥaddub* as a hendiadys, and then explicitly denies that Ḥunayn used *al-kuzāz* as its equivalent. This denial occurs with almost exactly the same formulation in bar ʿAli's entry as well. There, however, the fact that Ḥunayn did not use *al-kuzāz* as an equivalent for the Greek τέτανος is stated more clearly, without primary reference to the Syriac *zqātā* as an intermediary between the two.

Al-kuzāz is used as an equivalent for τέτανος several times in the Arabic version of Paul of Aegina's *Pragmateia*.[36] The explicit dismissal of Ḥunayn's use of *al-kuzāz* in this context is thus strong evidence against Ḥunayn's authorship of that work. The convergence amongst the three entries discussed above, along with the citation of Ḥunayn by the lexicographers for the distinctions they contain, is strong evidence for identifying Ḥunayn as the author of the entry at 789:8. In my opinion it is likely the case that the later compilers referred to Ḥunayn's discussion in that entry in writing their own entries for *zqātā.* Since the author of the entry there refers to 'the interpreter of the *Compendium* of Paul', meaning the translator of the *Pragmateia*, this attribution is strong evidence against Ḥunayn's authorship of that work.

---

34 Hoffmann (ed.), *Syrische-arabische Glossen*, 129:3559.

35 Although a distinction appears to be intended between these two phrases, their meanings are almost entirely indistinguishable. It may be that something has dropped out of the text.

36 Pormann, *Oriental Tradition*, 260–71.

From the perspective of the lexicographers' explicit attribution of some equivalents for τέτανος to Ḥunayn and their explicit refusal to attribute others to him, the remaining entries in bar Bahlul's *Lexicon* fall into two categories. One of these represents entries that contain equivalents for τέτανος linked to Ḥunayn, including the entries at 788:23 and 802:13. The other contains equivalents attributed to the commentator on Paul or 'the ancients'. This category has only one member, the entry at 789:11. Given the clear division laid out by the lexicographers, this unattributed definition probably should not be attributed to Ḥunayn, but could be associated with Paul. If so, this would be another example of Pauline material occurring in the lexicon without attribution, as was seen in the discussion of ἀπόστημα above (unit 1.3.8).

There exists an entry in bar Bahlul's *Lexicon* for the other Syriac equivalent given in these entries, *mqaysuṯā*, which also contains a definition attributed to Paul, and which further extends the account of these equivalents laid out in the entries above:

1146:5 **ܡܩܝܣܘܬܐ** ܒܨܚ̈ تشنّج. ܘܦܘܠ امتداد. ܘܒܪ ܣܪܘ التشبّك܀

Mqaysuṯā in a manuscript, *a spasm* (tashannuj). (According to) Paul, *rigours* (imtidād). (According to) bar Serošway, *perplexity* (al-tashabbuk).

Despite this quite consistent material, it is worth repeating that Ḥunayn did not use either of the equivalents attributed to him by the lexicographers in translating τέτανος in the *Aphorisms*, but instead preferred the word *al-imtidād.* While this equivalent was conservative in relation to *al-tashannuj* and *al-taḥaddub*, it is not dismissed in the lexicons in the same fashion as is *al-kuzāz*. Furthermore, the lexicographers' assertion that *al-kuzāz* belongs to an earlier stage of the translation movement is corroborated by al-Biṭrīq's use of that word to translate τέτανος in the early Arabic version of the *Aphorisms.*

2.7

φθίσις/φθισικοί

1560:14 **ܦܬܝܣܝܣ** ܐܝܟ ܒܪ ܣܪܘܫܘܝ، ܗ̄ ܒܨ̈ܪ ܐ النُّقصان السلّ܀

Piṯisis according to bar Serošway, this is diminution, *diminution, tuberculosis* (al-sill).

1645:19 **ܦܬܘܝ،** ܐܝܟ ܒܪ ܣܪܘ ܦܬܝܣܝܣ السلّ الدقّ܀

Ptway according to bar Serošway, tuberculosis (*pṯisis*), *tuberculosis* (al-sill), *hectic* (*fever*) (al-diqq).

1647:15 **ܦܬܝܣܝܣ** السلّ الدقّ السقيم العذاب الحمّى الدايمة مع نفث الدم وهي القرحة في الصدر.[37]
ܦܬܝܣܝܣ ܕܥܝܢܐ ܐܝܟ ܒܪ ܣܪܘ̈ هزال العين. **ܦܬܝܣܝܣ ܣܛܪ ܡܢ ܐܫܬܐ** ܒܨ̈ܚ الدم من قرحة الصدر بغير حمّى. **ܦܬܝܣܝܣ ܡܫܢܩܢܐ** السلّ⁘

Pt̲isis, tuberculosis, hectic (fever), the tormenting illness. Continuous fevers with spittle of blood, which is abscesses in the chest. Pt̲isis d-'aynē (tuberculosis of the eyes) according to bar Serošway, *consumption of the eyes, Pt̲isis sṭar men ešāt̲ā* (tuberculosis without fever) in a manuscript, *blood occurring from ulcers of the chest without fever. Pt̲isis*, tormenting (disease), *tuberculosis* (al-sill).

1648:21 **ܦܬܣܝܩܐ**[38] الذين بهم قرحة السلّ⁘

Pt̲siqē, those with the ulcers of tuberculosis (qarḥa al-sill).

1648:22 **ܦܬܣܝܣ** ܒܨ̈ܚ السلّ جاء به فولوس في علل عين. فقال إنّ السلّ علّة صبيّ العين اذا ضاق وضعف⁘

Pt̲sis in a manuscript, *tuberculosis* (al-sill). *Paul introduced it among the illnesses of the eye. He said tuberculosis is the illness of the pupil of the eye when it is weary and weak.*[39]

Forms of the disease-name φθίσις occur several times in the *Aphorisms*. The Syriac translation invariably gives a form of the self-same borrowed Greek word, while Ḥunayn's Arabic version translates regularly with a form of *al-sill* 'tuberculosis'. A translation of φθίσις exists in the fragments of the early Arabic version as well. In translating aphorism v. 9, al-Biṭrīq rendered the term with *al-ḍumr fī al-ri'a* 'emaciation in the lungs'. In the early Arabic version of aphorism v. 64, the related participial form φθινώδεσι is translated *man bihi ḍumr wa-qarḥ fī al-ri'a* 'he who was emaciation and ulceration in the lungs'.

Beside Ḥunayn's regular rendering of the disease *al-sill*, in several places the definitions from bar Bahlul's *Lexicon* given above agree with texts cited by Ullmann that use distinct terminology. In two texts from Dioscorides' *Materia Medica*, a form of the phrase *qarḥa fī al-ri'a* 'an ulcer in the lungs' translates the adjectival form φθισικός. The use of the word *qarḥa* relates these to the entries at 1647:22 and 1648:21. To translate the more general sense of φθίσις, 'diminution' and the related verb φθίνω, texts from the Arabic versions of Aristotle's *History of Animals* and *Generation of Animals*

37 Duval's manuscripts P and S add this text beginning from السقيم.

38 Duval: ܦܬܝܣܩܐ.

39 Cf. bar Bahlul's entry for *tarsāyt̲ā* at 2089:5 in the unit on ἀνάληψις in Chapter One (1.2.7).

use the word *al-nuqṣān* 'diminution'.[40] This word also figures in bar Bahlul's entry at 1560:14.

2.8

φρενός

1606:23 **ܦܪܐܝܐܣ** ܐܝܟ ܒܪ ܣܪܘ ܬܪܥܝܬܐ الفكر. **ܦܪܐܢܐܣ** ܒܨ حجاب ܦܘ صفاقات الصدر ܀

Prêyas according to bar Serošway, judgment, *thought*. *Prênas* in a manuscript, *diaphragm* (ḥijāb). According to Paul, *the peritoneum* (ṣafāqāt)[41] *of the chest*.

Forms of the noun φρήν occur three times in the *Aphorisms*. All of the extant texts from the Syriac version translate it with a form of the borrowed Greek word, while Ḥunayn's Arabic version utilizes forms of *al-ḥijāb* 'diaphragm' for two of these instances. However, in aphorism vi. 18, the word *al-kulya* 'kidney' appears in its place, in the context of a list of parts of the body prone to suffering mortal injury. The Syriac version of this aphorism follows the modern editions in placing φρένας in this place in the text, and no alternate readings appear for it in either Magdelaine's or Mimura's editions. The translation of this word in the early Arabic version of aphorism vi. 18 also exists. There al-Biṭrīq employed the word *ṣifāq* 'peritoneum'. Furthermore, Ullmann notes a text from Aristotle's *Parts of Animals* that makes *al-ḥijāb* and *al-ṣifāq* synonymous.[42]

Turning to the entry in bar Bahlul's Lexicon, we see that the two Arabic equivalents attested in the available literature both occur. Ḥunayn's usual equivalent in the Aphorisms, *al-ḥijāb,* is given in a definition referred to 'a manuscript', and which is thus relatively firmly attributable to the translator. A plural of al-Biṭrīq's equivalent *al-ṣifāq* in the single available example from the early Arabic version follows in a definition attributed to Paul. Although Ullmann's text shows that these two terms were known to be synonymous, the isomorphism obtaining between the Pauline definition and al-Biṭrīq's translation on the one hand and the unattributed definition and Ḥunayn's translation on the other is notable, and accompanied by other

40 Ullmann, *Wörterbuch zu den griechisch-arabischen Übersetzungen*, 728–9.

41 Although the sense of the word is clear, this particular plural is not attested with this meaning in Wehr and Freytag's dictionaries. Both agree that the word *ṣifāq* (pl. *ṣufuq*) carries the anatomical sense. This definition suggests that the plural *al-ṣafāqāt* was also in use in medical circles.

42 Ullmann, *Wörterbuch zu den griechisch-arabischen Übersetzungen*, 742.

evidence could bear further on the authorship of the Arabic version of the *Pragmateia*.

Section Three

In this section I discuss the translations and scholarly background of words for which there is evidence for a high degree of continuity between the earlier and later Arabic translations of the *Aphorisms*.

3.1

ἀήρ

7:13 **ܐܐܪ** ܐܝܬܘܗ ܐܝܟ ܒܪ ܣܪܘ̈ܫܘܝ ܠܘ ܒܠܚܘܕ ܕܕܟܪܘܬܐ ܐܠܐ ܢܩܒܘܬܐ ܕܠܐ ܪܘܚܐ. ܟܝܢܐ ܕܐܝܬ ܚܝܠܐ
ܕܩܪܝܪܘܬܐ ܡܕܒܪܢܝܬܐ. ܕܡܫܘܬܦ ܕܝܢ ܥܡܗ ܒܡܘܙܓܐ ܚܝܠܐ ܕܪܛܝܒܘܬܐ. ܗܢܘ ܕܝܢ ܫܡܐ ܕܡܕܒܪܢܝܬܐ ܥܠ
ܡܬܬܣܡܟܐ ܥܠ ܚܕ ܚܕ ܡܢܗܘܢ. ܗܘ ܓܝܪ ܕܠܝܬ ܟܝܢܐ ܕܐܝܬ ܠܗ ܚܕ ܡܢ ܗܠܝܢ ܚܝ̈ܠܐ ܐܝܟ ܚܕ.
ܡܢܗܘܢ. ܟܠܗܘܢ ܓܝܪ ܟܝܢܐ ܠܝܬ ܕܫܚܝܢ ܐܝܟ ܢܘܪܐ. ܘܠܝܬ ܕܪܛܝܒ ܐܝܟ ܡܝܐ. ܘܠܐ ܕܝܒܝܫ ܐܝܟ
ܐܪܥܐ. ܘܠܐ ܕܩܪܝܪ ܐܝܟ ܐܐܪ. ܐܠܐ ܐܣܘ̈ܬܐ ܒܕ ܚܙܝܢ ܕܕܡܐ ܕܐܝܬܘܗܝ ܚܡܝܡܐ ܘܪܛܝܒܐ. ܕܡܢ ܐܐܪ
ܐܝܬܘܗܝ ܩܘܡܗ. ܐܦ ܠܗ ܠܐܐܪ ܪܛܝܒܐ ܘܚܡܝܡܐ ܐܡܪܝܢ ܠܗ܀ ܡܠܦ̈ܢܐ ܕܝܢ ܕܥܕܬܐ ܡܛܠ ܕܚܙܘ ܘܚܙܘ
ܕܐܢ ܪܛܝܒܐ ܘܚܡܝܡܐ ܢܐܡܪܘܢܝܗܝ ܐܢܫ. ܠܐ ܡܫܟܚ ܡܕܒܪܢܝܬܐ ܢܬܬܝܠܝܬܐ ܕܕܝܠܗ ܗܝ. ܟܕ ܓܝܪ ܕܐܢ ܢܐܡܪܘܢܝܗܝ
ܚܡܝܡܐ ܐܢܫ. ܗܕܐ ܕܢܘܪܐ ܗܝ ܡܕܒܪܢܝܬܐ. ܘܐܢ ܪܛܝܒܐ ܗܕܐ ܕܡܝܐ ܗܝ. ܘܡܛܠ ܗܠܝܢ ܡܛܠ ܥܠܬܐ
ܕܕܐܝܟ ܗܕܐ ܩܪܝܪܐ ܐܡܪܘܗ̈ܝ ܡܕܒܪܢܝܬܐ. ܐܦ ܠܐ ܟܠܗܘܢ ܫܠܡܝܢ ܠܗ ܠܗܕܐ. ܕܩܪܘܝܐ ܕܝܢ ܐܝܬܘܗ.
ܐܝܕܐ ܕܟܠ ܕܫܦܝܪܐ ܠܗ ܢܩܒܠ. ܐܢ ܩܪܝܪܐ ܐܝܟ ܕܐܡܪܝܢ ܡܠܦ̈ܢܐ. ܘܐܢ ܪܛܝܒܐ ܘܚܡܝܡܐ ܐܝܟ
ܕܐܡܪܝܢ ܐܣܘ̈ܬܐ. ܐܐܪ الهوآء الجوّ ܀ ܘܐܝܟ ܚܢܝܢ **ܐܐܪ** ܡܬܐܡܪ ܕܕܟܪܘܬܐ ܘܢܩܒܘܬܐ. ܘܡܢ ܦܘ̈ܠܓܐ ܕܝܢ
ܐܐܪ ܡܬܩܪܐ. ܗܘ ܕܠܥܠ ܡܢ ܐܪܥܐ ܪܘܡܐ ܪܡܐ. ܗܘ ܕܝܢ ܕܡܬܚܙܐ ܡܢ ܗܠܝܢ ܡܬܩܪܐ ܡܬܩܪܐ الهواء الجوّ اخر
النسيم. ܘܐܣܬܝܐ الفضاء. ܒܝ ܢܘ ܐܬܐܡܪ **ܐܐܪ** ܡܛܠ ܡܬܬܕܡܝܘܬܗ܀

Ā'ar according to bar Serošway, it is neither only masculine or feminine, without spirit (*d-lā ruḥā*). A substance that has the power of coldness dominant, and that has associated with it in mixture the power of wetness. The sense of this is that the dominant one's (name) is applied to both of them, for there is no substance that possesses one of these powers simply. For all substances are not (solely) hot like fire, nor wet like water, nor dry like earth, nor cold like air. But because the physicians consider that blood is warm and wet, and that its constitution is of air, they also say of air that it is hot and dry. The doctors of the church, however, because they were observant, saw that if people called (air) wet and hot, no dominant power would belong to it specifically. For if people called it hot, that is the power of fire, and if wet, that is of water. And on that account, for these reasons they said cold is [its] power. But not all of them consent to that. So it is for the reader to accept which of all seems better to him, whether it is cold as the doctors say, or wet and hot as the physicians say. *Air, sky*. And according to Ḥunayn, *ā'ar*. It is said (both) masculine and feminine. The

Greeks call it *a'ayr*. This is below the tops of tall mountains. What is above this is called aether. *Air, the sky at the extremity of the clouds. Others, space (*al-faḍā'*).* In a manuscript it is written *ā'ar* with regard to its vocalization.

The Greek word ἀήρ occurs a single time in the *Aphorisms*. The Syriac gives the borrowed Greek word, which was present in the Syriac language for centuries prior to the period under consideration in this work. The Arabic translates with *al-hawā'* 'air'. The entry from bar Bahlul's *Lexicon* is of inherent interest. In it, bar Serošway contrasts the physical views of the physicians with those of the doctors of the church, while making no final judgment regarding their disagreement. A clear distinction is observable, furthermore, between the approach adopted by bar Serošway in this entry and that of the entry for the Syriac word *dmā* attributable to Ḥunayn given above (unit 1.3.1). Along with the entry for *ḥešoḵā* presented in chapter one (unit 1.3.14), this entry gives further evidence of tension between the authority of philosophical and religious sources in ʿAbbāsid-era Syriac thought.

As in the entry for *ḥešoḵā*, the religious and philosophical perspectives are allowed to stand side-by-side. In this case it is bar Serošway who clearly prefers the theological interpretation. While the writer prefers the churchmen's account, he leaves open to the reader the choice between the two interpretations, indicating a certain openness to speculative inquiry.

3.2

ἀκροχορδόνες

278:5 **ܐܩܪܘܟܘܪܕܘܢܝܣ** ܐܝܟ ܙܟܪܝܐ الثآليل المعلقة ܘܐܝܟ ܦܘܠܘܣ܀

Aqroḵordonês, according to Zakariya *hanging warts*, and according to Paul.

278:7 **ܐܩܪܘܟܘܪܕܘܢ** ܐܝܟ ܒܪ ܣܪܘ ܗ̄ ܪ̈ܝܫܝ ܝܬܪ̈ܐ قال و أصله ضيق حتى يظن أنه شيء متعلقة܀

Aqroḵordon, according to bar Serošway this is the extremities of tendons (*riši yaṯrē*). *He said its connection is thin, such that one would think it something attached.*

278:14 **ܐܩܘܟܘܪܕܘܢ** بثر يسمّى اقروخرذون ܗ̄ ܪ̈ܝܫܝ ܝܬܪ̈ܐ أطراف الأوتار܀

Aqoḵordon, a pustule called aqrūkhurdhūn. This is the extremities of tendons (*riši yaṯrā*), *the extremities of tendons (*aṭrāf al-awtār*).*

Ἀκροχορδόνες, the name of a type of skin disease, occurs once in the *Aphorisms*, in the list of disease-names in aphorism iii. 26. The Syriac gives the self-same word borrowed from the Greek, while Ḥunayn's Arabic translation gives *al-tha'ālīl al-mu'allaqa* 'hanging warts'. For its part, the early Arabic version of the *Aphorisms* simply gives *tha'ālīl* 'warts'.

Al-tha'ālīl is also a common element in the translations for this word mentioned by Ullmann, but the addition of *al-mu'allaqa* or *al-muta'allaqa* is significantly rarer in his citations.[43] In the second entry above, someone, presumably bar Serošway, provides a brief explanation of the reasoning behind adding *al-muta'allaqa*. At any rate it seems that the use of *al-tha'ālīl* in translating this word had achieved a level of consensus before Ḥunayn's time. In cases like this, the importance of earlier translation activity for Ḥunayn's work is emphasized.

Although Ḥunayn's definitions in 278:14 do not relate directly to the *Aphorisms*, there are interesting relationships between them and certain other sources noted by Ullmann. The Syriac translation *riši yaṯrā* is a calque of the Greek term, and the Arabic translations *aṭrāf al-awtār* is a near-calque. Ullmann notes that al-Rāzī's *Ḥāwī* contains the Arabic calque *ru'ūs al-awtār*, which Ullmann links to Iṣṭifān.[44] Furthermore, recalling the Arabic transliteration given in the entry at 278:14, three quotations from Dioscorides' *Materia Medica* translate ἀκροχορδόνες with *al-tha'ālīl allatī yuqāl lahā aqrukhurdūnis* ('the warts that are called *aqrukhurdūnis*').[45]

3.3

ἀσκαρίδες

241:10 ܐܣܩܪܝܕܣ ܥܠܩܐ ܕܩܛܝܢܐ ܘܙܥܘܪܐ ܕܗܘܝܢ ܒܟܪܣܐ ܒܪ ܣܪܘ الديدان الصغار التي في البطن❖

Asqārides, small, thin worms that are in the stomach. (According to) bar Serošway, *small worms that are in the stomach.*

The word ἀσκαρίδες occurs once in the *Aphorisms*, also in the list of disease-names in aphorism iii. 26. The Syriac gives the borrowed Greek word in its place, while in Ḥunayn's Arabic translation *al-dūd* 'worms' is employed. For the phrase containing two disease-names related to worms in the aphorism, ἕλμινθες στρογγύλαι, ἀσκαρίδες, the early Arabic version

43 Ullmann, *Wörterbuch zu den griechisch-arabischen Übersetzungen*, 90–1.

44 ibid.

45 There are slight variations in the transliterations amongst the three equivalents given by Ullmann.

gives three elements, *dūd 'irāḍ wa-dūd ṭiwāl wa-dūd mithla dūd al-khall* 'round worms, long worms, and worms like vinegar-worms'.[46]

In the entry from bar Bahlul's *Lexicon*, two almost identical sentences occur, one in Syriac and the other in Arabic. In this instance, the Syriac carries a single adjective, *qaṭinē* 'thin', that is not found in the Arabic. An entry for the Syriac equivalent given in the entry, *šušlē*, contains a direct citation of Ḥunayn's lexicographical activity:

1959:14 **ܫܘܫܠܐ** ܒܨ̤ **ديدان** حبّ القرع حيّات البطن الذي في الأعماء صحّحه حنين܀

Šušlē in a manuscript, *worms, ringworms,*[47] *worms of the belly which are in the intestines. Ḥunayn rectified it.*

The final element of this definition resembles a translation of the form ἀσκαριδάς cited by Ullmann in Galen's *On Simple Drugs* Book Seven, *al-ḥayyāt al-mutawallida fī al-baṭn* 'worms generated in the belly'.[48]

3.4

δυσεντερία

544:13 **ܕܘܣܢܛܪܝܐ** ܟܘܪܗܐ ܕܡܥܝܐ قرح الأمعاء وأيضاً الخلفة من قروح الأمعاء سحج.
ܕܘܣܛܣܪܝܐ ܗ̄ ܫܚܢܬܐ ܕܗܘܝܢ ܗܠܝܢ ܟܘܪܗܐ ܒܟܘܠܝܪܐ܀

Dusanṭareya, ulcers of the bowels, *ulcers of the bowels* (qarḥ al-am'ā'), *also diarrhoea* (khilfa) *because of ulceration of the bowels, dysentery* (saḥj). *Dusêṭsêria*, that is, the sores that are these ulcers in cholera.

Forms of the word δυσεντερία occur numerous times in the *Aphorisms*. The Syriac gives the self-same word borrowed from the Greek in every instance. In all but one case, Ḥunayn translates the word into Arabic with a version of the phrase *ikhtilāf al-dam* 'bloody diarrhoea'. The exception is found in aphorism iii. 30, where *saḥj al-am'ā'* 'abrasion of the intestines' is used instead. The early Arabic version of aphorism iii. 11 exists, and there δυσεντερίας is translated *ikhtilāf min al-a'fāj* 'diarrhoea from the large intestine'. In the extant early Arabic version of aphorism iii. 16, the translator specifies this interpretation somewhat further, giving *ikhtilāf min khurāj al-a'fāj* 'diarrhoea from abscesses of the large intestine'. Al-Biṭrīq's

46 Ullmann notes this usage with interest in his citation of this text, *Wörterbuch zu den griechisch-arabischen Übersetzungen*, 141.

47 The meaning of this phrase is obscure. The nearest suitable sense I have found is the word *qurā'* 'ringworm'.

48 Ullmann, *Wörterbuch zu den griechisch-arabischen Übersetzungen*, 141.

translations thus give more specific interpretations of the disease than do Ḥunayn's, while the latter's renditions are much more regular.

In the numerous texts from the Arabic versions of Book Six of Galen's *On Simple Drugs* cited by Ullmann, the usual translation of δυσεντερία in Ḥunayn's version is *qurūḥ al-am'ā'*.[49] However, in a citation from Book 10 of that work, the Greek word is transliterated. In the texts from Book Six, al-Biṭrīq preferred several different equivalents. Sometimes he used *ikhtilāf al-aghrās* 'diarrhoea with mucus', sometimes simply *al-aghrās* 'mucus',[50] and sometimes the same equivalent preferred by Ḥunayn in the *Aphorisms*, *ikhtilāf al-dam* 'bloody diarrhoea'.

The definitions attributable to Ḥunayn in the entry from bar Bahlul's *Lexicon* correspond only to the examples from the later version of Book Six of *On Simple Drugs* and the single exceptional translation in aphorism iii. 30. One way of interpreting the discrepancies between these translations follows on from a consideration of the different audiences for whom these works were intended. While the *Aphorisms* was often used as an introductory text to medicine, *On Simple Drugs* was a more advanced work meant for doctors with at least some training. Arguably, the aetiological translation found in the latter work is more appropriate for the specialist, while the symptomatological translation found in the former is more appropriate for students.

3.5

περιπλευμονία

1497:9 **ܦܪܝܦܠܐܘܡܢܝܐ** ܐܝܟ ܒܪ ܣܪܦܝܘܢ ܥܘܒܝܢܐ ܕܪܐܬܐ وجع الرئة. ܐܝܟ ܚܢܝܢ ܐܫܬܐ ܕܥܡ
ܥܘܒܝܢܐ ܕܪܐܬܐ. **ܦܪܝܦܘܠܘܡܝܐ** ܐܝܟ ܒܪ ܣܪܘ ܦܠܓܡܘܢ ܕܪܐܬܐ أورام الرئة. **ܦܪܝܦܠܐܘܡܢܝܐ**
ܐܝܟ ܒܪ ܣܪܘ ܟܐܒ ܪܐܬܐ ܘܥܘܒܝܢܐ ܕܪܐܬܐ وجع الرئة وورمها܀

Pêriplêumnyā according to bar Serapion, swelling of the lungs (*'ubbyānā ḏ-rāṯā*), *pain of the lungs*. According to Ḥunayn, fever with swelling of the lungs. *Pêripulumyā* according to bar Serošway, swelling of the lungs, *swellings of the lungs*. *Pêriplêumnyā* according to bar Serošway, pain of the lungs and swelling of the lungs, *pain of the lungs and their swelling*.

49 Ullmann, *Wörterbuch zu den griechisch-arabischen Übersetzungen*, 210–11.

50 This word is obscure. The only anatomical definition available for this form occurs in volume III, p. 269 of Freytag's dictionary. There he mentions the plural *aghrās* for the word *ghirs*, and defines it as *res ex utero muci instar prodiens cum foetu*.

1624:22 ܦܪܝܦܠܘܢܘܡܘܢܝܐ ܐܝܟ ܒܪ ܣܪܘܫܘܝ, ܥܘܒܝܢܐ ܕܪܐܬܐ ورم الرئة⁘

Priplunumunyā according to bar Serošway, swelling of the lungs, *swelling of the lungs*.

1634:7 ܦܪܦܠܓܡܘܢܝܐ ܐܝܟ ܒܪ ܣܪܘܫܘܝ, ܟܐܒ ܪܐܬܐ وجع الرئة⁘

Prplgmunyā according to bar Serošway, pain of the lungs, *pain of the lungs*.

Forms of this disease-name occurs some five times in the *Aphorisms*. The Syriac translation renders these instances in three different ways. For the occurrences in aphorisms iii. 23 and iii. 30, the borrowed Greek word is given as *pêriplumunyā*. In aphorism vi. 16, the phrase *'ubbyānā d-rāṯā* 'swelling of the lungs' is employed. Finally, in aphorisms vii. 11 and vii. 12 the phrase *ḥašā d-rāṯā* 'disease of the lungs' is given. Ḥunayn's Arabic translation consistently gives forms of *dhāt al-ri'a* 'disease of the lungs'.

Bar Bahlul's entry for the word at 1497:9 contains definitions written by several different authors, all of which are relatively similar. Ḥunayn's definition is distinguished mostly by the addition of the symptom of fever to the description of the disease, but since no Arabic text occurs in it, no comparison may be made between it and the text of his version of the *Aphorisms*. While one of the alternative Syriac translations *'ubbyānā d-rāṯā* 'swelling of the lungs' figures prominently in these definitions, the other, *ḥašā d-rāṯā* 'disease of the lungs', is not found there. In the absence of evidence from the early Arabic version, it is impossible to assume that Ḥunayn's translation in the *Aphorisms* represents any process of development in translation technique.

3.6

ποδάγρα

1489:3 ܦܕܓܪܐ ܒܨ̈ܚ ܘܒܪ ܣܪܘ النقرس⁘

Pdgrē in a manuscript and (according to) bar Serošway, *gout* (al-niqris).

1500:18 ܦܘܕܓܪܐ ܒܨ̈ܚ نقرس. ܦܘܕܓܪܐ ܦܘܛܓܪܐ ܘܐܚܪ̈ܢܐ ܦܘܕܢܓܐ النقرس⁘

Pudagrā in a manuscript, *gout* (al-niqris). *Pudagrā*, *puṭagrā*, and (according to) others *pudanga*, *gout*.

1534:5 ܦܛܓܪܐ نقرس⁘

Pṭagrā, *gout*.

1648:13 ܦܛܠܓܝܐ ܕܗܘ ܦܘܕܓܪܐ ܒܪ ܣܪܘ النقرس⁘

Ptlgya, which is *pudagrā*, (according to) bar Serošway, *gout*.

The disease ποδάγρα is mentioned several times in the *Aphorisms*. Both the Syriac version and Ḥunayn's translation adopt regular approaches to rendering the term. The former gives forms of the borrowed Greek word, while the latter uses *al-niqris* 'gout'. Beyond this, Ullmann cites a text mentioning a form of the related adjective ποδαγρικός from Book Six of Galen's *On Simple Drugs*. In translating it, both al-Biṭrīq and Ḥunayn again use *al-niqris*,[51] indicating that a stable equivalency between these two words had been established well before the beginning of Ḥunayn's career.

The entries from bar Bahlul's *Lexicon* also show a high degree of stability for the equivalence between ποδάγρα and *al-niqris*. However, no native Syriac equivalent is given, indicating that the borrowed Greek word had been thoroughly integrated into the language. On the other hand, the transcriptions of the Greek word in the *Lexicon* have a strong tendency toward irregularity, moderating somewhat this impression.

3.7

σατυριασμοί

1292:6 **ܣܛܘܪܝܣܡܘܣ** ܐܝܟ ܙܟ̈ أشياء تنتو من البدن. **ܣܛܘܪܝܐܣܡܘܣ** ܐܝܟ ܒܪ ܣܪܘ ܢܕ̈ܝܐ ܡܕܡ ܕܦܓܪܐ. ܒ̈ زواید تنتو من البدن. ܒ̈ إنعاظ من غير شهوة الجماع܀

Saṭurismu according to Zakariya, *things that protrude from the body*. *Saṭuriasmu* according to bar Serošway, certain protuberances of the body (*nḏāyē meddem d-pagrā*). In a manuscript, *excesses protruding from the body*. In a manuscript, *sexual excitement without desire for copulation*.

A form of this Greek word occurs a single time in the *Aphorisms*. The Syriac gives the self-same word borrowed from the Greek, while Ḥunayn's Arabic version gives *al-khānāzīr* 'scrofula'. The early Arabic version of this aphorism likewise gives this word, albeit in the indefinite. This indicates that a stable approach to translating this term into Arabic was established well before the beginning of Ḥunayn's career. Despite this, the entry in bar Bahlul's *Lexicon* has no trace of this Arabic equivalent and seems largely to refer to a different sense of the word. It is possible that this may bear on the question of the authorship of the Syriac *Aphorisms*. An entry in bar Bahlul's *Lexicon* for the word *nḏāyē* given in the entry above also does not contain Ḥunayn's Arabic equivalent:

---

51 Ullmann, *Wörterbuch zu den griechisch-arabischen Übersetzungen*, 543.

1218:23 **ܢܕܝܐ** ܐܝܟ ܒܪ ܣܪܘܫܘܝ ܕܗܘܝܢ ܒܓܒܪܘܬܐ القروح في القضيب ܘܐܝܟ ܙܟܪܝܐ ما ينتو من البدن مثل الثآليل وغيرها. **ܢܕܝܐ** ܒܨܚ تنضيح قفز شرارة ويقال منه ܢܕܐ ويكون نفر تفرّق اضطراب؞

Nḏāyē according to bar Serošway, that which occurs in the virile member, *abscesses of the penis.* And according to Zakariya, *that which protrudes from the body, such as worms and the like. Nḏāyā* in a manuscript, *splashing,*[52] *jumping, sparkling. Nḏā is derived from it, and it is fleeing, separating, disorder.*

3.8

σφάκελος

444:8 **ܓܢܓܪ** ܐܝܟ ܦܘܠܘܣ ܐܘܟܠܬ ܡܣܝܘܬܐ ܗܝ ܥܡ ܡܘܠܐ ܕܡܛܠܬܗ ܡܝܬ ܦܓܪܐ، ܠܓܢܓܪܢܐ. غغرانا وهو العفن. ܘܒܕܘܟ ܐܡܪ ܗܝ ܐܟܘܠܘܬܐ ܐܘܟܠܬ ܡܠܝܘܬܐ الآكلة الخبيثة. **ܓܢܓܪ ܘܐܣܦܩܠܘܣ** ܗܝ ܡܝܘܬܐ ܕܒܣܪܐ اللحم الميت؞

Gāngr according to Paul, this is decay with pus due to which the body dies. Ghanghranā, *which is decay* (ʿafan). In one place he says this is gangrene (*āḵuluṯā*), which is repletion,[53] *bad gangrenous sores* (al-ākila al-khabītha). *Gāngr w-aspaqelus*, this is death of the flesh, *dead flesh.*

This word occurs a single time in the *Aphorisms*, in aphorism vii. 50. There, both the Syriac *Aphorisms* and Ḥunayn's Arabic version reproduce the Greek word in transliteration. The Syriac translation gives the phrase *ḥšā ḏ-spaqêlos* 'the disease of sphacelus', while Ḥunayn's version gives *al-'illa allatī yuqālu lahā sfaqīlūs* 'the disease which is called sphacelus'. As we have seen in this chapter, it is quite rare for a technical Greek term to be thus reproduced without explanation in Ḥunayn's Arabic translation of the *Aphorisms*. Ullmann notes a single occurrence of this Greek term in Galen's *Anatomical Procedures*,[54] where the Arabic phrase *wa-mā yaḥduthu fīh min ta'affun al-'iẓām* 'that which occurs in it of decay of the bones' translates the Greek phrase καὶ σφακέλους τῶν ἐν αὐτοῖς ὀστῶν.[55] The Arabic definition of gangrene in bar Bahlul's entry corresponds partially with this translation.

An entry for bar Bahlul's Syriac equivalent of gangrene, *masyuṯā* 'decay', contains evidence of Ḥunayn's lexicographical work:

---

52 Neither this noun nor the second form of the root *nḍḥ* are attested in the dictionaries of Wehr and Freytag. I have translated it according to the sense of the root and the meaning of the Syriac word.

53 The sense of this is obscure. Noting it, R. Payne Smith wrote *sed vix recte*.

54 Ullmann, *Wörterbuch zu den griechisch-arabischen Übersetzungen*, 661.

55 Ibid.

1115:10 ... **ܡܣܝܘܬܐ** عفن صحّحه حنين. ܘܐܝܟ ܙܟܪܝܐ ܐܡܣܝܬ عفّنت ابتللت بللت. ܡܬܡܣܝܢܘܬܐ ܒܨܚܚܐ جمد܀

... *Masyuṯā*, *decay* (ʿafan), *Ḥunayn rectified it.* According to Zakariya *amsiṯ*, *I decayed, I became moistened, I moistened*. *Meṯmasyānuṯā* in a manuscript, *coagulation*.

3.9

τριταῖος

133:15 **ܐܡܛܪܝܛܐܘܣ** ܒܪ ܣܪܘܫܘܝ ܐܫܬܐ ܕܡܬܩܪܝܐ ܦܠܓܘܬ ܛܪܝܛܐܘܣ نصف حمّى الغبّ܀

Imṭriṭaus (according to) bar Serošway, a fever that is called half-tertian, *half-tertian fever* (niṣf ḥummā al-ghibb).

825:25 **ܛܪܝܛܐܘܣ** ܦܪܘܣܛܪܝܛܐܘܣ حمّى غبّ܀

Ṭriṭêus, *prosṭriṭêus*, *tertian fever* (ḥummā ghibb).

This type of fever is mentioned twice in the *Aphorisms*. In both cases the Syriac translates using the borrowed Greek word, but does so using slightly different forms. In aphorism iii. 21, the name occurs in the plural τριταῖοι, and the form of the Syriac borrowing of the Greek word reflects its plurality with the spelling *ṭriṭêo*. In aphorism iv. 59, the singular τριταῖος is found instead, and the Syriac correspondingly renders it *ṭriṭêos*. It would thus seem reasonable to call these usages transcriptions rather than borrowings. In both cases Ḥunayn's Arabic versions uses a form of the equivalent *al-ghibb* 'tertian fever', which is also the equivalent found in the entries from bar Bahlul's *Lexicon*.

Despite the consistency amongst the translations and the entries, a text from Ullmann's *Wörterbuch* demonstrates that the usage *al-ghibb* was not universal in the Greek-to-Arabic translation movement. In the Arabic version of the *Cyranides*, a description of the course of the fever reading *al-nāfiḍ alladhī min thalāth ilā thalāth* 'fits that run by threes' serves to translate a form of the related verb τριταΐζω.[56] This emphasizes the unanimity between the lexicons and Ḥunayn's translations, but does not constitute strong evidence for identifying any specific contribution from the translator.

56 Ullmann, *Wörterbuch zu den griechisch-arabischen Übersetzungen*, 684.

3.10

φλέγμα

1565:20 **ܦܠܓܡܐ** ܐܝܟ ܒܪ ܣܪܘ̄ ܐܝܬܘܗ̄ ܟܝܡܘܣ ܪܛܝܒܐ ܘܩܪܝܪܐ. ܕܐܝܬܘܗ̄ ܩܘܝܡܗ ܕܝܠܝܬܐ ܡܢ ܐܣܛܘܟܣܐ ܕܡܝܐ. ܘܐܝܬܘܗ̄ ܒܝܬܗ ܒܪܐܬܐ ܘܚܝܠܘܬܗ ܒܚܕܝܐ البلغم. **ܦܠܓܡܐ** ܬܘܒ ܘܦܠܓܡ̈ܛܐ ܀

Plegmā according to bar Serošway, this is a wet and cold humour. Its constitution is properly derived from the element of water. Its home is in the lungs and its power is in the chest, *phlegm (*al-balgham*). Plegmā* again, and *plegmāṭā.*

Forms of this Greek word occur four times in the *Aphorisms.* In each case the Syriac gives the self-same word borrowed from the Greek. The Arabic likewise uses a form of the borrowed Greek word *al-balgham* in each case. Ullmann cites a text for this word from Galen’s *On Simple Drugs* Book Six. There, the early Arabic translator al-Biṭrīq and Ḥunayn both translate using *al-balgham* as well, showing that the borrowing had occurred well before the beginning of Ḥunayn’s career. Bar Serošway’s entry from bar Bahlul’s *Lexicon* follows the same approach as that adopted in the several definitions found in the entry for *merṯā*, discussed in the discussion of μελαγχολία above (unit 1.7 in this chapter), as well as that found in the entry for *dmā* in the discussion of αἷμα (unit 1.3.1). Here, then, we may distinguish the Syriac as a full borrowing as opposed to a transcription, given that the lexicographers define it according to the conventions used in defining other Syriac humoural terms as opposed to those used in defining analogous Greek words.

3.11

φλεγμονή

1566:10 **ܦܠܓܡܘܢܐ** ܒܨܚܚ̈ البلغم ܘܐܝܟ ܙܟܪ̈ **ܦܠܓܡܘܢܝ** الورم الحارّ الذي يحدث عن الدم. ܘܐܝܟ ܒܪ ܣܪܘ̄ ܥܘܒ̈ܝܢܐ ܚܡܝܡ̈ܐ ورم حارّ ܀

Plêgmonê in a manuscript, *phlegm* (al-balgham). And according to Zakariya *plgêmonay, hot swellings that occur on account of blood.* And according to bar Serošway, hot swellings (*'ūbbyānē ḥamimē*), *a hot swelling* (waram ḥār).

The Syriac version of the *Aphorisms* adopts varying approaches to translating the forms of the Greek noun φλεγμονή and the participle of the related verb φλεγμαίνω that occur six times in the *Aphorisms*. Three of these instances are translated with the native Syriac equivalent *'ūbbyānā* ‘swelling’, while for the other three the borrowed Greek word is used. Ḥunayn’s Arabic version consistently employs a form of the equivalent *waram* ‘swelling’ to translate each instance. A slight variation occurs in aphorism v. 23, where the adjective *al-ḥāra* 'hot' is added to modify the plural *al-awrām*. This is almost certainly due to the context of that aphorism, which discusses the potential medicinal uses of the quality of coldness. This rendering is closer to the definitions for φλεγμονή found in bar Bahlul's entry at 1566:10.

Two translations of φλεγμονή from the early Arabic translation are also extant. In aphorism iii. 24, the same equivalent preferred by Ḥunayn, *waram*, is given. However, in another place aphorism al-Biṭrīq adopted a different approach, translating aphorism vii. 17 ἐπὶ φλεγμονῇ τοῦ ἥπατος, λύγχ with *man kharaja fī kabidih khurāj thumma taba'ah fuwāq fa-dhālika sharr* 'for the one upon whose liver an abscess comes out, then hiccups follow, that is a bad sign'. This contrasts with Ḥunayn's rendering of the text with *wa-'an waram al-kabid fuwāq* 'on account of swelling of the liver, hiccups'.

An entry for the Syriac equivalent *'ubbyānā* reads as follows:

1410:25 ܥܘܒܝܢܐ ܕܓܓܪܬܐ ܐܝܟ ܒܪ ܣܪܘ ورم اللهاة.[57] ܥܘܒܝܢܐ ورم. ܥܘܒܝܢܐ ܕܚܟܐ ورم الحنك. ܥܘܒܝܢܐ ܕܥܘܩܒܪܬܐ ورم عَضَل الحلق. ܥܘܒܝܢܐ ܚܡܝܡܐ ܕܗܘܝܢ ܠܦܘܬ ܥܩܪܐ ܕܛܦܪܐ الدواحس. ܥܘܒܝܢܐ ܕܗܘܝܢ ܡܢ ܬܪܥܝܬܐ ܘܠܥܠ ܚܠܒܐ ܗܘ ܕܦܪܝܣ الحجاب. ܥܘܒܝܢܐ ܕܡܬܩܪܐ ܒܪ ܬܐܬܐ ܐܝܟ ܒܪ ܣܪܘ ܗܘ ܗܘ ܕܗܘܐ ܒܕܩܢܐ الأورام التي تكون في موضع اللحية. ܥܘܒܝܢܐ ܒܨܚ̈ الورم. ܡܥܒܝ وَارِم܀

'Ubbyānā ḏ-gagarṯā according to bar Serošway, *swelling of the uvula. 'Ubbyānā, a swelling* (waram). *'Ubbyānā ḏ-ḥekkā, a swelling of the palate. 'Ubbyānā ḏ-'uqbarṯā* ('swelling of a muscle'), *swelling of the muscles of the pharynx. 'Ubbyānē ḥāmimē ḏ-hāweyn lpuṯ 'eqārā ḏ-ṭeprē* ('hot swellings that occur at the root of the fingernails'), *whitlow* (al-dawāḥis) *'Ubbyānē ḏ-hāweyn men tar'iṯā w-la'al ḥelbā haw d-pris* (swellings that occur from the brain to the outspread diaphragm), *the diaphragm* (al-ḥijāb). *'Ubbyānā ḏ-meṯqrā bar teṯā* ('the swelling that is called the son of the fig') according to bar Serošway, this is that which is on the chin, *swellings that occur in the place of the beard. 'Ubbyānā* in a manuscript, *swellings. Ma'bay, it swelled* (wārim).

Although bar Bahlul's Greek entry accurately conveys the sense of the term in question, the two main translations of the *Aphorisms* do not usually specify its sense to this same extent. That entry may therefore have been used more to explain the meaning of the Greek term, or it may itself derive from such an explanation. The Syriac entry, however, appears more to be focused upon the identification of day-to-day ailments.

---

57 Duval: سقوط اللهاة. I have followed the easier sense of the minority of Duval's manuscripts.

In this case, Ḥunayn's translations clearly relied in important respects upon prior Arabic and Syriac translations. However, neither the early Arabic translation nor the Syriac version of the *Aphorisms* followed an entirely regular approach to translating φλεγμονή. Ḥunayn's Arabic version stands out by virtue of its adoption of a single, regular, native equivalent.

3.12

χολέρα

876:5 **ܟܘܠܝܪܐ** هيضة تخمة ܒ̱ ܫܪܝܬܐ ܕܡܢ ܠܬܚܬ ܘܬܒܥܬܐ[58] ܕܡܢ ܠܥܠ܀

*Kolêrā, cholera (*hayḍa*), dyspepsia.* In a manuscript, diarrhoea from below and vomiting from above.

877:3 **ܟܘܠܐܪܐ** ܐܝܟ ܒܪ ܣܪܘ̈ܫܘܝ ܫܓܝܫܘܬܐ ܕܐܣܛܘܡܟܐ ܕܠܐ ܡܥܣܩܘܬܐ التخمة. ܘܟܘܠܐܪܐ ܬܘܒ܀

Kolêra according to bar Serošway, intense disturbance of the stomach, *dyspepsia*. Again, *kolara.*[59]

A form of χολέρα occurs once in the *Aphorisms*, in aphorism iii. 30. The Syriac version gives a form of the borrowed Greek word, while Ḥunayn's Arabic version gives *al-hayḍa* 'cholera'. The agreement between the entry at 876:5 in bar Bahlul's *Lexicon* and Ḥunayn's translation of the *Aphorisms* contrasts with the absence of the translator's equivalent *al-hayḍa* from bar Serošway's definition in the entry at 877:3. The presence of *al-hayḍa* in the entry at 876:5 indicates a relative degree of stability for this approach to translating the term, while the Syriac definition explains in greater detail the symptoms of the disease. This is further extended by the use of this Arabic word to translate χόλερα in Theomnestus of Nicopolis' *Horse-medicine.*[60]

Conclusion

Having provided these examples, several of the questions I posed in the introduction to this chapter may be answered. First, we may consider the extent to which the 27 Greek words discussed above were integrated into the

---

58 Duval: ܬܒܥ̈ܬܐ.

59 Duval also notes a definition for this Greek word at 544:15. I discuss the entry in which it occurs in the discussion of δυσεντερία in unit (2.3.4).

60 Ullmann, *Wörterbuch zu den griechisch-arabischen Übersetzungen* (supplement), II, 691.

Syriac language. To restate the question, how profound was the trend toward adoption of Greek vocabulary in Syriac medicine? In other words, did the Syriac glossographers treat these Greek words as fully native, or were etymologically-Syriac equivalents resorted to in order to explain them?

The entries in bar Bahlul's *Lexicon* and the translation of the *Aphorisms* give evidence of active Syriac equivalents for some of these words and not for others. Ḥunayn's Arabic translations of the eight words presented in section one display a high degree of instability. Four of these cannot be shown to possess a clear Syriac equivalent in the sources considered here, namely αἱμορροΐδες, εἰλεός, κίνδυνος and μελαγχολία. Conversely, the other four, ἐπίπλοος, κιρσός, λήθαργος and φρενῖτις, do correspond at least roughly to native Syriac equivalents.

Ḥunayn's translations of the nine words presented in section two evince a lower degree of instability than those in section one. However, they follow largely the same pattern in terms of the presence of active etymologically-Syriac equivalents in the translations and lexicons. Four of them, ἀθληταί, ἐπιληψία, φθίσις and φρενός, show no evidence of simple, active Syriac equivalents. The other five, ἀποπληξία, ἄρωμα, ἐπιληψία, καῦσος and τέτανος do show evidence for active Syriac equivalents. Although in certain cases the lexicographical entries for these Syriac equivalents may have been important loci for the establishment of Arabic terminology, evidence for the existence of these equivalents does not predict any particular level of order in Ḥunayn's Arabic translations.

Despite this negative conclusion, it may be fruitful to compare these examples with those presented in Chapter One. In the more or less arbitrary selection of the treatment of 29 Greek words in the translations of the *Aphorisms* presented there, significant explicative translations were only found in Ḥunayn's Arabic translation for a single instance, that of αὐτόματον (unit 1.1.3). In the present chapter, however, seven of the 28 terms presented were given explicative treatment by Ḥunayn in his Arabic version of the *Aphorisms*.[61]

61 Although other words discussed in Chapter One were translated in a variety of ways in the Arabic *Aphorisms*, like ἀγαθός (1.2.1) and ἀνάγκη (1.2.7), for example, I would argue that this variety is more stylistic than reflective of a need to interpret the sense of an unfamiliar term. For the same reason I have exluded κίνδυνος (2.1.4) from the tally of explicated terms treated in this chapter. Furthermore, in the set of Greek terms beginning with *alpha* found

A closer look at these examples should aid in explaining the source of the less orderly translations. In translating κιρσός (1.5), for example, Ḥunayn relied upon an Arabic word borrowed from the underlying Syriac equivalent *dalāyṯā*. It is possible to surmise that this word was somewhat unfamiliar to Ḥunayn's audience on the basis of his extant relevant lexicography. His approach to translating the word likewise appears to reflect this unfamiliarity. Rather than presenting the word simply without explanation, he provided an explicating translation to introduce the term to his readers. In later instances of the word in the text of the Aphorisms, however, he gradually reduces the amount of explication before finally allowing his preferred equivalent to stand by itself. A similar pattern is also observable in the case of εἰλεός (1.2).

In the example of μελαγχολία (1.7), it is more plausible that the absence of an established native Syriac equivalent for the Greek term had implications for Ḥunayn's Arabic translations. The evidence from the earlier Syriac translation of the Aphorisms attributed to Sergius indicates that the borrowed Greek word was not immediately adopted in Syriac medicine. The later Syriac translators, however, seem to have abandoned any attempt to render the complex sense of the Greek word, preferring to adopt it instead. Although Ḥunayn's preferred equivalent *al-sawdā'* eventually came to be a part of the Arabic lexicon with more-or-less an identical sense to that of the Greek word, the variety of approaches adopted for translating μελαγχολία in the Aphorisms reduce considerably the simple agreement between the source-text and the translation.

For terms presented in the second section, Ḥunayn's activity appears more to be that of an expert drawing upon the resources of his native tongue than that of the wordsmith innovating or borrowing lexical items. This is apparently the case in the discussion of ἐπιληψία in unit (2.4), for example. The terms so established may sometimes have resonance with native Syriac equivalents, as for example in the translations of ἀποπληξία (2.2).

---

both in the *Aphorisms* and bar Bahlul's *Lexicon*, Ḥunayn only translated two, αἱμορροΐδες and αὐτόματον, using a significant degree of explication. In a strict comparison of these words beginning with *alpha* with words translated with borrowings in the Syriac, the proportion of difference in explication would actually be greater than it is in the approach I have adopted here.

The bewildering swirl of terms surrounding τέτανος (2.6) gives strong evidence for the value of these sources for understanding the background of the Greek-to-Arabic translations. The regularity of Ḥunayn's translations of these terms combined with the evidence for the progressive development of Arabic translation techniques they provide shows clearly Ḥunayn's preference for simple and accurate translations of central technical terms of the medical art. Yet in considering the glossographical background for words like ἀθληταί (2.1), the rich background of potential Arabic equivalents available to Ḥunayn is emphasized as well.

The most important characteristic of the terms in the third section of this chapter is the degree of continuity between al-Biṭrīq's and Ḥunayn's Arabic translations they display. The Arabic translations for words like ἀκροχορδόνες (3.2), ἀσκαρίδες (3.3), δυσεντερία (3.4) and φλέγμα (3.10) were all established well before the beginning of Ḥunayn's career. This fact may be contrasted with several words, concentrated in section two, for which glosses attributed to Paul of Aegina agree better with al-Biṭrīq's translation than they do with Ḥunayn's. Ἀποπληξία (2.2), κίνδυνος (1.4), φρενός (2.8) and in particular τέτανος (2.6) all fit this description. The relevant lexicographical entries for the latter word provide strong evidence that the traditional ascription of the Arabic translation of Paul's *Pragmateia* is incorrect.

Furthermore, some important examples of more expansive discussions of medical and philosophical material appear in these examples. When compared with the material presented in Chapter One, descriptions in both Syriac and Arabic of concepts of medical theory appear more commonly in these examples. This is due to the fact that many more of these terms represent technical terms of art than do the words presented in chapter one. Although not written by Ḥunayn himself, bar Serošway's entry for ἀήρ (3.1) further extends the motif of tension between religious and philosophical authorities I noticed in the entry for *ḥešoḵā* in unit (1.3.14).

Although the evidence is mixed, important relationships between Syriac and Arabic in Ḥunayn's translation technique are displayed in several of these examples. In some cases it appears that Ḥunayn's Syriac usage may have differed from that found in the extant Syriac *Aphorisms.* The technical nature of several of the words considered allows for deeper insight into the specific contributions of Ḥunayn to Arabic medical translation. The evidence in these first two chapters thus provides firm ground for comparing the translations of the *Aphorisms* and their lexicographical background at a larger scale.

Part Two. Comparing the Syriac and Arabic Translations of the Hippocratic *Aphorisms*

Chapter 3

The Early Syriac Version of the *Aphorisms* Attributed to Sergius of Reš ʿAynā and ʿAbbāsid-era Syriac and Arabic Medical Translation: A Comparative Study

In the previous chapters, I treated the lexicographical relationships among the several translations of the Hippocratic *Aphorisms* on a word-by-word basis. In this chapter, I move to considering the translations at the sentence level of organization. Many of the trends observable in the previous chapter will also present themselves here, while other developments not noticeable at the level of individual words will also make their first appearances.

In particular, while the distinction between Ḥunayn's Arabic translation and the Syriac version in terms of adherence to the literal sense of the source-text has already been made clear in a general way, the key characteristics of the relationship between the early Arabic version and the other versions are not so easily discoverable at the lexical level. Furthermore, the very scanty remains of the early Syriac version require more concentrated attention in order to be made comprehensible in any general sense. For these reasons, I have chosen to consider several texts of the *Aphorisms* on the basis of their being represented in these earlier versions.

Although I shall not consider systematically all of the terminology present in these aphorisms, in several cases terminological variation makes consideration of the Greek entries in bar Bahlul's *Lexicon* useful. In these contexts I shall provide analyses of the relationship between these and the translations of the *Aphorisms*, following the same general approach as that adopted in the previous chapter. Furthermore, in several contexts there will arise opportunities to consider entries for Syriac terms that translate Greek words not represented in Duval's index to bar Bahlul's *Lexicon*. In this way our understanding of the usefulness of the *Lexicon* for studies of these translations will be further extended.

As discussed in the introduction, Grigory Kessel has extracted the text of seven aphorisms from the Syriac *Commentary on the Epidemics*. Of these seven aphorisms, four are also found translated in the fragments of the early Arabic version, as contained in the Arabic Palladius and/or al-Yaʿqūbī's *History*. Since these four allow for the fullest consideration of the Syro-Arabic translation tradition of the *Aphorisms*, I will consider these in Section One. I will then proceed to treat of the three that have no corresponding text in the *History* or in the Phoenix MS in Section Two.

For each aphorism, the texts will be presented in chronological order according to the current scholarly understanding of their periodization, except where otherwise noted. First, I shall provide the Greek text of the aphorism for reference. The early Syriac fragment will be presented next, followed by the early Arabic fragments. Then I will give the texts from the Syriac *Aphorisms*, followed by those from Ḥunayn's Arabic translation.

Section One

The following four aphorisms are represented in all both of the extant Syriac translations and the major Arabic translations of the *Aphorisms*.

Aphorism ii. 1

Ἐν ᾧ νοσήματι ὕπνος πόνον ποιεῖ, θανάσιμον· ἢν δὲ ὕπνος ὠφελῇ, οὐ θανάσιμον.

Syriac Commentary on the Epidemics (hereafter E)

ܐܝܟܐ ܕܫܢܬܐ ܠܟܐܒܐ ܥܒܕܐ ܡܡܝܬܢܝܬܐ ܗܝ. ܐܢܕܝܢ ܫܢܬܐ ܬܘܬܪ ܠܐ ܐܝܬܝܗ̇ ܡܡܝܬܢܝܬܐ.

When there is pain with sleep, it is deadly, but if sleep benefits it does not bring death.

Al-Biṭrīq's Version of Palladius' *Commentary on the* Aphorisms (hereafter P)

فى أيّ مرض كان إن جاءه النوم بوجع فذلك يموت وإن نفع النوم فليس بميّت.

In whatever disease it is, if sleep brings pain, that kills, but if sleep benefits it is not deadly.

Syriac *Aphorisms* (hereafter S)

ܟܘܪܗܢܐ ܕܥܒܕܐ ܒܗ̇ ܫܢܬܐ ܟܐܒܐ ܡܡܝܬܢܝܬܐ ܗܘ. ܐܢܕܝܢ ܡܘܬܪܐ ܫܢܬܐ ܠܘ ܡܡܝܬܢܝܬܐ ܗܘ.

Diseases in which sleep causes pain are deadly, but if sleep benefits it is not deadly.

Ḥunayn's Arabic *Aphorisms* (hereafter Ḥ)

إذا كان النوم في مرض من الأمراض يحدث وجعاً فذلك من علامات الموت، وإذا كان النوم ينفع فليس ذلك من علامات الموت.

When, in one of the diseases, sleep brings pain, that is (one of) the signs of death, but when sleep benefits, that is not (one of) the signs of death.

The Greek text of the aphorism consists of two conditional sentences resolved by predication. The adjective θανάσιμον has the same form in both instances. When comparing the four translations, one may note immediately that the two later versions preserve this symmetry while the two earlier versions do not. The predicate in the Syriac *Aphorisms* in both sentences is *d-mawta-w* '(it) is deadly', and in Ḥunayn's version both sentences conclude with *dhālika min 'alāmāt al-mawt* 'that is (one of) the signs of death'. This contrasts with the varying grammatical approaches of the earlier two aphorisms. The fragment from the Syriac *Epidemics* uses *d-mawta-y* '(it) is deadly' in the first sentence but *iṯēh d-mawta* 'it brings death' in the second. The early Arabic version gives *dhālika yumūt* 'that kills' for the first sentence but *(laysa) bi-mayyitin* '(is not) deadly' for the second. The two later translations thus appear to reflect a greater concern for rendering the style of the Greek original.

The version in the Syriac *Aphorisms* is the most literal translation of the four. Only a few particles of the Greek original are left unrendered, and no new text is added. Both of the Arabic versions add material, with Ḥunayn's version in particular making somewhat extensive expansions to the text. The early Syriac version in contrast does not translate the entire text, neglecting to translate the word ᾧ νοσήματι 'diseases'. The only substantive difference in the relatively simple terminology of the aphorism is found in the Syriac translations of the verb ὠφελῇ 'it benefits'. The early Syriac version translates this word with *tawtar*, while the later translates it with *mahnyā*, both of which carry the same general sense as the Greek.

Aphorism ii. 9

Τὰ σώματα χρή, ὅκου τις βούλεται καθαίρειν, εὔροα ποιεῖν.

E.

ܠܓܘ̈ܫܡܐ ܐܝܟܐ ܕܢܒܥܐ ܠܗ ܐܢܫ ܠܡܕܟܝܘ. ܦܫܝܩܝ ܡܪܕܝܬܐ ܢܥܒܕ.

For bodies, when someone desires that they be purified, he makes them easy of flowing.

P.

ينبغي لمن أراد تنقية الأجساد ان ينقّيها قبل ذلك أى بإذابة ما فيها من الكيموس الغليط.

It is necessary for the one who desires the purification of bodies that he purify them before that, that is, by liquefaction of whatever thick humours are in them.

S.

ܠܦܓܪܐ ܐܡܬܝ ܕܢܨܒܐ ܐܢܫ ܕܢܕܟܐ ܐܢܘܢ܆ ܕܠܬܠܝܠ ܠܪܕܝܐ ܢܪܕܘ ܠܡܥܒܕ ܐܢܘܢ܀

For bodies, when someone desires to purify them, he should make them easily flowing.

H.

كلّ بدن تريد تنقيته فينبغي أن تجعل ما تريد إخراجه منه يجري فيه بسهولة.

(For) every body that you desire to purify, it is necessary for you to make that (thing) whose expulsion you desire easily flowing in it.

In comparing these four texts, one notices immediately the substantial concord between the two Syriac versions and Ḥunayn's Arabic version against the early Arabic translation. All of the former three follow the source-text by beginning the aphorism with a phrase referring to the body, while the latter departs from the text by placing the word *al-ajsād* in the middle of the sentence instead. This appearance is even more noticeable in the treatments of the word εὔροα. The Syriac versions and Ḥunayn's version all translate εὔροα with various phrases signifying 'easily flowing'. The early Arabic version departs significantly from the Greek original, however. It translates εὔροα ποιεῖν with the causative form of the same verb already used to translate καθαίρειν, *naqiya* 'to purify'. Then follows the explication *ay bi-idhāba mā fīhā min al-kaymūs al-ghalīẓ* 'that is, by liquefaction of whatever thick humours are in them'. The introduction of the term *idhāba* heightens the level of lexical sophistication of the aphorism, but in general the translation's departures from the original tend to obscure the sense of the text. This lack of precision in translation was likely what made the explication appear necessary in the first place.

In some ways, Ḥunayn's version differs from the other three translations. Whereas the two Syriac versions and the early Arabic translation render the third-person verb βούλεται with third-person forms, it appears that Ḥunayn translated it with a second-person form. Although this judgment rests entirely upon small dots in the manuscripts that are often subject to variation, according to Mimura's apparatus the manuscripts are very consistent in making these verbs second person. Ḥunayn's translation is also somewhat more expansive in its treatment of the terminology in comparison with the Syriac versions, adding explicative phrases like *mā turīdu ikhrājahū minhu* 'that (substance) whose expulsion you desire'. This does not affect the clarity of his translation, however.

Each of the four translations gives a distinct equivalent for the Greek word σώματα. This word is strongly represented in bar Bahlul's *Lexicon*, and the entries for the Syriac terms provide very interesting background into the translation techniques used in producing these texts. I shall thus compare the translations of this word in the context of their lexicographical background, following a similar method to that adopted in the previous two chapters:

σῶμα/σώματα/σωμάτιον

218:4 ܐܣܘܡܛܐ ܕܣܪ ܠ ܠܓܘܫܡܐ ܕܝܢ ܦܪܨܘܦܐ ܘܩܢܘܡܐ ܠܘܬ ܚܕ ܡܢ ܝܘܢܝܐ ܚܢ: ܐܢܫ الأجسام الأشخاص الأقانيم ܀

Asomaṭā according to Sergius, bodies (*gušmē*), persons, and substances according to one of the Greeks. *Bodies (*al-ajsām*), persons, substances.*

1311:16 ܣܘܡܐ ܗ̄ ܦܓܪܐ ܀

Somā, this is the body (*pagrā*).

1311:26 ܣܘܡܛܐ ܘܐܣܘܡܛܐ ܠܓܫܝܡܐ ܘܠܐ ܠܓܫܝܡܐ. ܣܘܢܛܐ ܘܐܣܘܢܛܐ المتجسّمون و غير المتجسّمين. ܘܐܝܟ ܣܪ ܠܘܬ ܣܘܡܛܐ ܘܠܐ ܣܘܡܛܐ ܠܓܘܫܡܐ ܘܠܐ ܠܓܘܫܡܐ ܀

Somaṭā and *asomaṭā*, embodied (things) (*gšimē*) and unembodied (things). *Sonaṭā* and *asonaṭā, the embodied (*al-mutajassimūn*) and the unembodied.* According to Sergius *somaṭā* and *asomaṭā*, body (*gušmā*) and not-body.

Given that the body is the proper focus of the medical art, forms of the word σῶμα are found numerous times throughout the Hippocratic *Aphorisms*. Ḥunayn's Arabic version, the Syriac translation, and the early Arabic translation are all strongly consistent in their renderings of it. Save for one instance, and a few cases where he omitted it as superfluous to the sense of the text, Ḥunayn rendered the word with a form of *al-badan*. The only major exception occurs in his translation of vii. 40, where he translated τι τοῦ σώματος with *'uḍwin min al-a'ḍā* 'one of the parts'. For their part, the extant lemmas of the early Arabic translation consistently translate forms of σῶμα with forms of *al-jasad*. The Syriac translator employed *pagrā* in every translated instance of the term save one: for the first of the three occurrences of the word in aphorism ii. 15, the broadly synonymous word *gušmā* is given instead.

Three examples from the fragments of the Hippocratic lemmas in the *Syriac Commentary on the Epidemics* also exist. In aphorisms ii. 9 and iv. 13 the early Syriac version translates σῶμα with *gušmā* 'body', as discussed above. If these may be taken to indicate the translator's habitual translation of σῶμα, a clear contrast may thus be observed between the two Syriac versions. In aphorism ii. 6, the translator of this version renders the phrase ὁκόσοι πονέοντές τι τοῦ σώματος with *aylēn d-makebbin b-medem* 'those who feel pain in something'. It may be that a word has dropped out of the text.

The number of instances where Ḥunayn's Arabic omits the term σῶμα as superfluous to the sense of the aphorism is significantly greater than the number of instances where the Syriac version does so. This phenomenon occurs by my count five times in Ḥunayn's Arabic but only once in the Syriac version.[1] All of the occurrences in the Arabic version are near the end of the work. Also in a few places, despite choosing to translate an instance of σῶμα, Ḥunayn modifies its position in the aphorism.[2] This type of transposition generally does not occur in the Syriac version. Ullmann notices two translations of this word in Galen's *On Simple Drugs* Book Six. Although he indicates that one of the early Arabic examples is corrupt, the other translates with *al-abdān*, and so is close to Ḥunayn's translations of it in the *Aphorisms*.[3]

Although the entries for σῶμα extant in bar Bahlul's *Lexicon* contain several elements of interest, none of them relate directly to Ḥunayn's Arabic translation. The strong representation of Sergius' lexicographical material bears closer attention, however. In the entry found at 218:4, Sergius is cited for a three-word definition of the Greek term. This definition is then repeated in Arabic at the end of the entry. Since Sergius lived nearly a century before the Arab conquest of the Syriac-speaking lands, it is safe to assume that he was not the author of this Arabic definition. Thus we may note that bar Bahlul's *Lexicon* gives evidence that Sergius' lexicographical work was translated into Arabic. Further research may demonstrate whether or not this translation was systematic. In the entry attributed to Sergius, the equivalent for σῶμα used in the early Syriac translation of the *Aphorisms*, *gušmā*, is found. In the unattributed entry at 1311:16, the equivalent used in the later Syriac translation is found instead.

1 This occurs in Ḥunayn's translations of aphorisms vi. 56, vii. 28, vii. 60, vii. 61 and vii. 74. The Syriac omits any translation of σῶμα in aphorism ii. 7.

2 This occurs in Ḥunayn's translations of aphorisms ii. 51 and v. 69.

3 Ullmann, *Wörterbuch zu den griechisch-arabischen Übersetzungen*, 664–5.

The entries at 1311:16 and 1311:26 contain material likely attributable to Ḥunayn. One may imagine the former entry being drawn from a translator's working glossary. The latter entry allows Ḥunayn's (presumed) lexicography to be compared to Sergius' work. In that entry, a definition likely attributable to Ḥunayn glosses the plural noun σώματα and its negative ἀσώματα with the plural of the adjective *gšimā* 'embodied' and its negation. These are then rendered with an Arabic reflexive plural participle *al-mutajassimūn* 'those who are embodied' and its negation. The following definition attributed to Sergius adopts a somewhat less sophisticated approach, translating the Greek nouns with the literally equivalent Syriac noun *gušmā* 'body' and its negation. Thus here, in contrast to the preceding discussion, Ḥunayn's improvements to existing Syriac scholarship is noticeable.

An entry in bar Bahlul's *Lexicon* for the first equivalent given for σῶμα in the Syriac *Aphorisms, gušmā*, reads as follows:

476:6 **ܓܘܫܡܐ ܓܫܝܡܐ** ܐܝܟ ܒܪ ܣܪܘܫܘܝ ܐܝܬܘܗܝ ܠܐ ܡܫܬܟܚܢܘܬܐ ܠܗ ܠܐ ܡܫܬܥܒܕܢܘܬ ܠܘܬ ܪܓܫܐ ܘܡܚܘܝܢܘܬ
ܠܟܝܢܐ ܕܒܐܬܐܘܪܝܐ ܕܠܐ ܡܬܦܓܪܢܐ. جسم جسمانيّ جسدانيّ. **ܓܘܫܡܐ** جسم جسد. ܙܟܪܝܐ **ܡܬܓܫܡ** يتجسّم
يتجسّد. **ܓܫܝܡܐ** ذو جسد. ܐܝܟ ܒܪ ܣܪܘܫܘܝ **ܓܘܫܡܐ** ܗܘ ܡܐ ܕܦܝܫܐ ܬܠܬܐ ܢܦܫܢܐ ܐܝܬܘܗܝ ܡܬܡܫܚܘܬܐ
ܠܥܘܡܩܐ ܘܐܘܪܟܐ ܘܦܬܝܐ. جسم نفسانيّ❖

Gušmā, the body (*gšimā*) according to bar Serošway, it has no fixity, it is not subjected to the senses, and it displays the nature that is in the incorporeal idea, *body* (jism), *embodied, coporeal* (jasadānī). *Gušmā, body, corpus* (jasad). (According to) Zakariya *metgaššam, to be embodied, to be incarnate. Gšimā, one having a body.* According to bar Serošway *gušmā*, that which has three aspects (*napšānā*), (namely) extension in depth, length, and breadth. *Animate body* (jismun nafsānīyun).

Another longer entry that is left unattributed reads like this:

477:3 **ܓܘܫܡܐ** ܐܝܬܘܗܝ ܗܘ ܡܐ ܕܦܝܫܐ ܬܠܬܐ ܦ̈ܨܝܚܐ ܒܥܘܡܩܐ ܘܐܘܪܟܐ ܘܦܬܝܐ. ܟܠ ܓܒܪ
ܕ ܓܘܫܡܐ ܗܘ ܡܠܝܠ ܬܠܬܐ ܦ̈ܨܝܚܐ ܐܝܬ ܠܗ. ܘܟܠ ܕܡܠܝܠ ܦ̈ܨܝܚܐ ܐܝܬ ܠܗ ܓܘܫܡܐ ܐܝܬܘܗܝ.
ܡܬܬܚܝܕ ܓܒܪ ܓܘܫܡܐ ܐܦ ܡܚܒܠܐ: ܚܢܢܐ ܡܚܦܝܛ ܡܢ ܣ̈ܢܬܐ ܘܡܚܦܛܠܐ ܕ ܓܘ̈ܫܐ ܘܐܘܣܝܐ
ܡܣܝܒܪܬܐ. ܕܒܩܘܒܠܐ ܦܢܝܐ ܟܠ ܓܘܫܡܐ ܒܡܬܪܘܬܐ ܐ̈ܪܓܫܢܝܬܐ. ܘܡܬܬܦܠܓ ܡܕܡܐ ܠܬܪܝܢ
ܦܘܪ̈ܫܐ. ܠܪܘܫܐ ܘܠܕܠܐ ܪܘܫ. ܕܠܐ ܪܘܫ ܐܝܟ ܫܡܝܐ ܘܐܪܥܐ ܘܢܘܪܐ ܘܡܝܐ. ܕܪܘܫ ܕܝܢ ܡܬܦܠܓ
ܐܦ ܗܘ ܠܬܠܬܐ ܦܘ̈ܪܫܐ. ܠܚ̈ܝܘܬܐ ܡܠ̈ܬܢ ܒܝܫܬܐ. ܘܠܚ̈ܝܘܬܐ ܢܩܝܫܬܐ. ܘܠܢܩܝܫܘܬܐ ܒܠܚܘܕ.
ܚ̈ܝܘܬܐ ܡܠ̈ܬܢ ܒܝܫܬܐ. ܐܝܟ ܚ̈ܝܘܬܐ ܘܦ̈ܪܚܬܐ. ܚ̈ܝܘܬܐ ܢܩ̈ܝܫܬܐ. ܐܝܟ ܣ̈ܝܘܐ ܘܐܘܪ̈ܐ ܘܐܣܦ̈ܐ ܟܠ
ܘܐ̈ܠܦܬܐ. ܘܟܠܗܝܢ ܐܝܟ ܕܡܛܪ ܒܪ ܚ̈ܕ ܦܢܝܐ ܠܗܝܢ ܐ̈ܚܪܢܐ. ܚ̈ܕ ܥܒܝܕܐ ܕܡܢ ܕܪܘܝ ܠܕܪܝ ܠܒܬ ܠܗܝܢ.
ܢܩܝܫܘܬܐ. ܐܝܟ ܒܗܡܬܐ ܘܪ̈ܚܫܐ ܘܐ̈ܝܠܢܐ ܘܚܡܪ̈ܐ. ܘܟܠܗܝܢ ܐܝܟ ܕܪܘܚܐ ܕܡܬܚܒܠܐ قبل الجسد❖

Gušmā is that which possesses three aspects: depth, length, and breadth. Every body has these three aspects, and every thing that has these three aspects is a body. *Gušmā* is defined in this way: A nature consisting of powers, and a receptivity (*mqabblānā*) of colours and limited essences that doubly abide upon the body in an abundance of species. These are divided primarily into two types: That which is animate and that which is not animate. Those which are not animate are things like the heavens, the earth, fire and water. Those which are animate are divided into three further types: Perceiving living things, vegetative living things, and the simply vegetative. Perceiving living things are things like animals and birds. Vegetative living (things) are things like shellfish, sponges, and oysters and all things that sense when the hand is near to them, but do not move from place to place. The vegetative are things like grass, seeds, trees, and roots and everything that possesses the impulse of growth. *The body (*al-jasad*).*

This is an entry for *pagrā*, the main equivalent for σῶμα in the Syriac *Aphorisms*:

1487:23 **ܦܓܪܐ** جسد جسم. **ܦܓܪܐ** ܐܝܟ ܒܪ ܣܪܘ ܣܕܝܪܘܬܐ ܕܗܕܡܐ ܚܝܐ ܕܡܬܚܡܢܐ ܐܝܟ ܚܟܡܬܐ
ܕܡܬܚܡܢܘܬܗ الجسد وأقول البدن وجاء به اليّا أسقف بيت المقدّس المعروف بعليّ بن عبيد الفجر وعندي هو
الفغر. **ܦܓܪܐ ܡܣܝܛܐ** بدن مشيّط. **ܦܓܪܐ** ܐܝܟ ܒܪ ܣܪܘ ܬܘܒ ܣܕܝܪܘܬܐ ܘܡܛܟܣܘܬܐ ܕܗܕܡܐ
ܟܝܢܝܐ. ܟܠ ܓܝܪ ܕܦܓܪܐ ܗܘ ܣܕܝܪܐ ܘܡܛܟܣ ܒܗܕܡܘܗܝ ܐܝܬܘܗܝ. ܡܬܛܟܣܐ ܠܗ ܗܘ ܕܗܕܡܐ. ܡܛܠ
ܕܐܝܬ ܗܕܡܐ ܣܕܝܪܐ ܕܠܘ ܦܓܪܐ ܐܢܘܢ. ܐܝܟ ܗܕܡܐ ܕܐܕܪܝܢܛܐ الجسد. **ܦܓܪܐ** ܗ̄ ܝܘܢܝܐ ܒܚܕ
ܫܡܐ ܩܪܝܢ ܠܦܓܪܐ ܘܠܩܒܪܐ. ܘܦܓܪܐ ܣܘܡܛܐ ܡܬܩܪܝܢ. ܘܐܝܟܢܐ ܕܒܩܒܪܐ. ܗܟܢ ܚܒܝܫܢ ܢܦܫܬܐ
ܒܦܓܪܐ. ܘܬܘܒ ܩܪܝܢ ܠܢܦܫܐ ܦܣܘܟܝ. ܘܠܩܘܪܐ ܐܡܪܝܢ ܩܪܝܪܘܬܐ ܦܣܘܟܘܣ ܘܐܡܪܝܢ ܕܡܛܠ ܕܩܪܝܢ
ܢܦܫܬܐ ܡܢ ܡܫܒܚܘܬܐ. ܐܬܩܪܝ ܦܣܘܟܐ ܐܡܪܝܢ ܢܦܫܬܐ ܡܛܠ ܪܘܚܬܐ ܡܠܝܠܬܐ الجسد܀

Pagrā, corpus, body. Pagrā according to bar Serošway, the definite arrangement of the living members according to the wisdom of its Creator, *the body (*al-jasad*) and I say the body (*al-badan*). The bishop of the Holy House known as 'Alī ibn 'Ubayd suggested to me that it is* 'al-fajr' *but for me it is* 'al-faghr'*. Pagrā msayyṭā, flammable body. Pagrā* according to bar Serošway, the arrangement and order of the natural members, for every body that is has arrangement and order in its members. But there are ordered members which are not bodies, such as the members of a statue. *The body (*al-jasad*). Pagrā*, the Greeks call the body and the tomb by this single name. *Pagrē* are named *somāṭā*, and as though in tombs, thus are souls confined in the body. Again, the soul is called *psuḵê*, meaning cold, as coldness is *psuḵus*. They say that because souls are called by their best element, souls (*psuḵê*), meaning souls (*napšāṯā*), are so-called because of the rational spirits. *The body (*al-jasad*).*

These entries contain several important elements which deserve scrutiny. First among them is the presence of Ḥunayn's preferred translation of σῶμα in the *Aphorisms*, *al-badan*, in the entry for *pagrā* beginning at 1487:23. Although the definition in which it occurs is ascribed by bar Bahlul to bar Serošway, external evidence may be adduced to argue that it ought rather to be attributed to Ḥunayn. Consider the following entry from bar ʿAli's *Lexicon*:

ܦܓܪܐ. بدن جسد. ܣܘܪܓܬܐ ܕܗܕܡܐ ܚܝܐ ܕܒܬܚܘܡܐ ܐܝܟ ܚܟܡܬܗ ܕܡܒܪܝܢܐ.[4]

Pagrā, *body* (badan), *body* (jasad). The arrangement of the living members within limits according to the wisdom of the Creator.

The Syriac definition found here is almost identical to the first Syriac definition in bar Bahlul's entry at 1487:23. As discussed in the Introduction, according to his own testimony bar ʿAli relied in important respects on Ḥunayn's lexicon in the production of his own work, and there is no indication that he was familiar with bar Serošway's glossary. Thus it seems either that bar Serošway reproduced Ḥunayn's definition in his own lexicography or that the text of bar Bahlul's *Lexicon* is mistaken in its attribution of this definition.

It is somewhat surprising that the Arabic equivalent for σῶμα which Ḥunayn so systematically preferred in his translation of the *Aphorisms* should be so little represented in both the Greek and Syriac entries of bar Bahlul's *Lexicon*. This effect is heightened by the discussion of the two possible Arabic equivalents '*al-fajr*' and '*al-faghr*' mentioned near the beginning of 1487:23. These two words are both potential Arabizations of the Syriac word *pagrā*. The bishop's suggestion *al-fajr*, however, neglects the spirantisation of the medial *gāmal*, while the lexicographer's suggestion *al-faghr* apparently reflects the preference that the spirantisation be retained.

This indicates that these translators were unsatisfied with the usual Arabic equivalents for *pagrā* and were seeking alternatives. The reason for this is arguably that the Syriac words clearly express two different senses of the concept 'body', as may be seen in comparing the two entries translated above. *Gušmā* and related terms refer to objects having material extension broadly considered, while *pagrā* refers strictly to the bodies of living things. This entry thus allows us to observe some of the process by which medical Arabic was formed in relation to notions embedded in the Syriac lexicon.

4 Gottheil (ed.), *Syriac-Arabic Glosses*, II, 241:10.

Less attention is devoted to the Arabic equivalent of *gušmā*, since both *jasad* and *jism* may convey the broader meaning of 'body'. *Jism* is etymologically related to *gušmā* and accords with it in meaning very closely, and it is furthermore absent from the entry on *pagrā*.

Aphorism iv. 13

Πρὸς τοὺς ἐλλεβόρους τοῖσι μὴ ῥηιδίως ἄνω καθαιρομένοισι, πρὸ τῆς πόσιος προϋγραίνειν τὰ σώματα πλείονι τροφῇ καὶ ἀναπαύσει.

E.

ܒܐܠܒܪܘܢ ܐܝܠܝܢ ܕܠܐ ܦܫܝܩܐܝܬ ܡܬܕܟܝܢ ܙܕܩ ܠܡܩܕܡܘ ܘܠܡܪܛܒܘ ܠܓܘܫܡܐ.

In [giving] hellebore (*b-elebārun*) [to] those who are not purged easily, it is necessary beforehand to make the body moist.

P.

عند شرب الأدوية والخرْبَق ينبغي أن يرطِّب أجساد الذين لا تخفّ التنقية عليهم من فوق قبل الدواء بكثرة الطعام.

In [giving] purging drink and hellebore (*al-kharbaq*), it is necessary to make moist bodies for whom purging from above is not [borne] lightly, before the purging, with much food.

S.

ܒܫܩܝܐ ܕܚܘܪܒܟܢܐ ܠܗܢܘܢ ܕܠܐ ܦܫܝܩܐܝܬ ܡܬܕܟܝܢ ܡܢ ܠܥܠ ܕܢܩܕܡ ܙܕܩ ܩܕܡ ܫܩܝܐ ܕܢܪܛܒ ܠܦܓܪܝܗܘܢ ܒܡܐܟܘܠܬܐ ܣܓܝܐܬܐ ܘܒܢܝܚܐ.

In [giving] the hellebore drink (*šeqyā ḏ-ḥurbaḵnā*) to those who would not easily be purged from above from before, it is necessary before the drink that one make their bodies moist with much food and rest.

Ḥ.

من احتاج إلي أن يسقى الخربق وكان استفراغه من فوق لا يؤاتيه بسهولة فينبغي أن يرطب بدنه من قبل إسقائه إيّاه بغذاء أكثر وبالراحة.

One who needs to be given hellebore (*al-kharbaq*) to drink, but whose purging from above does not come easily, must have his body made moist, before his being given it to drink, with more food and rest.

Of these four translations, the version taken from the Syriac *Epidemics* stands out as abbreviated when compared with the other three versions. This could indicate that it was an *ad hoc* translation, or that it was for some other reason not intended to stand as a translation of the entire text. It omits any reference to 'from above' (ἄνω) or to food (τροφῇ) Whatever the reason for it, its abbreviation makes comparison of it with the other texts of limited utility.

The Syriac version and Ḥunayn's translation both follow the word order of the Greek original more closely than does the early Arabic translation. This is most evident in the early Arabic version's placement of the phrase 'to liquify bodies' before the phrase 'purging from above'. In the corresponding text of the original aphorism and of the two later translations, these phrases occur in the opposite order. In considering the translation of the first phrase, there is an example of the Syriac version's greater literalness when compared with Ḥunayn's translation. The Syriac's word order follows the source-text's as closely as possible, with almost every word translated literally. Although Ḥunayn's translation does not make any great departure from the source-text, the changes he introduced, such as introducting the aphorism with *man iḥtāj ilā* 'one who requires' instead of with a simple preposition, indicate less concern to follow the text literally.

The only terminological element of any interest is the translations of τοὺς ἐλλεβόρους. In the early Syriac version, the borrowed Greek word is employed, while in the later Syriac translation the native equivalent *ḥurbaḵnā* is used. For their parts, both of the Arabic translations employ the same word *al-kharbaq*. The Syriac translations thus show at least a superficial process of development, while the Arabic approach to translating this word appears to have been stable from the earliest period of Greek-to-Arabic medical translation.

Aphorism vi. 31

Ὀδύνας ὀφθαλμῶν ἀκρητοποσίη ἢ λουτρὸν ἢ πυρίη ἢ φλεβοτομίη ἢ φαρμακείη λύει.

E.

ܠܟܐܒܐ ܕܥܝܢܐ ܚܡܪܐ ܚܝܐ ܐܘ ܡܣܚܘܬܐ ܐܘ ܫܚܘܢܐ ܐܘ ܥܒܕ ܕܡܐ ܐܘ ܡܫܬܝܐ ܕܣܡܐ ܫܪܐ.

For pain of the eyes, pure wine, washings, fomentations, blood-letting, or a drink of medicine cures.

P.

شرب الخمر صرفاً والكماد الحارّ وقطع العروق وشرب الدواء يحلّ وجع العينين.

A draught of pure wine, hot fomentations, cutting the veins, and draughts of medicine resolve pain of the eyes.

S.

ܠܟܐܒܐ ܕܥܝܢܐ ܫܩܝܐ ܕܚܡܪܐ ܚܝܐ ܫܪܐ. ܐܘ ܒܢܐ. ܐܘ ܫܚܘܢܐ. ܐܘ ܦܨܕ ܘܪܝܕܐ. ܐܘ ܫܩܝ
ܣܡܐ ܫܪܐ.

For pain of the eyes, a draught of pure wine cures; a bath, a fomentation, venesection, or a draught of medicine cures.

Ḥ.

أوجاع العينين يحلّها شرب الشراب الصرف أو الحمام أو التكميد أو فصد العرق أو شرب الدواء.

Pains of the eyes are resolved by draughts of pure wine, baths, fomentations, venesection, or draughts of medicine.

Several points of contrast may be noted when comparing these translations. Both of the Syriac versions render the Greek text more literally than do either of the Arabic translations. This is especially true of the earlier Syriac translation, given that the later version does depart slightly from the source-text in that it repeats the verb *šrā* 'cures', while the Greek original gives the verb λυεί only once. Ḥunayn's Arabic translation for its part follows the source-text's word order slightly more closely than does the early Arabic version, in that the former text begins with 'pains of the eyes', as does the Greek original, while the latter places the corresponding phrase at the end of the aphorism. Ḥunayn however wrote the verb immediately following the introductory phrase. In this he appears to have preferred to conform to classical Arabic usage by introducing the main clause with the verb. The text of the early Arabic version from Houtsma's edition also neglects to translate λουτρόν.

Compared to the aphorisms treated above, this text contains a greater variety of vocabulary. Although the Greek words are rather thinly represented in bar Bahlul's *Lexicon*, a brief comparison of the variations observable in the Syriac terminology with their corresponding entries in the *Lexicon* should prove of interest.

First, we may observe that the Greek word λουτρόν is translated differently in the two Syriac versions. The early translation gives *masḥutā* 'washing'. An entry for this word in bar Bahlul's *Lexicon* reads as follows:

1115:3 ܡܫܚܘܬܐ أقول الغُسل܀

Masḥuṯā, I say washing.

For its part, the Syriac *Aphorisms* translates this word with *banā* 'bath'. Although this Syriac word does not appear to have its own entry in the

Lexicon, it is possible to discover it elsewhere. For example, consider these entries:

394:22 **ܒܠܐܢܝܢ** ܗ̄ ܒܢܐ الحمّام܀

Balanin, this is baths (*banā*), *baths (*al-ḥammām*)*.

399:20 **ܒܠܢܐ** ܐܝܟ ܪܒܢ ܝܘܢܐܝܬ ܒܠܐܢܝܢ ܗܘ ܗܘ ܚܕ ܗܘ حمّام. ܘܐܝܟ ܝܘܒܠܐ ܒܠܢܐ. ܘܐܚܪܢܐ ܒܠܢܣ.
ܒܢܝ ܚܒܢܪܐ حمّاميّ. **ܒܠܐܢܝ** الحمّام܀

Balanā according to our teacher, the Greek *balānin* (βαλανεῖον) is the same as *a bath (*ḥammām*)*. According to translations (*yuḇālē*), a bath (*balanā*). (According to) others a bath (*balanas*). *Banē ḥaḇnārā, a bath attendant (*ḥammāmī*). Balani, baths.*

403:1 **ܒܢܘܬܐ** ܒܢܣ الحمّامات. **ܒܢܝ** ܚܒܢܪܐ **حمّاميّ**◆

Bnawāṯā, baths (*banās*), *baths*. *Banē ḥaḇnārā*, a bath attendant (*ḥammāmī*).

The profusion of Syriac terms derived from the Greek βαλανεῖον makes it somewhat difficult to situate the specific word *banā* within the lexicographical tradition. However, the presence of Ḥunayn's Arabic translation of λουτρόν, *al-ḥammām*, in close proximity to *banā*, the translation of that word given in the Syriac *Aphorisms*, may be contrasted with the lack of correspondence between the equivalent given in the older Syriac translation and Ḥunayn's Arabic version. This suggests a closer relationship between Ḥunayn's Arabic translation and the later Syriac version.

Another significant difference between the two Syriac versions is found in the translations of the Greek word φλεβοτομίη. The fragment from the *Epidemics* gives *šḇāq dmā* 'blood-letting', while the text of the Syriac *Aphorisms* gives *psāq wariḏā* 'venesection'. The latter translation is more literal and more technical. In his translations of this and the related verb φλεβοτομέω in other places in the *Aphorisms*, the Syriac translator varies freely between phrases centered around *psāq wariḏā* and those centered around another equivalent, *tra' wariḏā* 'opening of veins, venesection'. Bar Bahlul's *Lexicon* appears to refer only to the last of these equivalents. However, a third phrase with the same meaning is referred to in the entry beginning at 2089:16 for the word '*trā'ā*', where this definition is found:

2089:18 … **ܬܪܥ ܘܪܝܕܐ** فصد العرق فصد العروق܀

… tra' wariḏā, opening of a vein, opening of veins.

This definition conforms to Ḥunayn's usage in his Arabic translation of the *Aphorisms*, where he gives *faṣd al-'urūq* 'venesection, opening of veins' for φλεβοτομίη. It contrasts, however, with the early Arabic translator's somewhat less technical equivalent of this Greek word *qaṭ' al-'urūq* 'cutting of the veins'. The contrast between these is lessened by the fact that a single exceptional rendition of the phrase χρὴ φλεβοτομεῖσθαι in Ḥunayn's translation of aphorism vii. 53 sees the use of the related phrase *yanbaghī an taqṭa' lahu al-' urūq* 'you should cut his veins'. Although Ḥunayn's regularity in translating this term does itself contrast with the variety found in the Syriac version, the difference is largely stylistic, more likely reflecting a greater wealth of relevant Syriac vocabulary than any substantive difference of interpretation between the two versions. Nevertheless it does contribute, however slightly, to the impression that the two versions were written by different authors.

Section Two

For the following three aphorisms, the early Arabic translation is not extant.

Aphorism ii. 6

Ὁκόσοι, πονέοντές τι τοῦ σώματος, τὰ πολλὰ τῶν πόνων μὴ αἰσθάνονται, τούτοισιν ἡ γνώμη νοσεῖ.

E.

ܕܐܝܠܝܢ ܕܡܬܟܐܒܝܢ ܒܡܕܡ ܘܣܘܓܐܐ ܠܟܐܒܐ ܕܟܐܒܐ ܠܐ ܡܪܓܫܝܢ: ܕܗܠܝܢ ܡܕܥܗܘܢ ܟܪܝܗ.

Those who suffer pain in some part, but do not sense most of the pain: the mind of these people is diseased.

S.

ܐܝܠܝܢ ܕܒܪ ܟܐܒ ܠܗܘܢ ܡܕܡ ܡܢ ܦܓܪܗܘܢ: ܐܝܟ ܕܣܘܓܐܐ ܠܟܐܒܐ ܠܐ ܡܪܓܫܝܢ ܒܟܐܒ̈ܐ: ܬܪܥܝܬܗܘܢ ܟܪܝܗܐ.

When part of some (peoples') body pains them, (but) mostly they do not sense the pains, their judgment is diseased.

Ḥ.

من يوجعه شيء من بدنه ولا يحسّ بوجعه في أكثر حالاته فعقله مختلط.

One to whom a part of his body causes pain, but he does not sense its pain in the majority of its circumstances, (this means that) his mind is confused.

The Syriac versions of aphorism ii. 6 differ from one another in several respects. In some ways, the later Syriac version is closer to the Greek original than is the earlier one. For example, in it the first word ὁκόσοι is translated with *kad*, but in the early translation that Greek word has no equivalent. The translations of the clause τὰ πολλὰ τῶν πόνων μὴ αἰσθάνονται also differ in that the early translator interpreted the genitive plural τῶν πόνων to refer back to τὰ πολλὰ in the sense of 'most of the pains', while the later translator read it as a genitive construct agreeing with the verb αἰσθάνονται, in the sense of 'not having perception of the pains most of the time'. Ḥunayn's Arabic translation agrees with the later Syriac translation in its interpretation of this element of the Greek text.

The most interesting differences amongst the three translations lie in their varying renditions of the noun ἡ γνώμη. Here I consider the lexicographical background to these translations:

γνώμη

504:3 **ܓܢܘܡܝ** ܗ̄ ܝ ܨܒܝܢܐ ܪܥܝܢܐ ܬܪܥܝܬܐ همة܀

Gnomê, this is will, mind (*re'yānā*), intellect (*tar'iṯā*), *will*.

Forms of γνώμη occur twice in the *Aphorisms*. For both of these instances the Syriac version gives the equivalent *tar'iṯā* 'intellect'. Ḥunayn's Arabic gives a different word in each case: in aphorism ii. 6, *al-'aql* 'reason' is employed, while in v. 16, *al-dhihin* 'mind' is found. The early Syriac version of ii. 6 exists, and there a different word, *madd'ā* 'mind', is used. Although the early Arabic version for v. 16 is also extant, it appears that the translation of γνώμη dropped out of the text Houtsma used in making his edition.

Considered by itself, the definition attributable to Ḥunayn in bar Bahlul's *Lexicon* links the translation from the Syriac *Aphorisms* with the translator's lexicographical work. If we look to the definitions of the Syriac words, a more complex picture emerges, however. The entry for *madd'ā* reads like this:

1014:18 **ܡܕܥܐ** ذهن فهم عقل. ܘܐܡܝܢ ܒܪ ܣܪܘ̈ܫܘ ܡܚܒܠܢܐ ܕܓܠܝܢܘܢ ܣܘܟܠܐ ܡܝܐ. ܘܐܝܬܘ̄ ܟܠܗ ܡܪܥܝܢܗ
ܟܠܟܐ. ܘܡܦܬܠܢܐ ܕܝܕܘܥܬܐ ܡܟܠܝܢܐ[5] ܕܠܘܬ ܐܘܣܝܐ. ܐܝܟ ܕܠܘܬ ܦܘܪ̈ܫܢܗܘܢ ܕܡܢ ܣܪܝܐ.
ܘܝܕܘܥܬܐ ܡܠܠܬܐ ܘܡܬܒܝܢܢܘܬܐ ܕܣܘܟܠܐ الفهم܀ ܡܕܥܐ ܐܝܬܘ̄ ܡܬܚܫܒܢܘܬܐ ܘܝܕܘܥܬܐ
ܕܡܠܬܐ ܕܢܦܫܐ ܕܐܝܬܘܗܝ ܡܠܬܐ ܕܝܠܗ ܘܡܬܬܥܝܢܬܐ ܘܬܪܥܝܬܐ. ܘܡܬܩܪܐ ܐܦ ܗܘܢܐ ܥܠ ܕܡܢܝ
ܡܠܝܠܘܬܐ ܡܢܗܪܬ ܡܢ ܗܘܝܐ ܕܗܘܐ ܕܡܠܟܬܐ ܕܪܘܚܐ ܠܐ ܡܬܐܡܪܢܝܬ ܘܠܐ ܡܬܦܫܩܢܝܬ ܒܥܘܠܐ

5 Duval: ܡܟܠܝܐ.

ܠܐ ܡܠܝܠܐ ܕܐܬܪܢܝܘܬܐ. ܠܡܬܝܕ ܒܟܠ ܡܐ ܕܝܕܥ ܘܟܠ ܡܐ ܕܡܬܝܕܥ. ܐܝܟ ܕܠܐ ܡܬܚܡܢܘܬܐ.
ܚܘܫܒܐ ܕܝܢ ܐܝܬܘܗܝ ܕܡܘܬܗ ܕܡܬܚܫܒܢܘܬܐ.[6] ܘܪܓܫܐ ܦܪܘܫܐ ܡܕܝܢܢܐ ܕܗܘܢܐ. ܡܠܝܠܘܬܐ ܗܟܢ
ܐܝܬܘܗܝ. [ܐܝܬܝ] ܐܝܠܝܢ ܕܠܗ ܠܡܕܥܐ ܕܢܦܫܐ ܡܦܪܫܝܢ. ܐܝܟ ܕܝܢ ܐܝܠܝܢ ܕܠܡܠܝܠܘܬܐ ܐܚܪܢܐ ܡܟܝܢܝܐ ܘܟܝܢܐ
ܕܢܦܫܐ ܡܟܝܢܝܢ ܡܠܝܠܘܬܐ. ܕܐܝܬܘܗܝ ܥܠܬܐ ܗܟܝܠ ܠܟܠ ܦܬܓܡܐ ܕܡܠܬܐ. ܐܚܪܢܐ ܕܝܢ ܚܠܦ ܗܘ ܕܡܠܝܠܘܬܐ
ܡܠܬܐ ܐܡܪܝܢ. ܚܝܠܐ ܕܢܦܫܐ ܕܐܝܬܘܗܝ ܨܒܝܢܝܐ. ܐܝܟܢܐ ܕܐܦ ܝܘܚܢܢ ܐܘܢܓܠܣܛܐ. ܟܕ ܨܒܐ ܕܢܚܘܐ
ܠܐ ܡܬܚܡܢܘܬܗ ܕܝܚܝܕܝܐ ܕܥܡ ܐܒܐ ܡܠܬܐ ܓܠܝܬܐ ܫܡܗܗ ܐܬܬܘܣܐܝܬ. ܘܠܐ ܗܘܐ ܡܠܝܠܘܬܐ. ܘܐܝܬ
ܗܠܝܢ ܕܝܢ ܕܠܒܪ ܠܗܠܝܢ ܡܫܠܡܝܢ. ܡܛܠ ܕܠܡܠܝܠܘܬܐ ܡܢܗܘܢ ܡܢܬܐ ܕܦܝܠܘܣܘܦܘܬܐ ܚܫܒܝܢ. ܘܡܢܗܘܢ
ܐܘܪܓܢܘܢ ܒܠܚܘܕ ܕܦܝܠܘܣܘܦܘܬܐ ܟܕ ܡܬܐܡܪ ܠܗ ܡܠܬܐ ܗܕܐ ܠܡ ܐܘܡܢܝܬܐ ܕܡܬܡܠܠܐ
ܕܡܬܬܚܘܝܢ ܒܬܚܘܝܬܐ ܬܪܝܨܬܐ. العقل المعرفة. **ܡܕܥܐ** ܬܘܒ ܐܝܬܘܗܝ ܗܘ ܡܕܥܬܐ ܚܕ ܡܢ ܚܝܠܐ ܕܢܦܫܐ
ܒܡܥܒܕܢܘܬܗ ܒܠܒܐ܀

Madd'ā, mind, understanding, reason ('aql). (According to) bar Serošway, it is the fount which possesses all thoughts. It has its dwelling-place in the heart, and it is that which receives exalted knowledge regarding the essences, according to their differences from one another, and rational knowledge, and the action of thoughts. *Understanding* (al-fahm). *Madd'ā* is thinking, and knowledge of the affair of the soul, which is the affair of speech, thought, and judgment (*tar'iṯā*). It is distinguished from intelligence (*hawnā*) in that it possesses the power of speech, free from the action of the voicing of the words of the current, unuttered, undivided in change, unlocalized (lit. 'a word of a place'). (It extends) into the future, in all who know and all that is understood, as though without limit. Thought (*ḥušāḇā*) is the likeness of that which is thought, and the discriminating, judging sense of the intellect. Thus is reason (*maliluṯā*). These distinguish the mind in the soul, for they produce reason by (means of) another natural power and the nature of the soul. Thus (the mind) is the cause of every utterance of a word. Others say that, instead of reason, the word is the willing power of the soul. So it is that John the Evangelist, when he desired to make clear the eternity of the only one who is with the Father, named him the word made manifest, and that is not (the same as) speech. And there are those beyond these who assent (as well). For some of them consider a portion of philosophy regarding speech, and of these the Organon alone of (the texts of) philosophy, when it states this argument, to wit, 'skillful words uttered with a correct manifestation'.[7] *Reason, gnosis. Madd'ā* again, it is mind (*idda'ṯā*), one of the powers of the soul in its activity in the heart.

This entry refers to both religious and philosophical texts to give specific definition to the faculty of the mind amongst the rich psychological

6 Duval: ܕܡܘܬܗ ܥܠܡܐ ܕܡܬܚܫܒܢܘܬܐ. Two of Duval's manuscripts give the reading I have preferred for clarity.

7 I have been unable to trace this reference.

terminology of Syriac. For our purposes, two aspects stand out. First, the Arabic terms given in the initial definition attributable to Ḥunayn include both of the Arabic equivalents for γνώμη to be found in the translator's version of the *Aphorisms*. Second, bar Serošway's detailed account of the term clearly makes the concept *tar'iṯā* a subsidiary product of the action of the mind. The implications of this may be seen more clearly when the entry for *tar'iṯā* itself is considered:

2090:6 **ܬܪܥܝܬܐ** روية رأي أو نيّة ܒ̣ܦ طويّة ܐܝܟ ܙܟ̈ الفكر. **ܒܢܝ̈ ܬܪܥܝܬܐ** أهل الرأي. ܒܪ ܣܪܘ̈ ܬܘܒ
ܬܪܥܝܬܐ ܥܠܝܐ ܕܡܚܫ̈ܒܬܐ ܒܡܛܫܝܘܬ ܒܓܘ ܠܒܐ ܘܥܒܕ ܒܗܘܢ ܒܘܚܢܐ. ܘܐܦ ܪܥܝܢܐ ܓܝܪ ܡܢ
ܬܪܥܝܬܐ ܡܫܬܚܠܦܐ الفكر والفهم والنيّة والرأي. **ܬܪܥܝܬܐ ܗܘܢܢܝܬܐ** ܐܝܟ ܒܪ ܣܪܘ̈ فهم عقليّ فكرة
عقليّة. ܒܦ̣ ܗܘ ܕܐܓܪܬܐ. ܘܐܦ ܟܠܐ ܠܗ ܬܪܥܝܬܐ ܕܫܛܝܘܬܐ وأمنع ذوي الالباب الرأي والفهم❖

Tar'iṯā, deliberation, opinion, or intention. In a manuscript *innermost conviction.* According to Zakariya *thought. Bnay tar'iṯā, people of opinion (*ahl al-ra'y*).* (According to) bar Serošway, again, *tar'iṯā*, the end of thoughts secretly within the heart upon which (one) makes examination. For *tar'iṯā* is distinct from *re'yānā* ('mind'), *thought, understanding, intention, or opinion. Tar'iṯā hawnānāyṯa, rational understanding, rational thought.* In the manuscript of an epistle, intellect. Intellect restrains folly, *it restrains those who possess understanding. Opinion, understanding.*

Drawing on this material, it is clear that to say that someone's *madd'ā* is disordered, as does the early Syriac translation of aphorism ii. 6, is quite different from saying that someone's *tar'iṯā* is disordered, as does the later Syriac version of that aphorism. The latter translation both is the more specific of the two and is represented in the short entry for γνώμη attributable to Ḥunayn provided at the beginning of this discussion. This constitutes a link between the translator's lexicography and the Syriac *Aphorisms*. On the other hand, the presence of Ḥunayn's Arabic equivalents for γνώμη taken from his translation of the *Aphorisms* in the entry for *madd'ā* and the concurrent absence of those equivalents from the entry for *tar'iṯā* rather suggest a link between Ḥunayn's Arabic translation techniques and the former Syriac term rather than the latter.

The source of this discrepancy could perhaps be located in the differing conceptual scope of these Syriac and Arabic psychological terms. Bar Bahlul's *Lexicon* does not provide an exact Arabic equivalent for *tar'iṯā*. In other words, the term's precise connotation of 'the faculty of mind that deals with the final products of thought, such as opinion or intention' is not represented in the lexicographical work presented here. When rendering *tar'iṯā* into Arabic without an exact equivalent, either the first element of this concept, i. e. 'faculty of mind', could be retained, or the second, i.e. 'intention or opinion'. In the context of aphorism ii. 6, it is clear that the element 'faculty of mind' is closer to the general sense of the text. For this reason, the Arabic terminology given in the entry for *madd'ā* better renders the Greek than that given for *tar'iṯā*.

The difference between the two translations' approaches to translating γνώμη in aphorism ii. 6 may also be due to the translators' responses to Galen's commentary on the aphorism. Ḥunayn rendered the end of Galen's commentary by writing '(I)n this place there is no difference between my saying mind (*'aql*), understanding (*fahm*), intelligence (*dhihin*), or thought (*fikr*)'.[8] Thus it may be that Ḥunayn preferred to employ the most general of the possible terms. Again, this approach renders Ḥunayn's translation closer to the earlier Syriac version than to the later.

Aphorism iii. 19

Νοσήματα δὲ πάντα μὲν ἐν πάσῃσι τῇσιν ὥρῃσι γίνεται, μᾶλλον δ' ἔνια κατ' ἐνίας αὐτέων καὶ γίνεται καὶ παροξύνεται.

E.

ܕܟܠܗ ܕܟܘܪ̈ܗܢܐ ܟܠܗܘܢ ܒܟܠܗܘܢ ܙܒ̈ܢܐ ܗܘܝܢ. ܠܬܪܐܬ ܕܝܢ ܚܕ̈ܚܕ ܡܢܗܘܢ ܒܚܕ̈ܚܕ ܡܢܗܘܢ
ܡܬܡܬܚܝܢ ܘܡܬܡܪܡܪܝܢ.

All diseases occur at all times. Some of these (diseases) in some of those (times) extend and exacerbate more.

S.

ܟܘܪ̈ܗܢܐ ܕܝܢ ܟܠܗܘܢ ܗ̇ܝ ܒܟܠܗܘܢ ܙܒ̈ܢܝܗ ܕܫܢܬܐ ܗܘܝܢ. ܡܢܗܘܢ ܕܝܢ ܒܙܒܢ ܕܟܘܪ̈ܗܢܐ ܒܡܢܗܘܢ
ܕܙܒ̈ܢܐ ܝܬܝܪ ܗܘܝܢ ܐܘ ܡܬܡܪܡܪܝܢ.

All diseases occur at all times of the year. However, some diseases occur or exacerbate more often at some of these times.

Ḥ.

والأمراض كلّها تحدث في أوقات السنة كلّها إلّا أنّ بعضها في بعض الأوقات أحرى بأن تحدث وتهيج.

All diseases occur at all times of the year, but at some of these times it is more to be expected that they occur or exacerbate.

8 Mimura (ed.), *Tafsīr Jālīnūs*, II, 11.

The Greek text of this aphorism is very concise. The early Syriac version strongly reflects this concision, while the later Syriac version and Ḥunayn's Arabic translation both add significant material to the text in order to clarify it for their readers. This is particularly the case in the translations of the phrase δ' ἔνια κατ' ἐνίας αὐτέων. In the Greek, both the substantives from the initial sentence, νοσήματα and ὥρῃσι, are subsumed under the pronouns in that phrase. The early Syriac translator preferred to translate the text literally without any explicitation, while the two later translations repeat one or both of the equivalent words. Ḥunayn in his Arabic translation chose to interpret the adverb μᾶλλον without reference to quantity, instead giving the word *aḥrā* 'more appropriate' in its place. In this the Arabic version contrasts slightly with both of the Syriac translations.

The verb παροξύνεται provides an opportunity to consider the very interesting Syriac and Arabic terminology for this medical phenomenon both in the *Aphorisms* and in bar Bahlul's *Lexicon.* I shall treat here the scholarly background to the translations of this and related terms.

Παροξύνει

1485:5 ܦܐܪܘܟܣܘܢܝ ܐܝܟ ܒܪ ܣܪܘ ܡܪܡܪ أغاظ܆

Paroksyunē according to bar Serošway, to exacerbate (*marmar*), *to exacerbate* (aghāẓ).

Forms of two quite distinct Syriac terms translate παροξυσμός and the related verb παροξύνω in the *Aphorisms*. The more common of the two, *'ḏāyā* 'paroxysm', is employed for eight of the nine occurrences of these words. In aphorism iii. 19, however, the verb *meṯmarmrin* serves to translate the verb παροξύνεται instead. Of these eight examples, iii. 19 is the only extant example from the early Syriac translation. There, the same word *meṯmarmrin* 'to exacerbate' is used in place of παροξύνεται as well.

For his part Ḥunayn employed a variety of words as equivalents for παροξυσμός in his Arabic translation, including *dawr* 'periodic exacerbation', *nawb* 'paroxysm', and the verb *hāja* 'to exacerbate'. In one of the three instances of these words in aphorism i. 11, he apparently interpreted παροξυσμός to be synonymous with ἀκμή, and gave the translation *waqt muntahā al-maraḍ* 'the time of the height of the disease'.[9]

9 See unit (1.2.4) above.

Several aphorisms containing these words survive from the early Arabic translation. These examples also display a variety of approaches to the translation of παροξυσμός. Generally in these translations the term *ihtiyāj* serves to render the Greek word. In cases where the phrase κατὰ περιόδους accompanies it, however, the translator interpreted the word to signify a particular type of fever, and so rendered it with phrases like *al-ḥummā allatī ta'rid ḥīna ba'da ḥīna* 'fevers that recur periodically'. In a single example in aphorism ii. 13, the phrase *ḥidda al-maraḍ* 'sharpening of the disease' translates the Greek word.

Several of these examples invite closer scrutiny, but before proceeding to that, I would like to examine the entries in bar Bahlul's *Lexicon* for the Syriac equivalents for παροξυσμός, as they will help greatly to clarify this relative variety of terminology. An entry for the word *murmārā* reads like this:

1042:1 **ܡܘܪܡܪܐ** اهتياج الحمّى إسخاط. ܐܝܟ ܚܢܝܢ احتداد. **ܡܬܡܪܡܪ** يحتدّ. ܡܘܪܡܪ̈ܐ ܘܥܕ̈ܝܐ
ܡܫܚܠܦܝܢ. ܥܕ̈ܝܐ ܓܝܪ ܥܠ ܚܘ̈ܡܐ ܡܬܐܡܪܝܢ ܒܟܐܢܘܬܐ ܕܒܙ̈ܒܢܐ ܦܘܫܩܐ. ܡܘܪܡܪ̈ܐ ܕܝܢ ܕܐܡܝܢܝܬܐ
ܐܡܝܢܝܬܐ ܡܬܐܡܪܐ ويقال للاوّل قلد[10] الحمّى ونوبة الحمّى ودَورها وللثاني اهتياج الحمّى. **ܡܘܪܡܪܐ**
ܐܝܟ ܒܪ ܣܪܘܫܘܝ ܗܘ ܕܪ̈ ܥܠ ܐܡܝܢܘܬܐ الغمّ الدائم صعوبة العلل الغيظ.÷

Murmārā, paroxysm of fevers (ihtiyāj al-ḥummā), *exacerbation* (iskhāṭ). According to Ḥunayn *exacerbation* (iḥtidad). *Meṯmarmar, to exacerbate (*yaḥtaddu*). Murmārē* and *'ḏāyē* differ, for *'ḏāyā* is properly used for periodic fevers, while *murmārē* is (used) mostly for continuous fevers. *The first is called* qild al-ḥummā, nawba al-ḥummā, *or* dawr, *while the second is called* ihtiyāj al-ḥummā. *Murmārā* according to bar Serošway, this is (said) of lasting anger, *lasting sorrow, the strengthening of illnesses, wrath.*

The following entries define words related to *'ḏāyā*:

1406:3 **ܥܕܝܐ** ܒܟܬ̈ܒܐ عبوق حُمّى غِب. ܘܐܝܟ ܒܪ ܣܪܘܫܘܝ ܚܘܕܪܐ الدور ÷

'ḏāyā in a manuscript, *the paroxysms of a tertian fever (*'ubūq ḥummā ghibb*).* And according to bar Serošway, a paroxysm (*ḥuḏara*), *paroxysms (*al-dawr*).*

1406:5 **ܥܕܝ ܥܠܘܗܝ** ܗ̄ ܟܒܫ̈ ܥܠܘܗܝ، مرّ به طرقه وأعربه زعم. **ܥܕܝܐ ܥܠܘܗܝ،** ܐܝܟ ܒܪ ܣܪܘܫܘܝ يتسلّط عليه
ويغلبه. **ܥܕܝܢ ܥܠܝ ܢܣܝܘܢܐ** تطرقني الآفات. **ܥܕܝܢ ܟܐܒ̈ܐ** تسلّط الاوجاع. ܥܕܝܐ ܘܡܘܪܡܪܐ ܐܝܟ ܒܪ
ܣܪܘܫܘܝ[11] ܡܫܚܠܦܝܢ. ܥܕ̈ܝܐ ܓܝܪ ܥܠ ܚܘ̈ܡܐ ܡܬܐܡܪܝܢ ܒܟܐܢܘܬܐ ܕܒܙ̈ܒܢܐ ܦܘܫܩܐ. ܡܘܪܡܪܐ ܕܝܢ ܥܠ ܐܡܝܢ̈ܝܬܐ
ܐܡܝܢܝܬܐ ܡܬܐܡܪܐ. يقال للاوّل قلد الحمّى ونوبة الحمّى آخر دور الحمّى عبوق الحمّى وللثاني اهتياج

10 Duval: قلّة. The word *qild* fits the sense and is supported by the analogous entry for *'ḏāyā* at 1406:5.

11 Duval's manuscripts F and S read ܐܝܟ ܪܒܢ 'according to our teacher' instead.

الحمّى. ܥܕ̈ܝܐ ܕܠܐ ܫܘܝܢ ܐܝܟ ܒܪ ܣܪܘ أدوار غير مستوية. ܥܕܝܐ ܘܬܘܒܐ المدّ والجزر. ܥܕܝܐ
ܕܐܫ̈ܬܐ الحمّى التي لا تنوب أدوار غير مستوية܀

'Āḏay 'alaw, this is 'passing it by', *he supposed he Arabicized it as 'he passed it by on his way'. 'Āḏāyā 'alaw* according to bar Serošway, *it overcame him and conquered him. 'Āḏên 'alay nesyunē, evils befell me. 'Āḏên ḥašē, pains overpowered. 'ḏāyā* and *murmārā* differ, according to bar Serošway, for *'ḏāyā* is used for periodic fevers, while *murmārā* (is used) mostly for continuous fevers. *The first is called* qild al-ḥummā, nawba al-ḥummā, *also* dawr al-ḥummā *and* ʿubūq al-ḥummā, *while the second is called* iḥtiyāj al-ḥummā. *'ḏāyē ḏ-lā šāwên* according to bar Serošway, *uneven paroxysms (*adwār ghayr mustawiya*). 'ḏāyā wa-tawbā, flow and ebb. 'ḏāyā ḏ-ešāṯā* ('paroxysm of a fever'), *fevers which do not exacerbate (*tanūb*), uneven paroxysms.*

Of central importance are the parallel definitions of *'ḏāyā* and *murmārā* which figure in the entries at 1042:1 and 1406:5. Besides the fact that bar Bahlul did not attribute the definition at 1042:1 to a specific lexicographer, the strong parallels between the terminology of the translations of παροξυσμός in the *Aphorisms* and that of these definitions should allow for their authorship to be attributed strongly to Ḥunayn. Although most of the manuscripts used by Duvaḷ attribute the version in the entry at 1406:5 to Bar Serošway, according to the editor's apparatus two of his manuscripts read *ayk rabban* 'according to our teacher (Ḥunayn)'. On the basis of the evidence presented below, I believe the alternate reading attributing the definition to Ḥunayn is likely the more accurate of the two. Such a reading is substantiated, furthermore, by an entry in bar 'Ali's *Lexicon*. There, the following entry is found:

ܡܘܪ̈ܡܪܐ. ܒܙܩܦܐ. ܡ̄. ܬܪ̄. ܘܥܕ̈ܝܐ ܡܫܚܠܦܝܢ ܥܕ̈ܝܐ[12] ܗܘ ܡܢ ܓܝܪ ܡܫܪܝܪܐܝܬ ܡܬܐܡܪܝܢ ܥܠ ܐܫ̈ܬܐ ܡܥܕ̈ܢܝܬܐ
ܩܘܫܝܐ: ܡܘܪ̈ܡܪܐ ܕܝܢ ܥܠ ܐܫ̈ܬܐ ܐܡܝܢܝܬܐ ܝܬܝܪܐܝܬ. ويقال للاوّل قلد الحُمى ونوبة الحُمى ودور الحُمى
ويقال الثاني اهتياج الحمى إسخاط احتداد.[13]

Murmārē, with long-a for the second *mim*, and *'ḏāyē* differ, for *'ḏāyē* is properly used for periodic fevers, while *murmārē* is (used) mostly for continuous fevers. *The first is called* qild al-ḥummā, nawba al-ḥummā, *or* dawr al-ḥummā, *while the second is called* ihtiyāj al-ḥummā. *Exacerbation, sharpening (*iḥtidād*).*

---

12 Hoffmann: ܥܕ̈ܝܐ.

13 Hoffmann (ed.), *Syrische-arabische Glossen*, 218:5585.

If we look closely at the examples from the *Aphorisms*, we see that the distinction introduced in the Syriac terminology between the paroxysm of recurrent fevers, *'ḏāyā* and that of the continuous fever, *murmārā*, is faithfully carried over into Ḥunayn's Arabic translation as well. In the vast majority of the instances where *'ḏāyā* or a related verb occur in the Syriac *Aphorisms*, Ḥunayn employed one of the words mentioned in the definition of that word in bar Bahlul's *Lexicon*. The only exception is found in aphorism i. 11, where *waqt muntahā al-maraḍ* 'the time of the height of the disease' is found instead, as mentioned above. However, as expected from his definition, in the one case where a verb related to *murmārā* is found, Ḥunayn translated it with the verb *hāja*, which is related to *ihtiyāj*, the word associated with *murmārā* in the entries from the lexicons.

Several points of interest may be noted in relation to these examples. Most importantly, the Syriac terminology had evidently developed a higher degree of terminological specificity relative to the Greek. Whereas the text of the *Aphorisms* refers to the exacerbations of periodic fevers and continuous fevers with the same term, παροξυσμός, the Syriac text introduces terms that immediately distinguish between the two. That such a distinction first makes its appearance in Syriac is evidenced by the fact that the entry for the Greek παροξύνει at 1485:5 makes synonymous Syriac and Arabic equivalents that refer respectively to the two types of paroxysm in the Syriac lexicography.

The correspondence between the terminology present in the translations of the *Aphorisms* and the definitions of *'ḏāyā* and *murmārā* strongly indicate Syriac influence upon Ḥunayn's Arabic translation of the *Aphorisms*. On the basis of this evidence, the distinction between the Syriac terms used as equivalents for παροξυσμός in the Syriac *Aphorisms* constitutes an important example of terminological innovation in Syriac medicine. As shown by comparing his entries for these terms in bar Bahlul's *Lexicon* and his translation of the *Aphorisms*, Ḥunayn's Arabic translations maintained this terminological distinction.

Although the evidence for translations of παροξυσμός from the early Arabic translation is partial, lacking in particular the crucial aphorism iii. 19, comparing these texts with the evidence taken from the other translations provides some opportunity for considering their relationships with one another and with the lexicographical tradition. Perhaps the most interesting element of these comparisons is the correspondence between Ḥunayn's simple definition of *murmārā* in the entry at 1042:1, *iḥtidad*, and the early Arabic version's rendering of παροξυσμός in aphorism ii. 13, *ḥidda al-maraḍ*. This may suggest that this equivalency of Ḥunayn's represents a continuation of an earlier stage of translation technique. In general, the early translator's approach to translating these terms was more haphazard than Ḥunayn's. Furthermore, he used the term reserved by Ḥunayn for the paroxysms of periodic diseases, *ihtiyāj*, in several aphorisms where the context refers the term to the paroxysms of acute diseases, and where the Syriac translation gives *'ḏāyā* and not *murmārā*. This suggests that Ḥunayn could have been responsible for the transferral of this distinction, and at the least that it was not established in Arabic at the time of al-Biṭrīq's translation. Furthermore, the link between the Syriac terminology and Ḥunayn's Arabic translation on the one hand contrasts with the dissimilarity between the Syriac terminology and al-Biṭrīq's Arabic translation on the other. This is a strong indication that Ḥunayn employed developments in Syriac medical terminology in order to modernize his Arabic translations.

Aphorism iii. 20

Τοῦ μὲν γὰρ ἦρος, τὰ μελαγχολικὰ καὶ τὰ μανικὰ καὶ τὰ ἐπιληπτικὰ καὶ αἵματος ῥύσιες καὶ κυνάγχαι καὶ κορύζαι καὶ βράγχοι καὶ βῆχες καὶ λέπραι καὶ λειχῆνες καὶ ἀλφοὶ καὶ εξανθήσιες ἑλκώδεις πλεῖσται καὶ φύματα καὶ ἀρθριτικά.

E.

ܕܒܐܕܪܐ ܗܘܝܢ ܟܘܪ̈ܗܢܐ ܕܒܢܝ ܡܪܬܐ ܐܘܟܡܬܐ ܘܕܫܢܝܘܬܐ [14] ܘܕܐܦܠܐܡܣܝܐ ܘܪܕܝܬܐ ܕܕܡܐ
ܘܚܢܘܩܝܐ ܟܠܒܝܐ ܘܟܘܪ̈ܙܐ ܘ ܓܪ̈ܒܐ ܘܣܪܘܬܐ ܘܫܚ̈ܢܐ ܘܡܦܩܬܐ ܫܘܚܢܢܝܬܐ ܘܚܫ̈ܘܟܐ ܘܟܐܒ
ܦܪ̈ܩܬܐ.

Those (things) that occur in spring are the diseases of the sons of black bile, madnesses, epilepsy, flow of blood, canine angina, catarrh, leprosies, ringworms, itches, ulcerous eruptions and pains of the joints.

S.

ܒܐܕܪܐܐ ܗ̈ ܟܢ ܗܟܢܐ. ܘܡܝܠܢܟܘܠܝܐ. ܘܡܢܝܩܘܣܐ. ܘܐܦܝܠܝܦܣܝܐ. ܘܡܪܕܝܬܐ ܕܕܡܐ.
ܘܣܘܢܩܐ. ܘܩܘܪ̈ܙܐ. ܘܣܪ̈ܢܟܐ. ܘܫܥܠܐ. ܘܓܪܒܘܬܐ. ܘܣܪܝܘܬܐ. ܘܚܡܘܡܬܐ. ܘܡܫܚ̈ܬܐ ܫܘܚܢܢܝܐ ܕܦܠ
ܗܦܟܝܢ. ܘܡܦܩܬܐ. ܘܟܐܒ ܦܪ̈ܩܬܐ.

14 Kessel: ܫܢܝܘܬܐ.

In spring there is mania, melancholy, epilepsy, apoplexy, flowing of blood, angina, catarrhs, quinsy, cough, scurf, ringworm, tetter, the greatest amount of ulcerous pustules, abscesses and pains of the joints.

Ḥ.

قد يعرض في الربيع الوسواس السوداوي والجنون والصرع وانبعاث الدم والذبحة والزكام والبحوحة والسعال والعلّة التي يتقشّر منها الجلد والقوابي والبهق والبثور الكثيرة التي تتقرّح والخراجات وأوجاع المفاصل.

There may occur in spring melancholic delusion, madness, epilepsy, flowing of blood, angina, catarrh, hoarseness, cough, the disease due to which the skin flakes off, tetter, herpetic eruptions, great amounts of pustules that ulcerate, abscesses and pains of the joints.

This aphorism consists entirely of a list of diseases which predominate in the springtime. The Syriac translations differ substantially from one another, both in the lists of diseases and, in the cases where lists overlap, in their respective terminologies. This is of particular interest in that the later Syriac version displays a much greater tendency to employ forms of the Greek words contained in the source-text as loan-words than does the earlier version.[15] I have already considered several of the Greek disease-names present in this aphorism in the first chapter of the work. These include μελαγχολικά (2.1.7), ἐπιληπτικά (2.2.4), ἀποπληξία (2.2.2),[16] ἀλφοί (1.3.3), and ἀρθριτικά (1.3.9). In the following pages, I shall provide lexicographical studies for those terms in this aphorism that I have not yet considered. I shall then return to consider the implications of these comparisons for our understanding of the relationship between the three translations presented above.

μανία

989:15 **ܡܐܢܝܐ** جنون ܘܐܝܟ ܦܘ ܘܒܪ ܣܪܘ ܫܢܝܘܬܐ ܟܠܒܘܬܐ܀

*Mānyā, madness (*junūn*),* and according to Paul and bar Serošway, madness (*šanyuṯā*), rabidity.

Forms of μανία, the related adjective μανικός, and the related verb μαίνομαι occur several times in the *Aphorisms*. Despite their close relationship, the Syriac version of the *Aphorisms* approaches these words quite differently. For the two instances of the adjective employed as a

15 This exemplifies well the broader trend discussed extensively in Chapter Two.

16 Although this word does not occur in the modern editions of this aphorism, it does occur in the later Syriac version of it.

substantive in aphorisms iii. 20 and iii. 22, the borrowed Greek word *maniya* 'madness' is employed. For the occurrences of the noun and the verb from book five on, however, forms of the native nouns *šnāyā* 'frenzy', *šānyuṯā* 'madness', and the verb *šnā* 'to go mad' are used instead.

In aphorism iii. 20, the early Syriac version gives *šānyuṯā* 'madness', contrasting with the later version's employment of the borrowed Greek word. For its part, Ḥunayn's Arabic version consistently translates all of these words with a form of *al-junūn* 'madness' adding a form of the verb *uṣīb* 'to be stricken' to render the verbs. Although most of Ullmann's examples also employ *al-junūn*, he notes one translation of a form of adjective μανικός from Dioscorides' *Materia Medica* that gives a transliteration of the word.[17]

The Greek lexicography in bar Bahlul's *Lexicon* matches well with both the Syriac and Arabic equivalents. An entry for the Syriac equivalent *šnāyā* adds more detail:

1993:1 **ܫܢܝܐ** مجنون معتوه مصاب. ܒܐܘܢܓܠܝܘܢ ܫܢܘ ܠܗܘܢ قد وسوسوا. ܫܢܝܘܬܐ الجنون. ܙܟ̄ خبل.
ܘܐܝܟ ܒܪ ܣܪܘ̄ الهيمان. ܘܒܨܚ̈ زوال. ܫܢܝܐ ܐܝܟ ܒܪ ܣܪܘ̄ جنون ܘܬܘܒ ܐܚܒܕܘܬ ܗ̇ܘܢܐ ذهاب
العقل... ويكون غير صورة العقلاء. او خالياً عن صورة العقلاء.

Šānyā, a madman, an insane person, one stricken. In the Gospel, *šnaw lahon, they were deluded. Šānyuṯā*, madness. (According to) Zakariya, *confusion*. And according to bar Serošway, *madly in love*. In a manuscript, *departure*. *Šnāyā* according to bar Serošway, *madness* and again annihilation of the reason, *departure of reason... Šani,* he fed him, *he nourished him, he fed him, he was lacking the form of the rational, absent from the form of the rational.*

κυνάγχη

1740:18 **ܩܘܢܢܟܐ** وجع الحلق والذبحة. ܘܐܝܟ ܒܪ ܣܪܘ̄ **ܩܘܢܟ̈ܐ** ܚܡܝܡܐ ܕܒܓܘܡܪ̈ܬܐ ܠܓܘܝܬܐ
ܕܓܓܪܬܐ ورم العضل الداخل في الحنجرة.

Qunnānḵê, pain of the throat, angina (al-dhibḥa). According to bar Serošway *qunāḵê*, a swelling in the innermost muscles of the throat, *swelling of the inner muscle in the throat.*

Forms of κυνάγχη occur six times in the *Aphorisms*. Both of the main translations are entirely consistent in their renderings of the term, the Syriac giving *ḥānoqā* 'angina', and Ḥunayn's Arabic giving *al-dhibḥa* with the same meaning. One aphorism from the early Arabic version containing

17 Ullmann, *Wörterbuch zu den griechisch-arabischen Übersetzungen*, 406.

κυνάγχη is extant, and there too *al-dhibḥa* is its translation. A single aphorism from the early Syriac version containing the word is also extant. The translation found there, *ḥānoqā kālbānā* 'canine angina', differs slightly from the later version's equivalent in that it gives reference to the etymological sense of the Greek word alongside the standard Syriac name for the disease.

The single entry in bar Bahlul's *Lexicon* for κυνάγχη contains two definitions of the term. The first, attributable to Ḥunayn, gives two Arabic equivalents for the Greek word, including *al-dhibḥa*, the translator's preferred equivalent in the *Aphorisms*. The second definition, attributed to bar Serošway, provides a brief symptomatological account of the disease first in Syriac and then almost identically in Arabic.

The definition in bar Bahlul's *Lexicon* for the Syriac equivalent of κυνάγχη runs as follows:

763:14 ܚܢܘܩܐ خنق. ܒܝ̈ ܐܕܫܐ ܕܚܢܘܩܐ أنواع الخوانيق. ܚܢܘܩܐ الذبحة܀

Ḥanoqā, strangulation (khanq). In a manuscript *edša d-ḥanoqā, types of strangulation. Ḥanoqā, angina* (al-dhibḥa).

It is clear from this evidence that this disease was clearly defined in both Syriac and Arabic. The presence of nearly univocal terminologies in both the Syriac and Arabic traditions, and the strong representation of these in both the Greek and Syriac entries in the *Lexicon*, makes it certain on the basis of this material that these terms were well-established long before Ḥunayn's career.

κόρυζα

1752:2 ܩܘܪܘܙܐ ܒܝ̈ برد ܘܐܝܟ ܒܪ ܣܪܘ̄ الزكام ܘܗܘܝܘ ܪܘܣܡܐ ܗܘ ܕܢܚܬ ܠܢܚܝܪܐ الزكام܀

Qoruzā, in a manuscript *a cold* (bard), and according to bar Serošway *catarrh* (al-zukām), which is a flux that goes down to the nostrils, *catarrh* (al-zukām).

1754:7 ܩܘܪܝܙܐ ܐܝܟ ܒܪ ܣܪܘ̄ خبطة من البرد܀

Qorizā according to bar Serošway *a catarrh* (khabṭa) *due to cold.*

Forms of the Greek word κόρυζα occur five times in the *Aphorisms*. The Syriac version in each case translates with a form of the word *qurārā* 'cold, catarrh'. In four of these five instances, Ḥunayn's Arabic translation gives forms of the word *al-zukām* 'colds', but in aphorism ii. 40, the nearly synonymous word *al-nazla* is found instead. Ullmann notes several other instances of this Greek word from various Arabic translations, all of which give forms of *al-zukām* as well.[18] The early Syriac version of iii. 20 is extant. As in the version of that aphorism found in the Syriac *Aphorisms*, it gives a form of *qurārā*.

The entries for the Greek word in Bar Bahlul's *Lexicon* corroborate only one of these three translations, that is, the more common Arabic equivalent *al-zukām*. Two other Arabic synonyms, *bard* and *khabṭa*, are also introduced there. Bar Serošway's definition at the end of the entry at 1752:2 gives a Syriac definition of the Arabic *al-zukām* in an interesting variation on the Syriac/Arabic bilingualism that characterizes these entries, which usually proceed in the opposite order of languages.

Turning to bar Bahlul's entry for the Syriac equivalent for κόρυζα in the *Aphorisms*, *qurārā*, we find the following text:

1757:13 ܩܘܪܪܐ ܐܝܟ ܙܟܪܝܐ ܢܙܪܐ. ܒܦ̈ܐ التبريد ويقال على النزلة. ܚܪܘܫܐ ܗܟܘܬ ܕܘܒ̈ܐ. ܐܠܐ ܗܕܐ
ܥܡ ܫܥܠܐ ܘܚܪܘܫܘܬܐ ܕܓܕܫܐ ܒܪܐܬܐ. نزلة وأيضاً خبطة. ܒܦ̈ النزلات التي يكون منها الزكام من البرد
والحرّ. ܘܐܝܟ ܒܪ ܣܪܘ ܕܘܒ̈ܐ ܕܢܚܬܝܢ ܡܢ ܪܝܫܐ ܕܗܘ ܩܘܪܝܙܐ الزكام܀

Qurārā according to Zakariya, catarrh (*nzārā*). In a manuscript, *chilling* (al-tabrīd), *which is said of catarrh* (al-nazla). Hoarseness (*ḥarušā*), that is catarrhs (*dawbē*). But this occurs with cough and hoarseness supervening in the lungs. *Catarrh* (al-nazla), *also catarrh* (khabṭa). (In) a manuscript *catarrhs* (al-nazlāt) *on account of which occur colds* (al-zukām) *due to* (*both*) *cold and heat*. According to bar Serošway fluxes which come down from the head, which is *qorizā*, *colds* (al-zukām).

By virtue of the prominence of forms of the word *al-nazla* in this entry, we find here a fuller representation of the vocabulary of the Arabic *Aphorisms*. Not only is *al-nazla* represented, but the author of this entry, presumably Ḥunayn because of the citation of 'a manuscript', has also placed that term in a causal relationship with *al-zukām*. This emphasizes the exceptional character of Ḥunayn's translation of κόρυζα with *al-nazla* in ii. 40. Whether his text differed from the Syriac translator's or he simply preferred another interpretation, this discrepancy is yet another example of variation between the two translations.

A further problem arises, however, in that the material attributable to Ḥunayn in this entry tends to make *al-nazla* rather than *al-zukām* the Arabic equivalent of the Syriac *qurārā*, while the reverse is the case in the

18 Ullmann, *Wörterbuch zu den griechische-arabischen Übersetzungen*, 363.

translations of the *Aphorisms*. This point is brought out further if we consider the translations of the Greek word κατάρροος 'catarrh' in the *Aphorisms*. In all four instances of that term, *al-nazl* or *al-nazla* is the equivalent given by Ḥunayn, while *dawbā* is the standard equivalent in the Syriac version. Here is an entry for *dawbā* in bar Bahlul's *Lexicon*:

536:19 **ܕܘܒܐ** الزكام السيلان والإمذاء الحيض. ܡܕܡ ܕܡܦܫܪ ܠܡܕܡ أقول يذيبه. ܐܝܟ ܒܪ ܣܪܘ الذوبان النزلة. **ܕܘܒܐ** النزف.܀

Dawbā, a cold (zukām), *flow* (*of bodily fluid*) *and excretion,*[19] *menstruation*. Something which melts something else, *I say* 'yudhībuhū (*it melted it*)'. According to bar Serošway, *liquefaction* (al-dhawabān), *catarrh* (al-nazla). *Dawbā, flows of blood* (al-nazf).

The material attributable to Ḥunayn in this entry makes *al-zukām* equivalent to *dawbā*, while the definition attributed to bar Serošway makes *al-nazla* its equivalent. That Ḥunayn held *al-zukām* equivalent to *dawbā* is further indicated by the following entry from bar ʿAli's *Lexicon*:

ܕܘܒܐ ܕܕܡܐ ܘܕܙܪܥܐ ܘܐܦ ܕܪܘܡܐ ܕܢܚܬܝܢ ܡܢ ܪܝܫܐ ويقال للأول النزف الحيض وللثاني الامذى وللثالث الزكام السيلان الذوبان.[20]

Dāwbā [is said] of menstrual blood, semen, or of fluxes that come down from the head. Al-nazf (*flows of blood*) (*and*) al-ḥayḍ (*menstrual blood*) *are used for the first,* al-imdhā (*excretion*) *is used for the second, and* al-zukām (*catarrhs*), al-saylān (*flows*), *and* al-dhawabān (*liquefaction*) *are used for the third.*

To recapitulate, in the Syriac translation κόρυζα is translated with *qurārā*, while κατάρροος is translated with *dawbā*. In Ḥunayn's Arabic *Aphorisms* and in other translations, κόρυζα is almost always translated with forms of *al-zukām*, while κατάρροος is generally translated with forms of *al-nazla*.[21] Yet in several examples of Ḥunayn's lexicographical writing, these Syriac and Arabic equivalents are reversed: *al-nazla* is associated with *qurārā*, while *al-zukām* is associated with *dawbā*. Based on the lexicons, it would seem reasonable to expect that Ḥunayn's Syriac translation would have used these two Syriac words in a corresponding way to these two Arabic words, yet the opposite is the case in the extant Syriac *Aphorisms*.

19 I take *al-imdhā'* to be the verbal noun of the fourth form of the root *mdhy as found in Freytag's dictionary. Otherwise it is not represented in the dictionaries I have consulted.

20 Hoffmann (ed.), *Syrische-arabische Glossen*, 109: 3054.

21 This equivalence also obtains in several translations of κατάρρους noted by Ullmann, *Wörterbuch zu den griechisch-arabischen Übersetzungen*, 333.

The close relationship between these terms makes firm argumentation solely on the basis of these variations difficult. With that said, the lexicographical evidence combined with the regularity of the translations indicates a rupture between Ḥunayn's Syriac to Arabic lexicographical activity as preserved by bar Bahlul and the equivalents for κόρυζα and κατάρροος in the Syriac *Aphorisms*. This contributes further to the impression that Ḥunayn was not the author of the latter work.

βράγχοι

The following word in the aphorism, βράγχοι, is not represented in Duval's Greek index to bar Bahlul's *Lexicon*. Furthermore, the early Syriac translation of it in the aphorism under consideration either was omitted by the translator or has dropped out of the text. The sense of βράγχοι is very close to that of κόρυζα, and the entries for the Syriac equivalents of it in bar Bahlul's *Lexicon* contain material relevant to the discussion of the latter term given above.

Ḥunayn's Arabic translation of the *Aphorisms* translates βράγχοι regularly with forms of the word *al-baḥūḥa* 'hoarseness', while the Syriac version gives as its equivalent forms *ḥurāšā* with the same meaning. If we consider the entries for the Syriac equivalent *ḥurāšā* in the lexicons, some notes of interest may be made:

734:1 ܚܘܪܫܐ عرفتُ أنّه نبات حارّ اذا أُكل أولد الذبحة زعموا. ܘܩܛܪ̈ܝܐ ܦܐܡ ܠܗ ܚܘܪܫܐ المنحر
والرقبة من الشاة. وقال لي سنان ابن ثابت أنّه الذبحة بعينها. ܚܘܪܫܐ نزلة زكام. ܚܘܪܫܐ ذبحة.

Ḥurāšā, I know it to be a hot plant. If it is eaten it produces angina, they claim. The people of Qatar say for *ḥurāšā, the neck and collarbone of the ram. Sinān ibn Thābit told me that it is specifically angina. Ḥurāšā, catarrh* (nazla), *a cold* (zukām). *Ḥurāšā, angina.*

Another entry for the term is found in bar ʿAli's *Lexicon*:

ܚܘܪܫܐ. البحوحة في الصوت النزلة يكون منها الزكام ويكون من حرارة وما كان من برودة يسمّى ܩܘܪܪܐ.[22]

Ḥurāšā. Hoarseness (al-baḥūḥa) *in the voice, catarrhs (*al-nazla*) due to which occur colds* (al-zukām). *They are produced on account of heat, and those which are produced from cold are called qurārā.*

This entry clarifies somewhat the material presented in the discussion of κόρυζα above. Two Syriac words for 'catarrh' *ḥurāšā* and *qurārā* exist with

22 Hoffmann (ed.), *Syrische-arabische Glossen*, 140:3762.

opposing senses; namely, the first is defined as 'hot catarrh', and the second as 'cold catarrh'. Two Arabic terms corresponding to these exist in the lexicons as well. According to this entry, the Arabic equivalent of *ḥurāšā* 'hot catarrh' is *baḥūḥa*. Although bar ʿAli's entry does not give an Arabic equivalent for *qurārā* 'cold catarrh', in the entry at 1757:13 the word *al-tabrīd* is given as its equivalent in a definition credited to 'a manuscript', which is thus strongly attributable to Ḥunayn. This latter Arabic word refers etymologically to the particular antithermic aetiology of the illness, as does the Syriac. *Al-tabrīd* would seem to be good candidate for a calque promoted by scholars who hoped to transfer Syriac etymological meaning into Arabic.

Although according to the lexicons this Syriac distinction was carried over into Arabic, it appears that Ḥunayn in his Arabic translation of the *Aphorisms* preferred to use more general terminology. Unlike *qurārā*, the Syriac equivalent for κόρυζα in the *Aphorisms*, neither word of the pair *al-nazla/al-zukām* refers to the heat or coldness of the congestion. Although the lexicographers attempted to maintain this element of the Syriac terminological apparatus, it does not appear to have found significant employment in the translations.

βήχιον

The Greek word βήξ has fully synonymous and etymologically interrelated equivalents in Arabic and Syriac, *al-suʿāl* and *šʿālā*, both meaning 'cough'. Forms of these words are used to translate all instances of forms of βήξ in all of the versions of the *Aphorisms* under consideration where an equivalent is extant. Notably, this word, like the preceding word βράγχοι, is not present in the early Syriac translation of aphorism iii. 20, either because of the translator's deliberate omission or because a word has dropped out of the text.

A single entry in bar Bahlul's *Lexicon* reflects the univocity of these translations:

1997:14 ܫܥܠܐ ܒܨܚ سعال✧

Šʿala in a manuscript, *cold* (suʿāl).

λέπρα

945:27 ܠܦܪܐ برص أسود✧

Lêpra, *black leprosy* (baraṣ aswad).

A form of this word occurs a single time in the *Aphorisms*, in aphorism iii. 20. The Syriac translation gives the term *qalāpitā* as its equivalent, while the fragment of the early Syriac version gives a different word, *garḇā*. Ḥunayn in his Arabic version used a five-word explicating translation, *al-'illa allatī yataqashsharu minhā al-jild* 'the disease due to which the skin' becomes scaled'. This same translation is also used in Ḥunayn's translations of occurrences of λέπρα in Galen's comment on this aphorism.[23]

Ullmann notes numerous examples of translations of this Greek word and the related adjective λεπρός.[24] A variety of Arabic equivalents may be found in these examples. The material recorded in the Syriac lexicons is also of significance for the variations observed in the translations, so here I will record Ullmann's examples serially.

In the occurrences of λέπρα in Book Six of Galen's *On Simple Drugs*, Ullmann cites three equivalents each from the versions of al-Biṭrīq and Ḥunayn. In all three of these cases the former translates λέπρα with *baraṣ* 'leprosy' while the latter gives *al-'illa allatī yataqashsharu ma'hā al-jild* 'the disease due to which the skin becomes scaled'. Although the overlap between Ḥunayn's translations and his translation of λέπρα in the *Aphorisms* is striking, Ullmann's next examples depart from this pattern. In the Arabic translation of the Hippocratic work *On Nutriment*, a form of λέπρα is translated with *al-baraṣ* 'leprosy', the same translation preferred by al-Biṭrīq in the example cited above. In each of two citations from Dioscorides' *Medical Material*, the word λέπρας is translated with the phrase *al-jarab al-mutaqarriḥ* 'ulcerous mange'. Again according to Ullmann, the Arabic translation of Artemidorus' *The Interpretation of Dreams* makes equivalent to the series of three disease-names ψώραν ἢ λέπραν ἢ ελέφαντα the two words *al-jarab aw al-baraṣ* 'mange or leprosy'. Finally, an example from Book 10 of Galen's *On Simple Drugs* translates a form of λέπρα with the hendiadys *al-jarab wal-waḍaḥ* 'mange and tetter'.[25]

---

23 Mimura (ed.), *Tafsīr Jālīnūs*, III 60–1. Λέπρα occurs twice in the context of Galen's repeating the disease-lists given in the lemma.

24 Ullmann, *Wörterbuch zu den griechische-arabischen Übersetzungen*, 387–8.

25 See Ullmann, *Wörterbuch zu den griechische-arabischen Übersetzungen*, 50 for a discussion of variations, including this one, between the translations of Books Six and 10 of *On Simple Drugs*.

Ullmann also records several translation equivalents for words related to λέπρα. For a participle of the verb λεπριάω, λεπριώντων, the translation of Dioscorides' *Materia Medica* gives *jarab* 'mange'.[26] In another example from the same work, a form of the word λεπρικός is again translated with *jarab* 'mange'.[27] Several translations of the Greek adjective λεπρός also occur in the *Wörterbuch*.[28] In one example from Galen's *On Simple Drugs* Book Six, the simple word λέπρας occurs, followed later in the text by the phrase λεπρούς ὄνυχας. The early Arabic translation of the work attributed to al-Biṭrīq gives for λέπρας *baraṣ* 'leprosy' and for λεπρούς ὄνυχας *al-baraṣ min al-aẓfār* 'leprosy of the fingernails'. Ḥunayn's later Arabic version translates λέπρας in a fashion similar to his other translations cited above, giving *al-'illa allatī yataqashshar ma'hā al-jild*', 'the disease with which the skin becomes scaled'. For λεπρούς ὄνυχας he used *al-aẓfār allatī tabyaḍḍ* 'fingernails which have whitened'.

In Arabic translations of the Gospels, words derived from *baraṣ* 'leprosy' are used to translate forms of λεπρός. In three citations from the Arabic translation of Dioscorides' *Medical Materials*, four translations of forms of the Greek word are found, each of them employing a different equivalent. Three of these translate the phrase λεπρούς ὄνυχας. Of these three, the first Arabic equivalent cited by Ullmann is *al-taqashshur al-'āriḍ fī al-aẓfār* 'scaling occuring in the fingernails', the second is *al-tashaqquq al-aẓfār wa-taqashshuruha* 'the splitting and scaling of the fingernails', and the third is *al-āthār al-bayḍ al-'āriḍ lil-aẓfār* 'white marks occurring on the fingernails'. In one of these citations, the simple word λέπρας is also found, and is translated into Arabic with *al-jarab al-mutaqarriḥ* 'ulcerous mange'.[29]

Turning to the lexicographical background in Ḥunayn's school, the single brief entry for λέπρα identified by Duval in bar Bahlul's *Lexicon* defines the disease as *baraṣ aswad* 'black leprosy'. This corresponds to a few of the translations, notably al-Biṭrīq's early translation of Galen's *On Simple Drugs* Book Six, the translations of the Gospels, and that of Artemidorus' *The Interpretation of Dreams*. When we consider the entries for the two Syriac terms *qalāpiṯā* and *garḇa* used in the translations,

26 Ullmann, *Wörterbuch zu den griechische-arabischen Übersetzungen*, 388.

27 Ibid.

28 Ullmann, *Wörterbuch zu den griechische-arabischen Übersetzungen*, 389.

29 Ibid.

however, much more significant information regarding the scholarly background lying behind the Arabic translations comes to light. First, this is an entry for *qalāpitā*:

1795:4 **ܩܠܵܦܹ̈ܐ** قشور. **ܩܠܵܦܝܼܬܵܐ** الحزاز القوابي. **ܩܠܵܦܬܵܐ ܕܣܲܝܦܵܐ** أقول أنّه توبال الفولاذ.[30] **ܩܠܵܦܝܼܬܵܐ**
ܐܝܟ ܒܪ ܣܪܘܫܘܝ ܗ̇ܝ ܕܢܳܬܰܪ ܒܗ̇ ܒܣܪܗ ܕܐܢܫ ܘܡܚܟ ܣܓܝ ܘܠܐ ܣܳܦܩ ܘܡܬܩܠܦ ܡܫܟܐ ܡܢ ܚܟܟܐ
القوابي التي تحكّ وتنقشر. ܬܘܒ **ܩܠܵܦܝܼܬܵܐ** ܕܡܬܩܠܦܐ ܘܡܬܢܬܪܐ القوباء التي تنقشر وتنتثر. ܒܨܚ̱ تقشير البدن
القوابي انتثار اللحم ويكون دوى. وجاء به حنين في البهق الذي ينقشر. المروزي الجرب اليابس القوباء
المتقشّرة. ܦܘܠܘܣ ܩܪܐ **ܠܩܠܵܦܝܼܬܵܐ** البرص. ܒܐܘܪܝܬܐ. ܢܡܚܝܟ ܡܪܝܐ ܒܫܚܦܘܬܐ ܘܒܩܠܵܦܝܼܬܐ. ܬܘܒ
ܩܠܵܦܝܼܬܵܐ ܚܘܪܬܐ ܥܒܘܫܬܐ ܕܝ̱ ܢܚܒ ܘܢܦܩ ܡܢ ܡܟܡܘܡܘܬܐ܀

Qlāpē, scales (qushūr). *Qalāpiṯā, itch* (al-ḥazāz), *tetter* (al-qawābī). *Qlāptā ḏ-saypa, I say it is the slag of iron* (tawbāl al-fūlādh). *Qalāpiṯā* according to bar Serošway, that in which a person's skin flakes (*naṯer bah besreh*), and he scratches much but it is not sufficient, and the skin scales off (*meṯqalap*) from the scratching, *tetter which itches and scales off* (tanqashir). Again *qalāpiṯā* which scales and flakes, *tetter which scales and flakes* (tantathiru). In a manuscript *the scaling of the body, tetter, the scaling of the flesh, which is a disease. Ḥunayn introduced it for tetter which is scaled.* (According to) al-Marwazī *dry mange* (al-jarab al-yābis), *flaking tetter*. Paul read for *qalāpiṯā leprosy* (baraṣ). In the Torah, 'the Lord strikes with torpor and with *qalāpiṯā*'.[31] Again, white, ulcerous *qalāpiṯā* which appears due to tetter.

A short definition of this Syriac word containing relevant material also occurs in bar ʿAli's *Lexicon*:

ܩܠܵܦܝܬܐ. الجراب اليابس أو القوباء المتقشّرة والحزاز والعلّة التي يتقشّر فيها الجلد. إنتثار اللحم. دواء.[32]

Qalāpiṯā, dry mange or flaking tetter, itch, the disease in which the skin flakes off (al-ʿilla allatī yataqashshar fīhā al-jild), *scaling of the flesh. A disease.*

An entry for *garḇā*, the equivalent given for λέπρα in the fragments of the early Syriac version of the *Aphorisms*, reads as follows:

512:15 **ܓܪܵܒܵܐ** بَرَص. **ܓܪ̈ܒܐ** أبرص. **ܓܪܒܐ** برص. **ܕܓܪܒ** الأبرص وضح البدن. ܐܝܟ ܒܪ ܣܪܘ
ܚܘܪܐ ܗܘ الوضح البَرَص. ܐܣܝܘܬܐ ܥܠ ܐܡܬܝ، ܘܐܝܟܢܐ ܕܡܬܒܠܬܐ ܥܠ ܦܘܡܐ ܒܪܫܐ ܓܪ̈ܒܐ ܐܬܬܘ
ܦܓܪܐ ܕ ܗ̄ ܓܪ̈ܒܐ. ܘܚܕ ܚܠܘܗܝ ܕܥܡܘܣܝܐ ܢܚܘܬ ܕ ܗ̄ ܓܪܒܐ. ܘܐܝܬܘܗ̇ ܡܢ ܡܬܬܘܬܐ ܕܒܣܪܐ ܢܝܫܐ
ܘܚܕܝܐ ܡܢ ܗܘ ܕܚܕ ܡܬܕܒܪܝ ܒܡܚܒܫܬܐ ܗܘ ܒܣܪܐ. ܠܐ ܢܦܩ ܡܢܗ ܕܡܐ. ܐܝܟ ܕܐܦܠܐ ܡܢ ܡܚܒܠܬܐ

30 Duval: الفولاذ.

31 Deut. 28:22.

32 Gottheil (ed.), *Syriac-Arabic Glosses*, II, 349:1

ܢܦܩ. ܘܐܝܬ ܡܢܗ ܕܦܫܝܐ ܒܓܘܫܡܐ ܘܐܝܬ ܕܠܐ. ܘܦܓܪܐ ܐܡܬܝ ܕܡܚܝܠ ܦܫܝܐ ܗܘ ܡܢ ܕܘܟܬܐ
ܠܕܘܟܬܐ. ܘܡܐܡܬܝ ܕܚܝܠܬܢ ܠܐ ܦܫܝܐ ܐܠܐ ܒܕܘܟܬܗ ܡܟܬܪܐ܀

Garḇā, leprosy (baraṣ). *Garbā, a leper. Garbē, leprosy. Da-greḇ, lepers, spotting of the body* (waḍaḥ al-badan). According to bar Serošway it is white, *spotting, leprosy.* (According to) others, whenever the word refers to the leprous individual it is pronounced without aspiration '*garbā*', and when it refers to the ulcers, it is pronounced with aspiration '*garḇā*'. It occurs due to the deadness of the living flesh, and it is known to be so, since where the flesh is pricked or dug out, no blood flows out from it, just as it does not flow out from the dead. Some (kinds) of it spread in the body, and some do not. When the body is weak it is spread from place to place, but when it is strong it does not spread, but remains in its place.

Before proceeding to a discussion of the relevance of these two entries for the Greek-to-Arabic translation movement, it should be noted that each of them appears to refer to a different skin disease. The interesting symptomatogical descriptions in Syriac differ clearly from one another. In particular, the disease *qalāpiṯā* is said to be accompanied by an intense sensory experience in the skin, namely itching, while in the disease *garḇā* the skin is said to have died.

Each one of these three entries contains important information concerning the variety of Arabic equivalents given for Greek words related to λέπρα in the literature surveyed above. Most prominently, Ḥunayn's translation activity is directly referred to in terms which link the entry for *qalāpiṯā* to the translations of λέπρα most strongly attributed to the translator in the scholarly literature. It appears from this material that the multi-word explicative translations in the *Aphorisms* and the later version of Galen's *On Simple Drugs* Book Six were developed in response to the sense of the Syriac word *qalāpiṯā*. It should also be considered very likely that *qalāpiṯā* served as Ḥunayn's equivalent for λέπρα in his Syriac translations. This example also serves well as an example of bar ʿAli's direct reliance upon Ḥunayn's work.

The Syriac word *qalāpiṯā* has a similar etymological sense-development to that of λέπρα, both words expressing the sense of 'scaling, flaking'. Ḥunayn's several Arabic definitions in the lexicons attempt to introduce a word related to an Arabic word for this general concept, *al-qishr* 'scales', to serve as an equivalent for *qalāpiṯā*. This etymology is not shared by any of the other equivalents discussed above. Also notable in this connection is the absence from the entry on *qalāpiṯā* of the otherwise commonly-used Arabic equivalent *baraṣ* save in a single brief reference to the translation of Paul of Aegina's *Pragmateia*. *Baraṣ*, however, figures prominently in bar Bahlul's entry for *garḇā*, the equivalent for λέπρα in the early Syriac version.

These distinctions are borne out by the accounts of skin diseases given in Thābit ibn Qurra's *Book of Treasures on the Science of Medicine*. Thābit divides his chapter on leprosy in that work into two parts. In the first part, *Fī al-judhām wal-bahaq al-abyaḍ wal-aswad* 'On leprosy and white and black tetter', he first describes the general aetiology of the various melancholic afflictions of the skin. He then goes on to cite Galen to the effect that at a late stage of the skin disease called *al-judhām*, the outer skin flakes off (*taqashshara al-jild al-ẓāhir*).[33] In a second section, *Fī al-baraṣ* 'On leprosy', Thabit gives a different aetiology which relies not on melancholy, but on phlegmatic blood.[34]

These sources indicate that a Syriac terminological distinction without an immediately obvious Arabic counterpart faced Ḥunayn. Less careful translators had rendered the Greek λέπρα with the term *baraṣ*. It is even the case that the single unattributed entry for that Greek disease-name in bar Bahlul's *Lexicon* defines the word as such. Yet in both his lexicographical work and in his translations, the least that may be said is that the etymological sense of the Syriac word *qalāpiṯā* urged upon Ḥunayn the introduction of new Arabic terminology centred around the word *al-qishr* 'scales'. Furthermore, the symptoms associated with *baraṣ* were not the same as those associated with *qalāpiṯā*, but rather were more closely associated with a different Syriac disease-name, *garḇā*. It is also possible that Thābit ibn Qurra's distinction between *al-baraṣ* and *al-judhām* corresponds to the distinction between these Syriac words. If that is the case, it would mean that Ḥunayn's terminological innovation did not entirely hold, even for the generations of medical authors immediately succeeding him. Yet at the same time, Ḥunayn's explicating translations appear to have given Galenic authority to a description of the symptoms of the disease that would

33 Thābit (d. 901) was an important figure in the development of Arabic philosophy and science. G. Sohby (ed.), *Kitāb al-Dhākhira fī 'Ilm al-Ṭibb Ta'līf Thābit ibn Qurra*, (Cairo 1928), ١٣٨-١٣٩.

34 Ibid., ١٤٠.

not necessarily have been present in the original Greek of whichever work Thābit consulted.

The various Arabic translations cited above may be divided into four categories. First are those works which translate λέπρα with *al-baraṣ*. These are either very early translations, such as those attributed to al-Biṭrīq, or non-medical works, such as the Gospels and Artemidoros' work on dream-interpretation. Second are those translations which use the multi-word explicating translation *al-'illa allatī yataqashsharu ma'hā al-jild* or a slight variation thereof. These examples are drawn from the works most strongly attributed to Ḥunayn, such as the *Aphorisms* and the later version of Book Six of Galen's *On Simple Drugs*, and to reiterate are strongly supported by Ḥunayn's entries for *qalāpiṯā* in the Syriac lexicons.

A third category includes translations which reflect somewhat Ḥunayn's lexicography by including a word related to *al-qishr* without using the identical explicating phrase. This category comprises some of the translations taken from Dioscorides' *Materia Medica*. These are particularly interesting in that they may give some insight into Ḥunayn's approach to modifying previous translations.[35] A fourth category includes medical works which translate neither with *al-baraṣ* nor with a word related to *al-qishr*. Included here are other translations from Dioscorides and the single example from Book 10 of Galen's *On Simple Drugs*. In most of these texts, the term *al-jarab* 'mange' is used. This word also figures in a definition of *qalāpiṯā* attributed by bar Bahlul to al-Marwazī. In the example from Book 10 of Galen's *On Simple Drugs*, the term *al-waḍaḥ* is employed alongside *al-jarab*.

What should be made of the single example of relevant Greek lexicography that appears in bar Bahlul's *Lexicon*? This definition, although unattributed, defines λέπρα with *al-baraṣ*, which as we have seen represents an older stratum of translation when compared with Ḥunayn's work. A potentially important clue may be found in bar Bahlul's entry for *qalāpiṯā*, where the authority of Paul is cited for the equivalence of that Syriac word and the Arabic *al-baraṣ*. As seen earlier, in Chapter One, material that closely tacks with Pauline definitions may be found without attribution in

35 The original Arabic translation of Dioscorides' *Materia Medica* is attributed to Iṣṭifān ibn Bāsil, and Ḥunayn is said to have rectified it. See Ullmann, *Wörterbuch zu den griechische-arabischen Übersetzungen*, 55.

bar Bahlul's *Lexicon*.[36] We may thus presume that Ḥunayn was not the source for the entry for λέπρα presented here. Given that at present Paul is the only other author besides Ḥunayn for whom there is evidence that bar Bahlul included his definitions without attribution, and given that *al-baraṣ* clearly represents a stage of the translation movement prior to Ḥunayn, the translation of Paul's *Pragmateia* is the most likely source of the short entry for the Greek word λέπρα.

To sum up this rather long discussion, it may be remarked that parallel developments regarding the translation of λέπρα occurred in the Syriac and Arabic medical traditions. In both the early Syriac and early Arabic translations, terms taken by the later lexicographers to be equivalent both to that Greek word and to one another were used, namely *garbā* and *al-baraṣ*. At some point in the centuries intervening between Sergius and Ḥunayn, the Syriac term *qalāpitā*, a word with a similar etymological sense as λέπρα, came to be preferred as the translation equivalent for that Greek word.

Ḥunayn, wishing perhaps to retain the nuances of the Syriac terminology and at any rate unsatisfied with *al-baraṣ*, attempted to introduce Arabic terminology that likewise agreed with the etymological sense of λέπρα. Although his terminology was not universally adopted, in the generations after Ḥunayn the distinction between these two types of leprosy persisted in various guises. Thus we see the Syriac and Arabic translation traditions undergoing parallel developments. That is to say, a distinction originating in the Syriac tradition was transferred into the Arabic translations in successive stages, with Ḥunayn's work playing a prominent but not ultimately decisive part in the process.

λειχήν/λειχηνικόν

965:24 **ܠܝܟܝܢܝܘܣ** قوابي. ܒ̈ **ܠܝܟܢ** ܚܙܙܝܬܐ ܕܟܐܦܐ حزازة الصخر صحّحه جبريل وحُنين في هذه النُسخة. **ܠܝܟܢ** حزازة الخيل ܐܝܟ ܪܒܢ. **ܠܝܟܢܝܣ** ܚܙܙܝܬܐ القوباء܀

Likinios, tetters. In a manuscript *ḥazāzitā d-kepā, lichen of stones.*[37] *Jibrīl and Ḥunayn rectified it in this manuscript. Likên, tetter of horses* according to our teacher. *Liknês*, tetter, *tetter.*

36 See the discussion of ἀποστήματα in unit (1.3.7) above.

37 Although *al-ḥazāza* does not carry this sense in the dictionaries of Wehr and Freytag, the sense here is clear.

966:3 ܠܝܟܢܝܩܘܢ دواء القوابي܀

Li<u>k</u>niqon, the disease 'tetters'.

The Greek word λειχῆνες occurs once in the *Aphorisms*, in aphorism iii. 20. Both the Syriac translations give *ḥazāzi<u>t</u>ā* 'ringworm, tetter' as its equivalent, while Ḥunayn's Arabic translation gives *al-qawābī* 'tetters'. Alongside this example, Ullmann notes others, including a text from Galen's *On Simple Drugs* Book Six. There, al-Biṭrīq employed *al-ḥazāz* to translate the Greek term, while Ḥunayn again translated it with a form of *al-qūbā'*.[38]

The entries for λειχήν and λειχηνικόν in bar Bahlul's *Lexicon* corroborate Ḥunayn's usage alongside definitions for other senses of these Greek words.[39] The entry for the Syriac equivalent does likewise:

737:1 ܚܙ̈ܙܝܬܐ ܐܝܟ ܒܪ ܣܪܘܫܘܝ، ܗܝ ܕܗܘܝܐ ܒܡܫܛܚܘܬܐ ܕܒܪܝܬܐ ܕܡܫܟܐ القوباء السعفة.
ܚܙ̈ܙܐ القوابي. ܚܙܙܐ ذو القوباء والحكّة والجرب. ܚܙܙܐ ܚܙܙ حزاز حكّة جرب ذو القوباء والحكّة.
آخر الصغير الالية. ܘܐܝܟ ܙܟܪܝܐ ܕܚܙܙ ذو القوباء. ܘܐܝܟ ܒܪ ܣܪܘ̄ܫ السعفة ܚܙ̈ܙܝܬܐ. ܚܙܙ ܗܘ ܐܬܪܐ
ܕܙܥܘ̈ܪܝ ܐܕܢܘܗܝ܂ ܘܐܝܬ ܕܐܡܪܝܢ ܐܬܪܐ ܕܕܢܒܐ ܐܠܝܬܗ. ܘܐܚܪ̈ܢܐ ܐܡܪܝܢ ܐܝܠܐ ܕܠܒܪ
ܒܙܥܘܪܗ ܚܙܙܝܬܐ الصغير الأذن܀

Ḥazāzi<u>t</u>ā according to bar Serošway, that which occurs on the surface of the outer skin, *tetter* (al-qubā), *ulcers* (al-saʿfa). *Ḥzāzē, tetters. Ḥzāzā, one suffering from tetter, itch, or mange. Ḥzāzā, ḥzāz, ringworm* (ḥazāz), *mange, one suffering from tetter, itch. Also, the small, the fat tail of a sheep* (al-ilya). According to Zakariya *da-ḥzāz, one suffering from tetter.* According to bar Serošway al-saʿfa, tetter (*ḥazāzi<u>t</u>ā*). *Ḥzāz*, this is the place of the smalls of the ears. And there are those who say the place where the fat tail of the sheep is small, and others say that which is on its exterior. *Ḥazāzi<u>t</u>ā, the small of the ear.*

It is of some interest, perhaps, that al-Biṭrīq used an Arabic word related etymologically to the Syriac equivalent, while Ḥunayn preferred a word from an entirely different root. This is the case despite the representation of *al-ḥazāz* in definitions of *ḥazāzi<u>t</u>ā* attributable to Ḥunayn in bar Bahlul's *Lexicon*. At least superficially, then, the Arabic translations of λειχῆνες represent a development away from terminological similarity with the Syriac.

38 Ullmann, *Wörterbuch zu den griechische-arabischen Übersetzungen*, 385.

39 Although several other entries for λειχήν and related words are noted in Duval's index, they refer to other senses of the term, so I shall not treat them here.

ἐξανθήματα

628:18 ܐܟܣܝܬܝܡܛܐ[40] ܗ̄ ܚܡܛܐ ܐܝܟ ܦܘ̄ البثر ❖

Êksānṯimaṭā, this is pustules (*ḥemṭē*), according to Paul, *pustules* (al-bathr).

Forms of this Greek word occur twice in the *Aphorisms*. Both Ḥunayn's Arabic translation and the Syriac version translate in the same way each time, the former with *al-buthūr* 'pustules' and the latter with *ḥemṭē*. These translations thus accord exactly with the entry in bar Bahlul given above. The early Syriac translation of aphorism iii. 20 gives a different word here, *mapqāṯā* 'eruptions of the skin'. This word figures prominently in the Syriac translations of the Greek word ἀπόστημα discussed above.[41] The entry in bar Bahlul for the Syriac equivalent *ḥemṭē* provides some additional information of interest:

758:5 ܚܡܛܐ وجدته الحصف. ܘܐܝܟ ܒܪ ܣܪܘ̄ ܚܡܛܐ ܕܗܘܝܐ ܒܠܡܦܬܐ. ܐܝܟ ܦܘ̄ البثر. ܘܐܝܟ ܒܪ ܣܪܘ̄
ܚܡܛܐ الحصف وايضاً قروح لم تنضج ܥܘܫܢܐ ܕܠܐ ܒܫܠܘ ❖

Ḥemṭē, I found it to be 'impetigo'. According to bar Serošway, *ḥemṭē* occurring on the eyelashes. According to Paul *pustules* (al-bathr). According to bar Serošway *ḥemṭē*, *impetigo, and also ulcers that are not concocted*, ulcers that are not ripe.

Two points of interest stand out regarding this entry. First is the repetition of Paul of Aegina's definition from the Greek entry above, which serves to emphasize again that material attributed to Paul occurs regularly in entries possessed of Syriac head-words. In this case, the Pauline Arabic definitions of the Greek word and its Syriac equivalent are identical with one another.

φύματα

1513:9 ܦܘܡܐܛܐ ܐܝܟ ܦܘ̄ ܢܦܩܐ خراجات❖

Pumāṭā according to Paul abscesses (*napqē*), *abscesses* (khurājāt).

Forms related to this Greek word occur several times in the *Aphorisms*. Both the translations of it in the Syriac *Aphorisms* and those in Ḥunayn's Arabic version of the work vary in their approaches to rendering it. The more common equivalent of the word in the Syriac version is *napqā* 'abscess', but the closely synonomous world *mapaqṯā* also may be found to represent it.

40 Duval: ܐܟܣܝܬܝܡܛܐ. Simply reading a *nun* in place of the *yoḏ* gives an exact transcription.
41 See unit (1.3.8).

Ḥunayn usually gave in its place *khurāj* 'abscess', but sometimes preferred *bathr* 'pustule' instead. In the extant examples of translations of this word in the early Arabic version of the *Aphorisms*, forms of *khurāj* are also employed. The early Syriac version of aphorism iii. 20 gives for φύματα a word with the consonantal skeleton *mg*ʾ, identified by Kessel as an *hapax legomenon*.[42]

Ullmann notes a variety of Arabic equivalents for φῦμα.Texts cited there from Ḥunayn's translations of Galen's *On Simple Drugs* Book Six likewise render φύματα with forms of *khurāj*. The equivalents given in the early Arabic version of that work attributed to al-Biṭrīq differ from those in the early Arabic version of the *Aphorisms*, however, in that they render φῦμα with forms of *waram* 'swelling' instead of *khurāj*. An example from the Hippocratic work *On Nutriment* translates φῦμα with *bathr*, while another from the Hippocratic *On the Nature of Man* gives for φύματα *khurāj*. Ullmann finally cites two translations from Dioscorides' *Materia Medica*. One of these translates φύματα with *al-khurājāt*, while the other translates that same form with the hendiadys *al-awrām al-khurājīya* 'protuberant swellings'.[43]

The definition attributed to Paul of Aegina in bar Bahlul's *Lexicon* notes the main equivalents for φύματα in Ḥunayn's translations and the Syriac *Aphorisms*. Somewhat unusually, however, I could find no entry in bar Bahlul's *Lexicon* Syriac that refers specifically to the sense of the main Syriac equivalent for φύματα, *napqā*. However, a few short entries in bar ʿAli's *Lexicon* do refer to it:

ܢܦܩ̈ܐ ܕܠܘܬ ܛܦܪ̈ܐ. البثر بقرب الاظفار.[44]

Napqē da-lwat taprē, pustules (al-bathr) *near the fingernails.*

ܢܦܩ̈ܐ. خراجات.[45]

Napqē, abscesses (khurājāt).

Although Ḥunayn or his students recognized the equivalence between this Syriac word and two of the three Arabic terms mentioned as translations of φῦμα in the sources mentioned above, when compared with the

42 Kessel, 'Sergius ar-Ra'sī', 3.

43 Ullmann, *Wörterbuch zu den griechische-arabischen Übersetzungen*, 747–8.

44 Gottheil (ed.), *Syriac-Arabic Glosses*, I 81:10.

45 Gottheil (ed.), *Syriac-Arabic Glosses*, I 81:13.

lexicographical activity for other Syriac words treated so far in this work, his extant treatment of *napqē* is very scant. The discrepancy is especially striking when the lexicographical material for the secondary equivalent for φῦμα, *mapaqṯa*, is considered.[46] This may indicate that Ḥunayn did not use this word often in his Syriac translations.

Conclusion

In Chapter Two, the absence of well-established Syriac technical equivalents for particular Greek words was shown to pose special challenges for Ḥunayn's Arabic translation technique. Building on this evidence, several examples presented in this chapter show the importance of Syriac lexicography as a scholarly locus for Ḥunayn's production of Arabic terminology. Often, extensive theoretical discussions in Syriac or broad-ranging excursions into the Arabic lexicon accompany Syriac words used as equivalents for Greek words in the *Aphorisms.* These Greek words, however, may be slightly represented in or absent from the lexicons. This is shown in the discussions of words like σῶμα (1., ii. 9), γνώμη (2., ii. 6), λέπρα (2., iii. 20), and παροξυσμός (2., iii. 19) above.

Parallel developments in Syriac and Arabic translation techniques may be observed when comparing the translations themselves. While it is still quite literal when compared with Ḥunayn's Arabic translation, the later Syriac version appears to be slightly more reader-oriented than does the earlier Syriac version. Ḥunayn's Arabic translation of the *Aphorisms* rather represents a movement towards both greater accuracy and greater ease of comprehension when compared with al-Biṭrīq's version.

At the same time, the development of these two languages' translation techniques displays some clear differences. In Chapter Two, I demonstrated the strong distinction between the Arabic and Syriac receptivity to Greek loan-words. In the present chapter, especially in the discussion of aphorism iii. 20, evidence of the progressive Graecization of Syriac vocabulary is observable in the higher number of Greek loanwords in the later Syriac version of the *Aphorisms* as compared with the earlier Syriac version. The later Syriac version and Ḥunayn's Arabic translation both display a higher

46 These entries are given in the discussion of ἀποστήματα in unit (1.3.7).

degree of sophistication when compared to the earlier examples of their respective traditions. Furthermore, given the background evidence available, both from Ḥunayn's *Risāla* and the material from the lexicons presented here, it is clear that Ḥunayn did not develop his Arabic translation technique in isolation from prior developments in the Syriac tradition.

The evidence presented thus far for Ḥunayn's Arabic version points to a combination of accuracy regarding the sense of the source-text combined with clear terminological influence from the Syriac scholarly background. The most obvious way to account for this is to posit that Ḥunayn produced his Arabic translation of the *Aphorisms* as an extension of his Syriac translation of the work. The material in this chapter thus specifies and emphasizes the importance of Syriac sources for Ḥunayn's translation praxis in the *Aphorisms* and beyond.

Chapter 4

The ʿAbbāsid-era Syriac and Arabic Translations of the *Aphorisms* and their Scholarly Background

In the previous chapter I compared the extant fragments of the early Syriac version of the *Aphorisms* with the translations of the corresponding texts in the broader Syriac and Arabic traditions. In this chapter, following a similar approach, I compare translations taken from the partially surviving early Arabic version of the *Aphorisms* attributed to al-Biṭrīq with the later Arabic version of Ḥunayn ibn Isḥāq and the ʿAbbāsid-era Syriac rendition of the work. Although the early Arabic version is of inherent interest in many respects, my primary intention in undertaking this comparison is to compare and contrast the techniques used in the Syriac translation with those adopted by Ḥunayn in his Arabic version in the light of the texts of al-Biṭrīq's translation. In doing so, the value of the Syriac *Aphorisms* for the study of the Greek-to-Arabic translation movement will be kept in focus. Because a much larger body of text is available from the early Arabic translation than from the early Syriac version treated in the previous chapter, it has been necessary to make a selection. I have chosen the texts presented below with the aim of discussing questions I perceive to be of interest for the study of these translations and their lexicographical background.

As discussed earlier, in the introduction to his edition of the Syriac *Aphorisms*, Henri Pognon contrasted the styles of the Arabic and Syriac translations contained in the Paris manuscript by describing the Syriac translation as more literal than Ḥunayn's Arabic version.[1] While including the early Syriac version in this type of comparison is difficult because of the paucity and brevity of the surviving fragments, the translations of the lengthiest lemmas of the *Aphorisms* survive from the early Arabic version, therefore allowing for extensive analysis. I have chosen a handful of aphorisms which I have found to be reasonably representative of the variations in style observable in the translations.

---

1 Pognon (ed.), *Une version syriaque*, iv.

Alongside a comparison of the varying styles and levels of sophistication of these translations, several themes and motifs prominent in earlier chapters of this work will be further extended in this one. Although I shall not be able to provide an exhaustive treatment of the lexicographical background for Ḥunayn's versions of these texts, I shall provide comparative studies for several terms of interest. In particular, key advances in translation technique, influential borrowings from Syriac and terms possessing extensive theoretical treatment in bar Bahlul's *Lexicon* will be given special attention.

Aphorism i. 1

(1) Ὁ βίος βραχύς, ἡ δὲ τέχνη μακρή, ὁ δὲ καιρὸς ὀξύς, ἡ δὲ πεῖρα σφαλερή, ἡ δὲ κρίσις χαλεπή.(2) Δεῖ δὲ οὐ μόνον ἑωυτὸν παρέχειν τὰ δέοντα ποιέοντα, ἀλλὰ καὶ τὸν νοσέοντα καὶ τοὺς παρεόντας καὶ τὰ ἔξωθεν.

P.

(1) العمر قصير والصناعة طويلة والزمان حديد والتجربة خطأ والقضاء عسير. (2) ينبغي للطبيب ألّا يقتصر على فعل ما ينبغي له أن يفعل دون أن يستعين بالمريض على نفسه وبمن يحضره وبالذين من خارج.

(1) Life is short, art is long, time is sharp, experience is mistaken, and judgment is difficult. (2) It is necessary for the physician that he not confine himself to doing what is necessary that he do without seeking the aid of the patient himself, those who serve him, and those who are outside.

S.

(1) ܚܝܐ ܟܪܝܐ. ܘܐܘܡܢܘܬܐ ܐܪܝܟܐ. ܙܒܢܐ ܚܪܝܦ. ܢܣܝܢܐ ܠܐ ܫܪܝܪ. ܒܘܚܪܢܐ ܥܣܩ (2) ܗܕܐ ܕܝܢ܆ ܠܘ ܐܢܬ ܒܠܚܘܕ ܬܬܠ ܢܦܫܟ ܠܡܥܒܕ ܐܝܠܝܢ ܕܘܠܝܢ. ܐܠܐ ܐܦ ܗܘ ܕܟܪܝܗ܆ ܘܐܝܠܝܢ ܕܩܪܝܒܝܢ ܠܗ܆ ܘܐܝܠܝܢ ܕܠܒܪ.

(1) Life is short, and the art is long. The moment is sharp. Experience is not sure. The crisis is difficult, (2) therefore, it is necessary not only for you that you give yourself to doing what should be done, but also he who is ill, those nearby him, and those outside.

Ḥ.

(1) العمر قصير والصناعة طويلة والوقت ضيّق والتجربة خطر والقضاء عسر (2) وقد ينبغي لك أن لا تقتصر على توخّي فعل ما ينبغي دون أن يكون ما يفعله المريض ومن يحضره كذلك والأشياء التي من خارج.

(1) Life is short, the art is long, the moment is narrow, experience is dangerous, and judgment is difficult. (2) It may be necessary for you not to content yourself with putting your mind to doing what is necessary without that (also) being what the patient does, or those who serve him likewise, or the things that are outside.

As by far the most famous of the Hippocratic *Aphorisms*, this text has received a correspondingly larger amount of scholarly attention. Most important for the purposes of this discussion is Franz Rosenthal's 'Life is Short, the Art is Long'.[2] Before proceeding to his overview of the Arabic commentaries, Rosenthal made some brief comparisons of the terminology of the three translations presented above. Most of his attention was given to the difference between the translations of the Greek phrase ὁ δὲ καιρὸς ὀξύς, for which Ḥunayn's Arabic version represents a significant advance in accuracy over al-Biṭrīq's. Rosenthal characterized this as an advance due to the fact that the Arabic *ḥadīd* 'sharp' does not carry the same idiomatic sense of urgency as the Greek ὀξύς does.[3] This account may be supplemented by remarking that the Syriac *ḥarrip* does carry this idiomatic sense, so the Syriac translation does not suffer from the same awkwardness despite its employing a broadly analogous technique.

The relative obscurity of the second half of the aphorism allows for the description of the varying approaches to handling difficult material observable in these translations. Of the three, Ḥunayn's translation is by far the most complex, and adds the most material. The early Arabic version adds some interpretative elements, but does not explicate to the extent that Ḥunayn's translation does. At the same time, there are some interesting overlaps between the two versions. In translating the verb παρέχειν, for example, both Arabic translators employed the same form of the verb *iqtaṣara* 'to confine oneself, to content oneself', although the contextualized senses of the word are slightly different between the two versions. In contrast, the Syriac version, which of the three follows the source-text most closely in general, preferred to render a much more basic and obvious sense of the Greek verb, translating it *teṯel napšāḵ* (*l-maʿbeḏ*) 'give yourself (to doing)'.

Although several of the lexical variations are interesting, the approaches to translating the Greek word κρίσις are of particular importance for our purposes. This importance derives from the fact that the Syriac translation of the word *buḥrānā* was borrowed into Arabic with the sense of 'medical crisis' in certain contexts, but was not used to translate other, more general senses of κρίσις. Here I shall consider the translations of this word along with their scholarly background.

---

2 F. Rosenthal, 'Life is short, the art is long: Arabic commentaries on the first Hippocratic aphorism', *Bulletin of the History of Medicine* 40: 3 (1966), 226–45.

3 Ibid., 227–8.

κρίσις/κρίνω

1844:1 ܩܪܝܢܘܢ ܕܐܢ يحكم:

Qrinon, to judge, to judge.

1844:9 ܩܪܝܣܝܣ ܐܝܟ ܒܪ ܣܪܘ̄ ܕܝܢܐ الحكم:

Qrisis according to Bar Serošway, judgment, *judgment*.

As one of the more important motifs of the *Aphorisms*, discussion of the prognostic construct of the crisis in fevers occurs in several places in the work. Forms of the noun κρίσις, the verb κρίνω, and various related words occur numerous times in the work. In all cases, the Syriac version translates these words with a form derived from the root **bḥr*, either the noun *buḥrānā* 'crisis' or the verb *bḥar*. Reference to the Syriac summary of Book III of Galen's *On Critical Days* attributed to Sergius of Res Ayna shows that these equivalents were well established long before Ḥunayn's lifetime.[4]

Ḥunayn's Arabic translation is less regular. Although the most common equivalent is the noun *al-buḥrān* 'crisis', either singly or, when translating verbs, with accompanying verbs such as *atā* 'to come', there are several exceptions. A handful of examples from the early Arabic translation of the *Aphorisms* also exist. The translations in that version tend to be based on forms related to the word *al-faraj* 'relief'. These are often extended by the words *qaḍā'* or *yaqḍī* 'conclude/judge'. For example, in aphorism ii. 23, the verb κρίνεται is translated by the phrase *yaqḍī 'alayhā bil-faraj* 'conclude with relief'.

Several of Ḥunayn's exceptions to these techniques deserve further scrutiny. Perhaps most interesting of these are the translations of the noun κρῖνον in aphorism v. 22. The relevant Greek sentence admits of multiple interpretations, and here Ḥunayn and the translator of the Syriac version have each chosen a different one. The Greek sentence and the two translations run like this:

τούτοισι τὸ θερμὸν φίλιον καὶ κρῖνον, τὸ δὲ ψυχρὸν πολέμιον καὶ κτεῖνον.

For these, heat is a friend and a crisis, but cold is an enemy and a harm.

S.

ܠܗܠܝܢ ܚܡܝܡܘܬܐ ܓܝܪ ܪܚܡܬܐ ܐܝܬܝܗ̇ ܘܩܪܝܪܘܬܐ ܒܘܚܪ̈ܢܐ ܕܝܢ ܩܛܘ̈ܠܐ ܘܒܥܠܕܒ̈ܒܐ.

For these, heat is a friend, but cold crises are deadly opponents.

4 E. Sachau (ed.), *Inedita Syrica*, (Vienna 1870), ܦܐ-ܦܕ, *passim*.

Ḥ.

فالحارّ لأصحاب هذه العلل نافع شاف والبارد لهم ضارّ قاتل.

For those suffering from these illnesses, heat is a benefit and a cure, but cold is for them a deadly harm.

The two translations clearly reflect different readings of the Greek text. Ḥunayn's translation of κρῖνον with *shāf* 'cure' reflects a reading close to that of the modern editions, with κρῖνον referring back to θερμόν. On the other hand, the Syriac text reads κρῖνον as a substantive introducing a new clause, and translates it with *bāḥurē* 'crises'. Furthermore, the Syriac translation renders the words φίλιον and πολέμιον literally, while in Ḥunayn's version they are given a medical interpretation. This example strongly contributes to the argument against Ḥunayn's authorship of the Syriac translation.

Another interesting exception to Ḥunayn's translation of κρίσις with *al-buḥrān* occurs in the aphorism under consideration here, aphorim i. 1. There both Ḥunayn and the early Arabic translator translate κρίσις with *al-qaḍā* 'judgement', while the Syriac translator's choice *buḥrānā* is consistent with his other translations of the term. In aphorism iv. 59 as well, Ḥunayn's translation of the verb κρίνεται with *takūn tanqaḍī* 'conclude' hearkens back to the preference of the older translator and contrasts with the Syriac translator's continued consistency expressed by his translation *meṯbaḥrā* 'come to a crisis'.

A further exception occurs in aphorism i. 19. At the end of that text the phrase πρὸ τῶν κρισίων 'before the crisis' is found. Although there is nothing in the text of the aphorism itself to suggest that anything other than the usual medical crisis is intended, Ḥunayn in this place gives *min qabl awqāt al-infiṣāl* 'before the time of separation', while the early Arabic translator gives *qabla an ta'khudhahum al-ḥummā* 'before the fever seizes them'. The Syriac translator again follows his normal technique, translating the phrase with *qḏām buḥrānē* 'before the crises'.

Although it has long been clear that the Arabic word *al-buḥrān* was borrowed from the Syriac *buḥrānā*,[5] the examples above show that the borrowing was quite limited in its grammatical scope. At least for Ḥunayn, *al-buḥrān* could only be used as a noun with the limited sense of 'medical crisis'. For the broader sense of the Greek term κρίσις, as found for example in the first aphorism, the Syriac borrowing could not be expected to be understood as an equivalent.

5 G. Cooper, *Galen, de Diebus Decretoriis, from Greek into Arabic* (Farnham 2011), 18.

Furthermore, although *al-buḥrān* could be employed in translations of the verb κρίνω, the term itself was never allowed to exert verbal force. Rather, auxilary verbs had to be used to support the sense. One might speculate that the inelegance of such constructions led Ḥunayn to prefer the Arabic verbal equivalent *tanqaḍī* in aphorism iv. 59, where the Greek source-text is very concise. These phenomena stand in contrast to the Syriac examples, where *bḥar/buḥrānā* was used to represent all of the complex senses of this Greek word. Ullmann's examples for κρίσις taken from the Arabic translation of the Hippocratic *Epidemics* likewise contain both of the main Arabic equivalents. In the first of these, *al-buḥrān* is given, while in the second, *waqt al-inqiḍā'* occurs instead.[6]

Even in this well-known and broadly accepted example of Syriac influence, close attention to the details of these translations suggests a nuanced account wherein the Syriac borrowing was forced to compete with other, better established Arabic usages. The combined circumstances of terminological instability in the Arabic and terminological stability in the Syriac clearly did make the borrowing attractive, but this was by no means a mechanical transfer from the Syriac lexicon into the Arabic. On the other hand, by resorting to the Syriac term, the Arabic translator introduced further complexity into his lexical apparatus. The effect of this was to eliminate the one-to-one correspondence between *bḥar* and κρίνω evidenced in the Syriac *Aphorisms*, and thus to reduce the degree of similarity between the source-text and the translation.

The two brief entries for κρίνον and κρίσις in Bar Bahlul's *Lexicon* presented at the beginning of this discussion refer only to the element of 'judgment' in the sense of these words, and not at all to their medical senses. Some relevant information is found in the definitions for the Syriac terms, however. The following entry is one example:

365:8 ܒܘܚܪܢܐ امتحان وأقول تبحّر تفتيش. ܒܚܘܪܘܬܐ استشفاف اختبار امتحان. ܒܚܝܪܐ ممتحن مختار
مصفّا منتجب منتخب. ܒܚܘܪܐ ناظر ممتحن مفتّش منتقد حزّار. ܒܘܚܪܢܐ ܐܝܟ ܒܪ ܣܪܘܫܘܝ البحران. ܒܘܚܪ̈ܢܐ
الامتحانات܀

*Buḥrānā, trial, and I say deep study (*tabaḥḥur*), inquiry. Bḥurutā, discernment, examination, trial. Bḥirā, examined, chosen, ordered, selected, elected. Bḥurā, observer, examiner, inquirer, assessor. Buḥrānā* according to bar Serošway, *crisis (*al-buḥrān*). Buḥrānē, inquiries.*

6 Ullmann, *Wörterbuch zu den griechisch-arabischen Übersetzungen*, 369.

According to modern standards of lexicography, the relationship between the words in the Arabic lexicon derived from the root **bḥr* and those words in the Syriac lexicon derived from the same is very obscure at the least. The Arabic words tend to display a relationship with the noun *baḥr* 'sea', while the senses of the Syriac words proceed from the verb *bḥar* 'to try (metal by fire)'. Developing from each of these two senses, however, both languages came to signify a certain similar concept, which we may call 'mastery of learning', with words derived from this root. The sense of the Arabic *tabaḥḥur* is that of learning as deep as the sea, while the Syriac verb may carry the meaning of expertise in a field of knowledge, such as is gained by intense effort and trial. The lexicographer's awareness of this overlap in meaning between the two languages is indicated in the entry at 365:8. Reference to this happenstance etymology could have served to suggest or to justify the borrowing of the Syriac word *buḥrānā* into Arabic.

Although Ḥunayn's use of the Arabic *al-buḥrān* to translate κρίσις is not reflected in the Syriac entries in bar Bahlul's *Lexicon* attributable to the translator, a definition from bar ʿAli's *Lexicon* does contain it:

ܒܘܚܪܢܐ. البحران والمحنة القضا تفتيش.[7]

*Buḥrānā, crisis (*al-buḥrān*), inquiry, judgment (*al-qaḍā*), discrimination.*

Aphorism i. 3

(1) Ἐν τοῖσι γυμναστικοῖσιν αἱ ἐπ' ἄκρον εὐεξίαι σφαλεραί, ἢν ἐν τῷ ἐσχάτῳ ἔωσιν· (2) οὐ γὰρ δύνανται μένειν ἐν τῷ αὐτῷ οὐδὲ ἀτρεμεῖν· (3) Ἐπεὶ δὲ οὐκ ἀτρεμέουσιν, οὐκέτι δύνανται ἐπὶ τὸ βέλτιον ἐπιδιδόναι· λείπεται οὖν ἐπὶ τὸ χεῖρον. (4) Τούτων οὖν εἵνεκεν τὴν εὐεξίην λύειν συμφέρει μὴ βραδέως, ἵνα πάλιν αρχὴν ἀναθρέμψιος λαμβάνῃ τὸ σῶμα. (5) Μηδὲ τὰς συμπτώσιας ἐς τὸ ἔσχατον ἄγειν, σφαλερὸν γάρ, ἀλλ' ὁκοίη ἂν ἡ φύσις ᾖ τοῦ μέλλοντος ὑπομένειν, ἐς τοῦτο ἄγειν. (6) Ὡσαύτως δὲ καὶ αἱ κενώσιες αἱ ἐς τὸ ἔσχατον ἄγουσαι σφαλεραί· καὶ πάλιν αἱ ἀναλήψιες αἱ ἐν τῷ ἐσχάτῳ ἐοῦσαι σφαλεραί.

P.

(1) عند تكشيف الصحّة القصوى أخطأ إن كانت في المنتهى (2) لأنّها لا تستطيع أن تثبت على حالها ولا تقيم على غير انتقال، (3) وإذا كان لا بدّ لها من الانتقال وليس تقدر على أن تنتقل إلى خير ممّا هي عليه فقد بقي أن تنتقل إلى ما شرّ. (4) من أجل ذلك هو أمثل أن تطلق الصحّة بلا إبطاء كيما يبتدئ الجسد

7 Hoffmann (ed.), *Syrische-arabische Glossen*, 81:2284.

بالتربية من ذي قبل. (5) وألّا يفرط في التنقّص فإنّ ذلك خطأ ولكن على قدر ما تحتمل طبيعة الذي يفعل ذلك به. (6) قال: وكذلك أيضاً الفرغ إذا بلغ المنتهى خطأ والملء إذا بلغ المنتهى خطأ.

(1) In stripping, extreme health is mistaken, if it be to the utmost, (2) because it is not possible that it can be established in its state, and does not remain without change. (3) If there is no escape for it from change, and it cannot change to better than that which it currently is, there only remains that it can change to that which is worse. (4) Because of this it is preferable that you disengage health without delay, to the point that the body begins with training as before. (5) Let it not be lax in diminution, for that is a mistake, but rather (let it be done) to the extent that the nature to which it is done can bear. (6) He said: And likewise, again, purging when it reaches the limit is a mistake, and repletion that reaches the limit is a mistake.

S.

(1) ܠܡܬܕܪܫܢܐ ܡܦܛܡܘܬܐ ܓܡܝܪܬܐ ܠܐ ܙܗܝܪܐ. ܐܝܢܘ ܕܒܣܟܐ ܐܚܪܝܐ ܐܝܬܝܗܘܢ. (2) ܠܐ ܓܝܪ ܡܫܟܚܝܢ ܕܢܩܘܡܘܢ ܒܗ̇ ܒܗ̇ ܘܠܐ ܕܢܫܠܘܢ. (3) ܡܛܠ ܕܝܢ ܕܠܐ ܫܠܝܢ ܠܐ ܡܟܝܠ ܡܫܟܚܝܢ ܠܡܬܩܕܡܘ ܠܘܬ ܗ̇ܝ ܕܡܝܬܪܐ. ܫܪܟܐ ܡܕܝܢ ܕܠܘܬ ܗ̇ܝ ܕܒܝܫܐ ܢܫܢܘܢ. (4) ܦܩܚܐ ܡܕܝܢ ܡܛܠ ܗܠܝܢ܆ ܠܡܫܪܝܘܗ̇ ܠܡܦܛܡܘܬܐ. ܠܐ ܡܬܡܗܠܢܐܝܬ. ܐܝܟܢܐ ܕܬܗܘܐ ܢܫܪܐ ܦܓܪܐ ܬܘܒ ܠܡܬܩܒܠܢܘܬܐ ܕܬܘܪܣܝܐ. (5) ܐܦܠܐ ܬܘܒ ܠܣܦܝܩܘܬܗܘܢ ܢܝܬܘܢܝܗ̇ ܠܣܟܐ ܐܚܪܝܐ. ܠܐ ܙܗܝܪܬܐ ܗܝ ܓܝܪ ܐܦ ܗܕܐ. ܐܠܐ ܟܡܐ ܕܡܛܝܒ ܟܝܢܗ ܕܦܓܪܐ ܠܡܣܝܒܪܘ ܣܦܝܩܘܬܐ ܥܕܡܐ ܠܗܕܐ ܢܝܬܝܘܗ̇. (6) ܗܘ ܗܟܘܬ ܕܝܢ: ܘܐܦ ܣܦܝܩܘܬܐ ܗܢܝܢ ܕܠܣܟܐ ܐܚܪܝܐ ܡܬܝܬܝܢ ܠܐ ܙܗܝܪܢ. ܘܬܘܒ ܐܦ ܡܬܚܕܬܢܘܬܐ ܕܬܘܪܣܝܐ ܗܝ ܕܒܣܟܐ ܐܚܪܝܐ ܠܐ ܙܗܝܪܐ.

(1) For those who exercise, complete fattening which is in the furthest extreme is unsafe, (2) for it is not possible that they persist in it, nor that they be still. (3) Then, because they cannot be still, and it is no longer possible to advance to that which is better, it remains therefore that they pass to that which is worse. (4) It is advantageous, therefore, because of this, not slowly to relax the fattening, until the body begins again to receive nourishment, (5) but also not to bring their evacuation to the furthest extreme, for this is unsafe. Instead, to the extent that the body's nature is prepared to endure evacuation, one should bring it as far as that. (6) Likewise, then, both evacuations brought to the furthest extreme are unsafe, and, again, renewed nourishment that is in the furthest extreme is unsafe.

Ḥ.

(1) خصب البدن المفرط لأصحاب الرياضة خطر إذا كانوا قد بلغوا منه الغاية القصوى. (2) وذلك أنّه لا يمكن أن يثبتوا على حالهم تلك ولا يستقرّوا. (3) ولمّا كانوا لا يستقرّون وليس يمكن أن يزدادوا إصلاحاً، فبقي أن يميلوا إلى حال أردأ. (4) فلذلك ينبغي أن ينقص خصب البدن بلا تأخير كيما يعود البدن فيبتدئ في قبول الغذاء. (5) ولا يبلغ من استفراغه الغاية القصوى فإنّ ذلك خطر لكن بمقدار احتمال طبيعة البدن الذي يقصد إلى استفراغه. (6) وكذلك أيضاً كلّ استفراغ يبلغ فيه الغاية القصوى فهو خطر. وكلّ تغذية أيضاً هي عند الغاية القصوى فهي خطر.

(1) Excessive abundance of body for the people of exercise is dangerous, when they have reached the furthest limit of it. (2) This is because it is not possible that they be stable in that state of theirs, nor that they be established. (3) Because they cannot be established, and it is not possible that they increase in health, it remains for them to tend to a worse state. (4) Because of this it is necessary to decrease abundance of body without delay, to the extent that the body reduces and begins to accept nourishment. (5) But one should not reach the furthest limit in purging it, for that is dangerous, but (purge) only to the extent that the nature of the body that you intend to purge can bear. (6) And likewise, again, all purging that reaches the furthest limit is dangerous, and again, all nourishment that goes to the furthest limit is dangerous.

This aphorism presents a relatively straightforward example of the different translators' approaches to rendering the lengthier prose sections of the *Aphorisms*. Although they display several notable variations in technique, Ḥunayn's translation and the Syriac version accurately communicate the meaning of the source-text. The early Arabic version, however, appears to suffer from a fundamental miconstrual of the Hippocratic author's intended subject of discussion. Despite this, all three display a high degree of consistency.

The two Arabic renditions overlap in some places. For example, in sentence (3), both Arabic translations render the verb λείπεται with the same word, *baqiya* 'it remains'. Ḥunayn's version tends to be much more fluid and concise, and to utilize a much greater variety of grammatical strategies to translate the text. In that same sentence, Ḥunayn used an inner accusative *(an) yazdādū iṣlāḥā* '(that) they increase in betterment' to translate ἐπὶ τὸ βέλτιον ἐπιδιδόναι, whereas al-Biṭrīq used a simpler verbal construction *(an) tantaqil ilā khayr* '(that) they change for the better' in place of it. Ḥunayn's version both translates ἐπιδιδόναι more literally and uses more elegant Arabic. To the final clause of this sentence, which in the Greek is a simple nominative construction, moreover, Ḥunayn added the verb *yamīlū* 'they tend to', while al-Biṭrīq simply repeated the verb *tantaqil* 'they change'. Although both made additions, Ḥunayn introduced stylistic variation, while al-Biṭrīq's approach employs stylistic repetition.

In considering the Syriac version, elements of the text tend to confirm Pognon's initial judgment that the translation proceeds in a more literalistic way than does Ḥunayn's version. One example of this is found in the translations of the verb ἄγειν in sentence (5). The Syriac version renders both of these in a very literal way with word *naytē* 'to bring', but neither Arabic version provides a literal translation of the first occurrence, nor any translation at all of the second.

Several terminological notes of interest may be made as well. Most importantly, the early Arabic version's translation of the Greek ἐν τοῖσι γυμναστικοῖσιν with *'inda takshīf* 'in stripping' is very obscure. Although this aphorism is only attested in the single Phoenix manuscript of Palladius' *Commentary on the Aphorisms*, some sense can be made of this reading in that the Greek word derives from the word γυμνός 'nude'. If this explanation holds or may be supplemented with other evidence, the word *takshīf* carrying this sense would be a significant new addition to the Arabic lexicon. Whatever the case, this is at best a very vague and unclear rendition of the sense of the aphorism. Ḥunayn's Arabic and the Syriac translation both render the word γυμναστικοῖσιν in a way closer to the mainstream interpretation of the aphorism as reflected in Galen's commentary on the text.[8]

The three translations of εὐεξίαι may also be fruitfully compared. The interpretation underlying the equivalent in the Syriac translation *mpaṭmuṯā* 'fattening' largely accords with Ḥunayn's rendering *khiṣb al-badan* 'abundance of the body'. Both of these, however, are both less literal and more accurate than the early Arabic version's *al-ṣiḥḥa* 'health', which is simplistic to the point of misconstrual.

The word with the broadest theoretical relevance by far in this aphorism is ἡ φύσις 'nature', which occurs in sentence (5). Here I provide below a study of that term as it occurs in the *Aphorisms* and the Syriac lexicons:

φύσις

1518:9 **ܦܘܣܝܣ** ܐܝܟ ܒܪ ܣܪܘ ܐܘܣܝܐ الأسّ الجوهر ܙܟܪܝܐ ܪܘܚܢܝܘܬܐ ܒ̈ ܩܘܡܬܐ ܕܒܪܢܫܐ܀

Pusis according to bar Serošway, essence, *essence, substance (*al-jawhar*)*. (According to) Zakariya, spirituality. In a manuscript, the stature of mankind.

1555:13 **ܦܝܣܝܣ** ܒ̈ ܟܝܢܐ ܘܐܝܟ ܒܪ ܣܪܘ الجوهر. **ܦܝܣܝܣ** الطبيعة ܘܬܘܒ الجوهر. **ܦܝܣܝܣܝܐ** ܟܝܢܝܐ الجوهريّ܀

Pisis in a manuscript, nature (*kyānā*), and according to bar Serošway, *substance (*al-jawhar*)*. *Pisis*, *nature (*al-ṭabīʿa*)*, and again, *substance*. *Pisisāyā*, naturalness, *substantiality*.

1588:15 **ܦܣܝܣ** ܐܝܟ ܒܪ ܣܪܘ ܐܘܣܝܐ ܕܡܕܡ أسّ الشيء جوهره܀

Psis according to bar Serošway, the essence of something, *the essence of something, its substance (*jawharuh*)*.

8 Mimura (ed.), *Tafsīr Jālīnūs*, I, 21–2.

Forms of the word φύσις occur several times in the *Aphorisms*. Ḥunayn's Arabic translation, the early Arabic version, and the Syriac translation all use regular equivalents to translate them. The Syriac version employs *kyānā* 'nature', while the two Arabic translations both use forms related to *al-ṭabīʿa* 'nature, character'.[9] Ullmann notes examples from other Arabic translations as well. All of these also use forms related to *al-ṭabīʿa* as well, except for two examples Galen's *On Simple Drugs* Book Six for which Ḥunayn uses *al-jawhar* 'essence' instead.[10] For one of these examples, the early Arabic version exists as well, and gives a form of *al-ṭabīʿa*. Thus Ḥunayn in this case moved away from what appears to have been a wide consensus preferring *al-ṭabīʿa* as the equivalent for φύσις.

The etymological patterns of sense-derivation for these words display some interesting features. The Greek verb φύω, from which φύσις derives, has several senses, including prominently 'to give birth to', 'to grow', and 'to become'. The Syriac *kyānā* is related to the verb *kān* 'to be', and so shares with the Greek term a similar sense-development. The Arabic *al-ṭabīʿa*, however, derives from the verb *ṭabaʿa* 'to stamp, to impress'. Its sense development is thus closer to that of the English 'character', which derives ultimately from the Greek χαρακτήρ 'impress, stamp'.

This etymological distinction has figured interestingly in at least one modern debate around language reform in the modern Muslim world. The following passage was written in Turkey during the twentieth century in response to the official introduction into Turkish of the neologism *doğa* 'nature', derived from *doğmak* 'to be born', as a replacement for *tabiat*, the borrowed Turkish form of *al-ṭabīʿa*:

> The Western languages have 'nature', which comes from a Latin word meaning birth. According to our belief, however, what is called 'nature' is not born but created, which means that this [word *doğa*] is wrong, conceptually and semantically. We cannot say *doğa*, for *tabiat* was not spontaneously born; it was divinely created.[11]

---

9 Although *al-ṭabīʿa* is usually translated into English with 'nature', and is broadly synonymous with that English word, I have sometimes preferred to use 'character' to emphasize the differing etymological senses of the various terms treated here.

10 Ullmann, *Wörterbuch zu den griechisch-arabischen Übersetzungen*, 750.

11 G. Lewis, *The Turkish Language Reform: A Catastrophic Success* (Oxford 1999), 115.

From the material considered here it seems that *al-ṭabī'a* was the established translation of φύσις from a very early date. However, Ḥunayn was perfectly capable of introducing new lexical approaches in his Arabic translations at least partly in response to etymological congruencies between Greek and Syriac vocabulary, as I have already shown in the discussion of the translations of λέπρα (3.2., iii. 20), for example. Furthermore, as I shall show below, entries for the Syriac equivalent *kyānā* demonstrate that the translators were well aware of Arabic equivalents which share a similar sense-development to the Greek and Syriac words under discussion. Not only, then, has the peculiar Arabic approach to the concept of 'nature' resisted change in modern times, the word *al-ṭabī'a* and its etymological derivation also seems to have proved resilient in the face of two of its most prominent intellectual forebears as well. The only exception to this is the Arabic word *al-jawhar*, which appears roughly to have a similar sense-development to φύσις and *kyānā*.[12] This usage is the only substantial evidence that Ḥunayn preferred an Arabic usage closer to the Greek and Syriac terms in question.

Entries for the Syriac equivalent *kyānā* in bar Bahlul's *Lexicon* provide important context for these translations. They also contain interesting material showing the prominence of Aristotelian logic in the Syriac scholarly background to the Syriac and Arabic translations of Ḥunayn and his successors:

888:18 **ܟܝܢܐ** ܗܘ ܕܩܐܡ ܠܢܦܫܗ ܘܐܝܬܘܗܝ ܡܩܒܠܢܘܬܐ ܕܡܕܡ الطبيعة الجوهر. **ܟܝܢܐ** الطبيعة الجوهر الطبع.
ܟܝܢܐܝܬ بالطبيعة.[13] **ܟܝܢܝܐ** الطبيعيّ الجوهريّ. **ܟܝܢܝܘܬܐ** الطبيعيّة. ܘܐܝܟ ܙܟܪܝܐ ܐܟܝܢ هيّأ وطرّز وكوّن
وخلق. **ܡܟܝܢ** يقوّم يوبّخ يعظ.

Kyānā, that which exists of itself, and is the receptivity of a thing, *nature (*al-ṭabīʿa*), essence (*al-jawhar*). Kyānā, nature, essence, character. Kyānā'iṯ, by nature. Kyānāyā, characteristic, essential. Kyānāytā, characteristicness.* And according to Zakariya *aḵin, to form, to style, to bring into being (*kawwan*), or to create. Mḵawwen, to correct, to reprimand, to admonish.*

At the end of this entry, a definition of the *ap'el* verb *a̲k̲in* attributed to the lexicographer Zakariya gives several Arabic equivalents. Among these we find the verb *kawwana* 'to bring to into being', the presence of which demonstrates

12 This word derives from the Pahlavi *gōhr*, which means 'essence' but may also mean 'bloodline'. It is related to the Sanskrit *gōtrá* 'clan'.

13 Duval: (*sic*) الطبيعة. For several places in the *Aphorisms* which the Syriac translates with the adverbial form *kyānā'iṯ*, Ḥunayn's Arabic translation reads *bil-ṭabī'a*, thus making this the best supposition for the otherwise strange collocation in this entry.

awareness of the etymological relationship between these Syriac and Arabic words. Despite this, again, Ḥunayn preferred to rely upon the previously-established equivalence between the Greek φύσις and the Arabic *al-ṭabī'a* rather than to seek a more semantically exact term by resorting to the resources of Syriac.

Another related entry runs as follows:

889:3 **ܟܝܢܐ ܡܬܘܡܝܐ** ܕܒܕܘܟ ܠܐ ܡܣܬܝܟ ܐܘ ܥܠܬܐ ܕܟܠ. ܐܘ ܣܦܩ. ܐܘ ܐܘܣܝܐܣ ܠܟܠ ܛܒ̈ܬܐ
الطبيعة الجوهر الازليّ وهو الله عزّ وجلّ. ܟܝܢܝܬܐ ܐܝܬܝܗ̇ ܗܘ ܡܐ ܕܐܝܟܐ ܕܐܝܬ. ܡܕܡ ܥܡܗ ܐܝܬܝܗ̇.
ܐܝܟ ܡܠܝܠܘܬܐ ܠܒܢܝ̈ܢܫܐ. ܘܚܡܝܡܘܬܐ ܠܢܘܪܐ الطبيعيّة. **ܟܝܢܐ** ܐܝܬܝܗ̇ ܗܘ ܡܐ ܕܩܐܡ ܒܝܘܬܗ. ܘܐܝܬܝܗ̇
ܡܩܒܠܢܐ ܕܡܕܡ. ܩܐܡ ܠܢܦܫܗ ܒܪ ܡܬܚܡ. ܡܛܠ ܕܡܬܦܪܫ ܡܢ ܓܘܫܡ̈ܐ ܕܠܐ ܢܦܫܐ ܠܢܦܫܗܘܢ. ܗܘ ܕܝܢ
ܕܡܩܒܠܢܐ ܕܡܕܡ. ܡܛܠ ܕܒܗ ܦܢܝܢ ܚܝ̈ܠܐ ܘ ܓܘܫܡ̈ܐ ܘܡܬܒܕܪܢܘܬܐ. ܡܬܬܚܝܡ ܕܝܢ ܐܦ ܗܟܢܐ. ܡܕܡ
ܕܩܐܡ ܒܗܘ ܘܟܠܗ̇ ܡܘܡܝܬܐ. ܗܘ ܕܡܘܡܝܬܐ. ܡܛܠ ܕܠܐ ܟܝܢܐ ܕܠܐ ܡܘܡܝܐ. ܐܠܐ ܟܠ ܟܝܢܐ ܕܐܝܬ.
ܡܘܡܝܐ ܕܝܠܗ ܦܝܐ. ܗܘܝܬ ܕܝܢ ܐܦ ܡܛܠ ܕܡܣܝܡܢܐ ܐܝܬܘܗܝ. ܡܬܦܠܓ ܠܐܪܒܥܐ ܦܘܪ̈ܫܢܐ. ܠܡܬܚܫܚܢܐ
ܘܠܡܬܪܓܒܝܐ. ܘܠܦܓܪ̈ܢܝܐ. ܘܠܡܫܚܠܦܢܐ. ܡܬܚܫܚܢܐ ܐܝܟ ܡܠܐܟ̈ܐ ܘܢܦܫܬܐ. ܡܬܪܓܒܝܐ ܕܝܢ ܐܝܟ
ܟܠܗܘܢ ܓܘܫܡ̈ܐ ܡܬܚܫܚܢܐ. ܓܘܫܡܐ ܐܝܟ ܟܝܢܐ ܐܝܬܘܗܝ ܕܗܘ. ܐܢ ܕܒܫܝܛܐ ܘܐܢ ܕܪܟܝܒ ܡܢ ܐܪ̈ܒܥܐ
ܐܣܛܘܟܣܐ. ܗܢܐ ܕܡܬܚܫܚܬܐ ܒܠܫܢܐ ܡܬܬܪܝܐ ܦܣܝܩܬܐ. ܘܐܘܣܝܐ ܕܡܬܪܬܝܢ ܡܬܩܪܝܢ ܠܗ ܢܚܘܬܐ.
ܢܚܘܬܐ ܐܝܟ ܚܕ ܟܝܢܐ ܡܢ ܟܠܗܘܢ ܟܝܢ̈ܐ. ܐܘ ܚܕ ܡܘܡܝܐ ܡܢ ܟܠܗܘܢ ܐܪ̈ܒܥܐ. ܐܝܟ ܦܠܛܘܢ ܘܦܠܛܘܣ.
ܗܢܐ ܕܐܘܣܝܐ ܡܪܚܒܬܐ ܘܡܕܒܪܢܘܬܐ ܩܐܡ ܠܗ ܢܚܘܬܐ. ܢܦܩ ܕܝܢ ܘܟܠ ܟܝܢܐ ܐܝܬܘܗܝ ܕܗܘ ܕܢܟܝܘܬܐ ܥܠ.
ܐ̄. ܗܘ ܕܠܐ ܢܣܒܐ ܒܡܕܡ. ܐܠܐ ܟܠ ܒܗ. ܒ̄. ܗܘ ܕܢܦܠ ܡܢ ܥܘܡܗ ܘܡܢ ܬܫܒܘܚܗ ܠܟܠ ܡܐ ܕܡܬܐܡܪ
ܟܠܗ̇. ܓ̄. ܗܘ ܕܝܢ ܕܢܣܒܐ ܡܦܩܘܕ ܗܢܐ ܡܕܡ ܕܐܝܬ. ܕ̄. ܗܘ ܕܠܝܬ ܠܗ ܕܠܡܘܡܝܐ. ܗ̄. ܗܘ ܕܠܝܬ ܒܗ
ܟܝ ܢܛܪܬܐ ܘܡܬܛܪܬܐ. ܘ̄. ܗܘ ܕܒܗ ܚܕ ܗܘ ܗܘ ܒܗ ܐܝܬܘ̈. ܘܢܣܒܐ ܡܩܒܠܢܐ ܕܩܢܝܢ ܕܠܡܘܡܝܐ.
ܘܐܘܣܝܐ ܕ ܓܒ̈ܐ. ܘܦܘܪܫܐ ܕܩܐܡ ܒܢܦܫܗ ܘܟܠܗ̇ ܡܘܡܝܬܐ. ܘܐܘܣܝܐ ܦܢܝܬܐ ܠܢܦܫܗ. ܕܡܓܒܪܐ ܟܝܢܬܗ
ܡܬܓܫܡܢܘܬܐ ܕܡܕܡ طبيعة. **ܟܝܢܐ** ܡܩܒܠܢܘܬܐ ܕ ܓܒܝܘܬܐ ܦܪܝܫܬܐ ܕܡܬܢܛܪܐ ܒܬܪ ܚܘܬܐ ܘܡܬܚܬܐ
ܕܡܬܝܚܕܬ ܠܐܘܣܝܐ ܡܢ ܡܣܬܥܢܘܬܐ ܚܝܘܬܐ ܕܠܐ ܡܩܒܠܢܐ ܒܟܠܗܝܢ ܡܬܓܫܡܢܘܬܐ ܗܝܘܠܢܝܬܐ ܘܡܣܝܡܢܐ
ܕܬܘܣܦܬܐ ❖

Kyānā mṯumāyā ('eternal nature'), which, in one place, is the Infinite, or the Cause of all, or the Sufficient, or the essences of all good (things), *nature (*al-ṭabīʿa*), the eternal essence, who is God, the Noble and Majestic (*wa-huwa Allāh ʿazz wa-jall*). Kyāniṯā* is that which, wherever something is, it accompanies it, such as reason for men, and heat for fire. *Characteristicness. Kyānā* is whatever exists of itself, and is the receptivity (*mqabblānā*)[14] of a thing. It is defined as self-existent

14 As a technical term, *mqabblānā* is somewhat difficult to translate. In direct conjunction with the word *kyānā*, the word refers to 'receptive nature' (*natura receptiva*) in opposition to 'effective nature', (*kyānā ma'bdānā*, *natura effectrix*). See R. Payne Smith, p. 3475. In that light, the discussion translated here would seem to place 'receptive nature' as opposed to 'effective nature' closer to 'nature' simply considered by identifying nature with 'the receptivity of a thing'.

because it is distinguished from the accidents which do not exist of themselves, and from that which is of the receptivity of the thing. Because powers, accidents, and actions exist of it, the thing which exists substantially due to it and on account of it is distinct from that which exists substantially (of itself). There is no nature that is not a substance, and each nature that is possesses substance of itself. Again, because it is an existent, it is separated into four types: The intelligible, the sensible, the general, and the particular. The intelligible is, for example, the angels or the souls. The sensible is, for example, the visible bodies. The universal is, for example, a nature, whatever it is, whether of men or of one of the other species, which occurs to the judgment exercised alone and simply. The wise named these conceptions 'essence' (*usiyā*). The particular is, for example, one nature out of all of the natures, or one substance out of all of the species, like Paul or Peter. The wise said of this that it is the vehicle and principle part of the essence. Accompanying and belonging to each nature, whatever it is, are six attributes. 1. That it is not in the thing, but all (of the thing) is in it. 2. That it gives from its name and from its definition all of what is said of (the thing). 3. That it indicates this thing expressly. 4. That it does not have that which the contrary has. 5. That there is not in it lack or excess. 6. That when it is one, at the same time it is. The receptivity of these is that which the contrary has, the common essence, the stature which exists due to it and on account of it, and the essence existing of itself, which is an indication of itself for the engenderedness of the thing. *Nature*. *Kyānā*, a state of generality that is near to (the state of) being understood in the mind. And in the reckoning of the sense[15] of the definition, an individual state that does not accept along with (the others) plural enumeration, nor, analogously, increase.

This entry displays clearly the importance of Aristotelian logic for the terminology of Syriac philosophy. Several elements of the unattributed, encyclopaedic definition strongly resemble discussions found in Aristotle's *Categories*, for example.[16] Thus, the Peripatetic account of the concept of 'nature' colours unavoidably the scholarly background to the Syriac translations of φύσις in the Hippocratic *Aphorisms*. In this way, the historical diversity of Greek philosophy collapses into a single Syriac idiom dominated by Attic and Hellenistic understandings of key theoretical concepts.

15 The sense of this is somewhat obscure. The word *haniyuṯā* (translated here 'sense') literally means 'pleasure, sweetness', which makes little sense in this context. For this reason I have translated according to the evident meaning of the passage.

16 Several Syriac translations of and commentaries on the *Categories* were performed at various stages between the sixth and ninth centuries. The study of this tradition has received important scholarly attention, notably in D. King, *The Earliest Syriac Translation of Aristotle's* Categories (Leiden 2010). According to King, Ḥunayn later composed a translation of this work, which is lost.

Finally, it may be remarked that the absence of an analogous Arabic text penned by Ḥunayn or one of his successors, coupled with the strongly independent cast of the Arabic equivalent for φύσις *al-ṭabīʿa*, indicates a certain degree of rupture even at the heart of the translation movement. Of course, Ḥunayn could not have foreseen the extent to which Arabic would come to dominate philosophical discourse at the expense of languages like Syriac over the following centuries. As this process continued, however, the important elements of the endeavour of Greek-to-Arabic translation that were written in Syriac came to be relatively inaccessible to many scholars who sought to use the translations as independent works. Lacking knowledge of Greek, many scholars must have remained generally unaware of the tension between the etymological senses of φύσις and *al-ṭabīʿa* and the implicit challenge represented thereby, for example. Yet even a passing acquaintance with the Syriac versions of Greek philosophical works could have afforded such scholars an opportunity to consider the significance of this terminological variation. At least in some senses, then, the transition from the bi-lingual Syriac-Arabic scholarly culture of Ḥunayn to the monolingual Arabic one of later centuries entailed a significant loss of intellectual and cultural wealth and value.

Aphorism i. 4

(1) Αἱ λεπταὶ καὶ ἀκριβέες δίαιται, καὶ ἐν τοῖσι μακροῖσιν αἰεὶ πάθεσι, καὶ ἐν τοῖσιν ὀξέσιν, οὖ μὴ ἐπιδέχεται, σφαλεραί. (2) καὶ πάλιν αἱ ἐς τὸ ἔσχατον λεπτότητος ἀφιγμέναι δίαιται χαλεπαί, (3) καὶ γὰρ καὶ αἱ πληρώσιες αἱ ἐς τὸ ἔσχατον ἀφιγμέναι χαλεπαί.

P.

(1) الأطعمة اللطيفة لطافة دقيقة جداً ليست تحتمل لا في الأمراض المزمنة ولا في الحادّة (2) الأطعمة التي أيضاً على حدّ اللطافة رديئة (3) مثل أنّ الملء[17] الذي على الحدّ الأقصى رديء يعني الممزوج.

Thin feedings of a thinness seriously thin and established are not borne, neither in chronic illnesses, nor in acute. Again, feedings upon the limit of thinness are harmful, just as fillings which are upon the furthest limit are harmful, meaning mixed.

S.

17 The ms. here reads *al-māʾ* 'water'. Biesterfeldt corrects to *al-milʾ* 'repletion', which is clearly preferable. However, it appears a later scribe added to the end of the aphorism the phrase *yaʿnī al-mamzūj* 'he means mixed' in response to the copyist's mistake, which then came to be integrated into the manuscript tradition.

(1) ܕܘܒܪ̈ܐ ܩܛܝ̈ܢܐ ܘܡܫܬܪ̈ܪܐ܆ ܒܟܘܪ̈ܗܢܐ ܐܪ̈ܝܟܐ ܒܣܘܟܐ܆ ܘܒܚܪ̈ܝܦܐ ܐܝܟܐ ܕܠܐ ܡܫܠܡܝܢ ܠܗܘܢ܆

(2) ܕܘܒܪ̈ܐ ܕܡܛܝܢ ܥܕܡܐ ܠܣܘܟܐ ܐܚܪܝܐ ܕܩܛܝܢܘܬܐ ܥܣܩܝܢ܀

Regimens thin and established, in illnesses of extreme length, and in acute where they are not appropriate; regimens that go unto the furthest limit of thinness harm.

Ḥ.

(1) التدبير البالغ في اللطافة عسر مذموم في جميع الأمراض المزمنة لا محالة (2) والتدبير الذي يبلغ فيه الغاية القصوى من اللطافة في الأمراض الحادّة إذا لم يحتمله القوة عسر مذموم.

Regimens extreme in thinness are a blameworthy harm in all chronic diseases without exception. Regimens that go to the furthest extreme of thinness in acute diseases, if they do not maintain the patient in strength, are a blameworthy harm.

The Greek text of this aphorism consists of three complete nominal sentences, the latter two compounded into a single sentence. The first sentence describes 'restricted and rigid' regimens of feeding as 'treacherous' in certain cases. Specifically, in chronic diseases (μακροῖσιν… πάθεσι) such regimens are called 'always' (αἰεί) treacherous, while in acute (ὀξέσιν) diseases they are called treacherous 'where they are not called for' (οὗ μὴ ἐπιδέχεται). The latter two sentences together make an analogy between regimens that 'reach' (ἀφιγμέναι) the states of being 'extremely thin' (ἔσχατον λεπτότητος) and 'extremely full' (πληρώσιες αἱ ἐς τὸ ἔσχατον).

Both Ḥunayn's Arabic translation and the Syriac version of this aphorism reflect a significantly different Greek text than that given by modern editors. Most importantly, the third sentence referring to 'repletion' (πληρώσιες) is omitted entirely. Notably, a sentence carrying much the same meaning occurs at the end of aphorism i. 3, discussed above. In Ḥunayn's translation, furthermore, the differentiation between the appropriateness of thin regimens for different kinds of diseases is made with two contrasting sentences, rather than a single sentence as in the Greek edition. The translation of the word 'extreme' (ἔσχατον) with the phrase 'the furthest extreme' (*al-ghāya al-quṣwā*) colours the qualified impermissibility of thin regimens in acute diseases, while in the modern Greek edition the word takes its sense from its opposition to 'extremely full' regimens.

The Syriac translation may be read either as employing an extended *casus pendens*, both clauses being predicated by the final word 'are grievous' (*'asqīn*), or alternatively as having suffered the loss of the predicate of the first sentence through scribal error. Importantly, the text follows the same general outline as Ḥunayn's Arabic translation in its omission of the third sentence. Unlike in

Ḥunayn's translation, however, the distinction between the appropriateness of thin regimens for chronic and for acute diseases is carried out entirely in the first sentence. In the notes to his French translation of the Syriac translation, Pognon speculates that the Greek manuscript tradition used by the translator likely did not include some parts of the text, in particular καὶ πάλιν and καὶ γὰρ αἱ πληρώσιες.[18]

The fact that both of the later translations appear to refer to the same variant of the Greek text would appear at first glance to give evidence that the two works were produced by the same author. However, the subtle but clear differences between the two versions substantially vitiates this line of argumentation. Given that Galen does not discuss the omitted sentence in his commentary on this aphorism,[19] it is possible that both Ḥunayn and the author of the Syriac translation each chose to translate in a way reflecting Galen's understanding of the text rather than to provide a more complete text along the lines of those preferred by modern editors.

Regarding the terminology of this aphorism, I shall now consider the scholarly background for the translations of the Greek word δίαιται with the translations of that word in the works under consideration here:

δίαιται (-ης)

559:16 ܕܝܐܛܝܣ ܗ̄ ܕܘܒܪܐ التدبير ✣

Diêṭis, this is regimen (*dubbārā*), *regimen (*al-tadbīr*)*.

Forms of this Greek word and the related verb διαιτάω occur several times in the *Aphorisms*. The instances of these words are mostly concentrated in Book One of the work. The Syriac version translates all of these with a form of the word *dubbārā* 'regimen' or the related verb *dabbar* 'to manage'. Both of the Arabic versions are less regular in their approaches. Ḥunayn translated these instances in two distinct ways. In all but two of these cases, he employed forms of the word *al-tadbīr* 'regimen' and the related verb *dabbar* 'to manage'. In some cases, however, he used an alternative word, *al-ghidhā'* 'feeding, nourishment', for example in aphorism i. 9. In the early Arabic version attributed to al-Biṭrīq, these Greek words are usually translated with forms of *al-aṭ'ima* 'feeding', *al-ṭa'ām* 'food', and the related verb *aṭ'ama* 'to give food'. In aphorism i. 16, however, the word *al-tadābīr* 'regimens' is employed instead.

18 Pognon (ed.), *Une version syriaque des Aphorismes*, ii. 4, note 1.

19 Mimura (ed.), *Tafsīr Jālīnūs*, i. 25–8.

There is a strong resemblance and clear etymological relationship between the Syriac equivalent *dubbārā* and Hunyan's usual preference *al-tadbīr*. However, the presence of this Arabic word's plural *al-tadābīr* in the early Arabic version of the *Aphorisms* demonstrates that it was used to translate δίαιται at an earlier stage of the translation movement. Nonetheless, it is possible that the very well-established Syriac usage evidenced both in the *Aphorisms* and in bar Bahlul's *Lexicon* influenced Ḥunayn's Arabic translations by making *al-tadbīr* seem a more natural choice. A brief entry for the Syriac equivalent further extends this pattern of agreement:

537:4 **ܕܘܒܪܐ ܡܣܘܣܝܢܐ** تدبيرات العليل الناقة أقول تدبير ترفّق. **ܕܘܒܪܐ** تدبيرات سير وأقول مذاهب وزاد المروزي إعمال. **ܡܕܒܪܢܐ** مدبّر سائس.[20] ܐܝܟ ܒܪ ܣܪܘܫܘܝ **ܕܒܪ ܕܘܒܪܐ** ܗܘ ܐܝܟ ܗܘ ܕܡܕܒܪ ܐܠܗܐ ܠܥܡܐ دبّر ܀

Dubbārā msawsyānā (caretaking regimen), *regimens (*tadbīrāt*) for the ill, convalescence. I say, caretaker's regimen (*tadbīr taraffuq*). Dubbārē, regimens, modes of conduct, and I say methods (*madhāhib*). Al-Marwazī adds practices. Mḏabbrānā, director, leader (*sā'is*).* According to bar Serošway *dāḇar, dubbārā*, that according to which God directs the people, *to direct.*

Aphorism i. 12

(1) Τοὺς δὲ παροξυσμοὺς καὶ τὰς καταστάσιας δηλοῦσιν αἱ νοῦσοι καὶ αἱ ὧραι τοῦ ἔτεος καὶ αἱ τῶν περιόδων πρὸς ἀλλήλας ἀνταποδόσιες, (2) ἤν τε καθ' ἡμέρην, ἤν τε παρ' ἡμέρην, ἤν τε καὶ διὰ πλείονος χρόνου γίνωνται· (3) Ἀτὰρ καὶ τοῖσιν ἐπιφαινομένοισιν. οἷον ἐν πλευριτικοῖσι πτύελον ἢν αὐτίκα ἐπιφαίνηται ἀρχομένου μὲν βραχύνει, ἢν δ' ὕστερον ἐπιφαίνηται, μηκύνει. (4) Καὶ οὖρα καὶ ὑποχωρήματα καὶ ἱδρῶτες, καὶ δύσκριτα καὶ εὔκριτα καὶ βραχέα καὶ μακρὰ τὰ νοσήματα, ἐπιφαινόμενα, δηλοῖ.

(1) الأدلّة على اهتياج الأمراض وإشكالها الأمراض أنفسها وساعات السنة وتداول الاهتياج بعضه بعضاً (2) إن كان يكون في كلّ يوم أو كان يكون يوماً بعد يوم وإن كان في أكثر ذلك يكون. (3) قال أبقراط: الدليل على حال الأمراض ما يظهر من لفظ الجسد فيها مثل من به ذات الجنب إن ظهر به نفث عاجل من أوّل المرض قصر مرضه، وإن ظهر ذلك متأخّراً طال مرضه. (4) والبول والبراز والعرق وإذا ظهر على الوجه الذي يجري عليه القضاء بالفرج أو على خلاف ذلك دلّ على قصر الأمراض وطولها.

(1) The indications of the excitations of diseases and their shapes are the diseases themselves, the times of the year, and the alternations of the excitations relative to one another, (2) if they are occurring every day, or occurring day after day, or if they are occurring [at intervals] greater than that. (3) Hippocrates said: The indication of the state of diseases is what appears of the emissions of the body on account of them. For example, in one suffering from pleurisy, if spittle appears

---

20 Duval: سايس.

quickly from the beginning of the disease, his disease is short, but if that appears in a delayed fashion, his disease is long. (4) And urine, faeces, and sweat, when they appear in such a way as to bring about the crisis or in an opposed way, indicate the brevity of the disease or its length.

(1) ܥܠ ܟܘܪ̈ܗܢܐ ܕܝܢ ܘܥܠ ܛܘܟܣܐ ܡܫܘܕܥܝܢ: ܗܢܘܢ ܟܘܪ̈ܗܢܐ. ܘܙܒܢܐ ܕܫܢܬܐ. ܘܬܘܣܦܬܐ ܕܚܘܕܪ̈ܐ. (2) ܐܢ ܥܠ ܝܘܡ: ܘܐܢ ܚܕ ܝܘܡ ܘܚܕ ܠܐ: ܘܐܢ ܚܕܐ ܠܙܒܢܐ ܕܝܬܝܪ ܐܪܝܟ ܗܘܝܢ. (3) ܐܠܐ ܘܐܦ ܐܝܠܝܢ ܕܒܬܪܟܢ ܡܬܚܙܝܢ ܐܝܟܢܐ ܕܒܕܘܪܬܐ. ܐܢܗܘ ܓܝܪ ܕܒܪ ܫܥܬܗ ܢܦܩ ܡܬܚܙܐ ܪܘܩܐ ܡܢ ܫܘܪܝܐ: ܒܪܝܐ ܗܘ. ܐܢܕܝܢ ܠܫܪܬܐ ܡܬܚܙܝܐ ܢܓܝܪܬܐ ܗܝ. (4) ܘܬܦܫܘܪܬܐ ܬܘܒ ܘܡܦܩܬܐ ܘܕܘܥܬܐ ܟܕ ܢܦܩ ܡܬܚܙܝܢ ܡܫܘ̈ܕܥܢ ܕܐܢ ܒܥܛܠܐܝܬ ܐܘ ܒܦܫܝܩܐܝܬ ܡܬܟܪܝܢ ܟܘܪ̈ܗܢܐ ܘܐܢ ܐܪܝܟܝܢ ܐܘ ܟܪܝܢ.

(1) The diseases are indications of paroxysms and orders, as are the times of the year and the intervals of the cycles, (2) if they occur each day, or occur one day and one day not, or are some time of greater length. (3) But so also is that which is seen afterwards, for example in pleurisy. For if simultaneously accompanying it spittle is seen from the beginning, it is short, but if it is seen at length it is long. (4) And urine also, and faeces, and sweat, when they are seen to accord, they indicate whether the diseases come to crisis with difficulty or with ease, and if they are long or short.

(1) إنّه يدلّ على نوائب المرض ونظامه ومرتبته الأمراض أنفسها وأوقات السنة وتزيّد الأدوار بعضها على بعض نائبة (2) كانت في كلّ يوم أو يوماً ويوماً لا أو في أكثر من ذلك من الزمان والأشياء التي تظهر بعد. (3) ومثال ذلك ما يظهر في أصحاب ذات الجنب فإنّه إن ظهر النفث فيهم بدياً منذ أوّل المرض كان المرض قصيراً، وإن تأخّر ظهوره كان المرض طويلاً، (4) والبول والبراز والعرق إذا ظهرت بعد فقد تدلّنا على جودة بحران المرض ورداءته وطول المرض وقصره.

(1) The diseases themselves indicate the paroxysms of the disease and its order and its degree, as do the times of the year and the increase of the periodic exacerbations alternating relative to one another, (2) whether they are each day, or are one day and one day not, or are greater than that in time, as do the things which appear afterwards. (3) An example of that is what appears in sufferers from pleurisy, for if spittle appears in them immediately from the beginning of the disease, the disease is short, but if its appearance is delayed, the disease is long. (4) And urine, faeces, and sweat, when they appear afterwards, may indicate the good or bad quality of the crisis of the disease, and the lengthiness of the disease or its brevity.

Several points of interest may be observed in comparing these translations. In translating ἀτάρ in sentence (3), each of the three versions takes a different approach. Due to the division of the commentary in which it occurs, the early Arabic translation resumes with ‘Hippocrates said’ followed by a restatement of the subject of the aphorism, thus adding an entire clause to the text. The Syriac interprets ἀτάρ in a relatively strong sense, reading the word as an indication of contrast with the first part of the aphorism, and thus translates it *elā wa-ap* ‘but, however'. Ḥunayn in his Arabic version interpreted this Greek word in its weaker sense, and so passed over it without giving a translation. This is another example both of the more literal approach of the Syriac version compared with Ḥunayn's translation and in general of the fact that the two translations often approach the Greek text in distinct ways.

Similarly, later in the third sentence, the Syriac again adopts a much more literal technique in translating the two verbs βραχύνει 'it is abbreviated' and μηκύνει 'it is prolonged' when compared with both of the Arabic versions. In the source-text, the subject of these verbs is not stated explicitly. In the Syriac version, the phrases *karyā-y* 'it is short' and *nagirtā-y* 'it is long' are likewise employed without the subject being made explicit. In both of the Arabic translations, however, the subject *maraḍ* 'disease' is introduced to specify the sense. Ḥunayn's uses of the inner accusative, for example in the phrase *kāna al-maraḍu qaṣīran* 'the disease is short', add a certain Arabic stylistic flair that is lacking in al-Biṭrīq's translations here, for example in the latter's corresponding phrase *qaṣura maraḍuh* 'his disease is short'.

The translations of δύσκριτα and εὔκριτα in sentence (4) are also notable beyond the phenomena I described above in the discussion of κρίσις in the context of aphorism i. 1. Al-Biṭrīq's version adopts a significantly different interpretation of the text in translating these words than do Ḥunayn's translation and the Syriac version. The Greek text proceeds by listing first three types of bodily excretions: οὖρα 'urine', ὑποχωρήματα 'faeces', and ἱδρῶτες 'sweat'. Following these, four qualities of diseases are listed: δύσκριτα 'having an ill crisis', εὔκριτα 'having a good crisis', βραχέα 'shortness', and μακρά 'length', which modify τὰ νοσήματα. All seven of these words are simply coordinated by the repeated conjunction καὶ. Following these are the plural participle ἐπιφαινόμενα 'appearing', and the plural verb δηλοῖ 'they show'.

Due to their having the neuter gender, there is no obvious reason to place δύσκριτα and εὔκριτα with either the words preceding or the words following them. That is to say, these two words could equally well be among the things that show, or the things being shown. Al-Biṭrīq evidently considered them to be among the things that show, along with the bodily excretions preceding them in the text. Ḥunayn's translation and the Syriac version, however, both interpret these to be among the things shown by the excretions. In doing so they follow the same interpretation as that adopted by Galen in his commentary on the aphorism.[21] In this case the earlier and later Arabic translations of the *Aphorisms* are distinguished by the fact that Ḥunayn translated according to Galen's interpretations.[22]

Whoever was the author of the Syriac version, in this case that text and Ḥunayn's translation are largely in accord regarding their following the authority of Galen. However, even here a certain difference between the two is noticeable. Ḥunayn's Arabic translates δύσκριτα and εὔκριτα more literally than does the Syriac version. The former translation renders these two with *jawda buḥrān (al-maraḍ) wa-ridāʾatih* 'goodness of the crisis (of the disease) and its badness', while the latter gives '*(en) ʿasqāʾiṯ wa-pšiqāʾiṯ mṯbḥarin (kurhānē)* '(if) the diseases come to crisis with difficulty or with ease'.

Having already discussed the lexicographical background for several of the terms found in this aphorism, including παροξυσμός (3.2., iii. 19) and κρίσις (above, i. 1), the word in this aphorism with the most varying and interesting approaches across the three versions is καταστάσιας. I shall consider here its scholarly background:

κατάστασις

1691:23 **ܩܐܛܣܛܣܝܣ** ܐܘܟܝܬ ܠܫܘܝܘܬܐ ܦܣܣܐ ܛܟܣܐ ܘܛܘܟܳܣܐ اعتداد قوام. آخر المرتبة الموقّف
ܒ̱ ܫܘܠܚܦܐ ܕܐܐܪ. ܘܬܘܒ **ܩܐܛܣܛܣܝܣ**. ܫܝܢܐ ܐܘ ܕܘܒܳܪܐ܀

Qaṭasṭasis, this is fitness, permission, rank, and arrangement (*ṭukkāsā*), *reliance, support. Elsewhere, degree, position.* In a manuscript, alteration of the air (*šuḥlāpā ḏā-ʾar*). Again, *qāṭasṭāsis*, peace or order (*dubbārā*).

1760:8 **ܩܛܣܛܣܝܣ** ܐܘ **ܩܛܣܝܣ** ܒܟܬܒ ܦܪܕܝܣܐ ܛܘܟܳܣܐ ܒ̱ ܫܝܢܐ ܐܘ ܕܘܒܳܪܐ܀

Qaṭasṭasis or *qṭsis* in the Book of Paradise, arrangement (*ṭukkāsā*). In a manuscript, peace or order.

1761:7 **ܩܛܘܣܛܣܝܣ** ܐܝܟ ܣܪ ܓ̱ ܛܘܟܳܣܐ܀

Qṭusṭasis according to Sergius, arrangement (*ṭukkāsā*).

1765:16 **ܩܛܣܛܣܝܣ** ܘ**ܩܛܣܝܣ** ܐܝܟ ܟܬܒ ܦܪܕܝܣܐ ܠܫܘܝܘܬܐ ܚܒܝܒܘܬܐ ܒ̱ ܫܝܢܐ ܐܘ ܕܘܒܳܪܐ.
ܩܛܣܛܣܝܣ ܗ̄ ܛܘܟܳܣܐ ܕܐܚܐ܀

Qaṭasṭasis and *qṭsis* according to the Book of Paradise, fitness, familiarity. In a manuscript, peace or order. *Qṭsṭāsis*, this is a fraternal order.

21 Mimura (ed.), *Tafsīr Jālīnūs*, I, 40.

22 For several more examples of Ḥunayn's translations and the Syriac version's use of Galen in their renditions of the *Aphorisms*, see Overwien, 'Paradigmatic Translator', 165–77.

Forms of κατάστασις and related words occur several times in the *Aphorisms*. The Syriac version of the work takes a largely uniform approach to translating these instances by employing forms of the noun *ṭukkāsā* 'arrangement' for κατάστασις and the related verb *ṭakkes* 'to arrange' for the verb καθίστημι. Ḥunayn in his Arabic version regularly adopted two different approaches for translating two different senses which these Greek words carry in the *Aphorisms*. For the sense of 'order of a fever', Ḥunayn basically employed the word *al-niẓām* 'order'. For example, in the aphorism under consideration here, i. 12, this term forms part of the hendiadys *niẓāmih wa-martabatih* '(the disease's) order and degree'. This translation may be contrasted with the early Arabic version's rendition *ishkālihā* '(the diseases') shapes'. In another aphorism, iii. 8, Ḥunayn translated two instances of the word ἀκατάστατος 'irregular' with *ghayr muntaẓim* 'without internal order' and '*ghayr lāzima l-niẓāmihā* 'without adhering to its order'. Κατάστασις also occurs with the sense of 'condition of the atmosphere' in other places in the work; for these, Ḥunayn employed phrases like *ḥālāt al-hawā'* 'states of the air', as for example in aphorism iii. 15.

The relationship between the standard Syriac equivalent *ṭukkāsā* and the entries for κατάστασις in bar Bahlul's *Lexicon* are of some interest, in that the former word is a slightly modified loan-word itself based on the Greek word τάξις 'arrangement'. The entries identified by Duval as relevant to κατάστασις for the most part define senses of the Syriac loan-word *qaṭasṭasis*, rather than senses of the Greek word itself. An important exception to this occurs in the entry at 1691:23. There, bar Bahlul refers to 'a manuscript' for the definition *šuḥlāpā ḏ-ā'ar* 'alteration of the air'. Considering that Ḥunayn showed a sensitivity to the difference between the medical and meteorological senses of κατάστασις in his Arabic translation of the *Aphorisms* while the extant Syriac translation does not, it is interesting to see a reference to this sense of the Greek word in a Syriac definition attributable to Ḥunayn.

The Greek entries identified by Duval are not strongly representative of Ḥunayn's Arabic equivalents for κατάστασις as given in the translator's version of the *Aphorisms*. The closest match occurs in entry 1691:23, where the second element of the hendiadys *niẓāmih wa-martabatih* is found. The translator's approach is better reflected in parts of bar Bahlul's entries for the Syriac equivalent *ṭukkāsā*:

793:17 ܛܘܟܵܟܵܣܐ ܐܝܟ ܙܟܪܝܐ التقرير التدبير. ܛܟܣ هيّا قرّر. ܝ ܛܘܟܵܟܵܣܐ ترتيب܀

Ṭukkāsā according to Zakariya, *establishment, regimen (*al-tadbīr*). Ṭakkes, to form, to establish.*

In a manuscript *ṭukkāsā*, *arrangement.*

807:1 **ܛܟܣܐ** ܗ̄ ܝ̣ ܦܐܬܐ ܐܬܐ ܗ̇ܘ ܕܗܘ ܩܐ ܕܩܒܝܥ. ܕܐܝܟ ܢܝܫܗ ܕܡܛܟܣܢܐ[23] ܪ̈ܕܐ. ܐܝܟ ܒ̣ ܟܝܢܐܝܬ
ܟܠܗܝܢ ܟ̈ܝܢܬܐ. ܘܡܫܡܠܝ ܠܬܘܩܢܬܐ ܕܐܝܟܢܝܘܬܗ ܕܐܘܣܝܐ الترتيب والرتبة. **ܛܟܣܐ** ܐܝܬܘܗ̄ ܗ̇ܘ ܡܐ
ܕܣܥܘܪܘܬܗ ܕܡܬܚܙܝܐ ܥܠ ܡܕܡ ܐܚܪܢ ܡܚܘܐ ܘܐܝܬܘܗ̄ ܫܘܡܠܝܐ ܙܕܩܐ ܕܐܝܟܢܝܘܬܐ ܕܐܘܣܝܐ
الترتيب والرُتبة. **ܛܟܣܐ ܕܕܘܡܣܛܝܩܘܢ** ترتيب الأمور. ܒ̣ ܘܒܐܓܪܬܐ. **ܘܢܟܦ ܘܡܛܟܣ** عفيفاً ذو مروة. **ܛܟ̈ܣܐ**
مراتب درجات رسّوم. **ܛܟܣܐ** منزلة رسم درجة نظام. **ܛܟܣܐ ܒܝܫܐ** منزلة سوء. **ܡܛܟܣܢܐ** ܙܟܪܝܐ مرتّب
معبّا. **ܡܬܛܟܣ ܐܪܙܐ** أقول ܐܬܐܟܠ جل. **ܐܬܛܟܣܝܘܗ̄** ܐܬܐܟܠܬܝܘܗ̄. **ܛܟܣܝܣܛܐ** ܗ̄ ܥܡܐ ܠܛܟܣܐ܀

Ṭeḵsā, a fitting aim that is established, which, according to the intention of the one who orders, proceeds for all things naturally, to the completion of the fashioning of the quality of the essence, *arrangement, degree*. *Ṭeḵsā* is something whose action indicates figuratively something else, and is the rightful completion of the quality of the essence, *arrangement, degree*. *Ṭeḵsā ḏ-ḏumesṭiqun*, *the arrangement of affairs.* In a manuscript and in an Epistle, *wa-nḵep wa-mṭakkas* ('chaste and orderly'), *one chaste and having virtue.*[24] *Ṭeḵsē*, *grades, degrees, limits*. *Ṭeḵsā*, *position, limit, degree, order (*niẓām*)*. *Ṭeḵsā bišā*, *an evil position*. *Mṭakksānā* (according to) Zakariya, *one who arranges, one who prepares*. *Mtṭakkas rāzā* ('the sacrament was received') *I say*, it was eaten. *Tṭakkesiw*, you ate it. *Ṭaksisṯā*, this is the people of an order.

In these examples, the presence of Ḥunayn's preferred Arabic equivalent for κατάστασις *al-niẓām* in the entry at 807:1 makes the Syriac lexicography much more strongly representative of the Arabic *Aphorisms* than the Greek lexicography. Again, the important evidence for Ḥunayn's Syriac activity in the entry for κατάστασις at 1691:23 is also the only information relevant to the atmospheric sense of this Greek term in the entries presented here. This again tends to indicate the importance of both Greek and Syriac in Ḥunayn's lexicographical work.

Aphorism i. 13

(1) Γέροντες εὐφορώτατα νηστείην φέρουσι, δεύτερα οἱ καθεστηκότες, ἥκιστα μειρακία, (2) πάντων δὲ μάλιστα παιδία, τούτων δὲ ἣν τύχῃ αὐτὰ ἑωυτῶν προθυμότερα ἐόντα.

P.

(1) الشيوخ يحتملون الصوم ويخفّ عليهم ومن بعدهم على الذين انتهى شبابهم فأمّا الأحداث فاحتمالهم له يسير
(2) والصبيان أقلّ احتمالاً لذلك ولا سيّما الأكياس منهم لكثرة الحرارة فيهم.

(1) The elderly bear fasting, as it is light upon them, and after them upon those at the limit of

23 Duval: ܡܛܟܣܢܐ.

24 1 Tim. 3:2.

youth, and then juveniles, whose bearing of it is slight. (2) Children are the least in bearing that, and especially the most appetitive (*al-akyās*) of them, due to the great heat in them.

S.

(1) ܣܒܐ ܛܒ ܕܠܝܠܐܝܬ ܡܣܝܒܪܝܢ ܨܘܡܐ. ܦܠܓܝ ܫܢܝܐ ܬܢܝܢܐܝܬ. ܠܥܕܘܪܐ ܛܒ ܒܨܝܪ ܡܨܝܐܝܬ.

(2) ܠܛܠܝܐ ܝܬܝܪ ܡܢ ܟܠܗܘܢ ܛܒ ܒܨܝܪ ܡܨܝܐܝܬ. ܘܡܢ ܗܠܝܢ ܐܝܠܝܢ ܕ ܠܒܥܝܐ ܕܡܛܝܪ ܐܢ ܐܝܟ ܡܢ ܫܘܝܐ ܕܒܢܝ ܩܘܡܬܗܘܢ.

(1) The elderly very easily bear fasting. The middle aged are second. Youths are less well-able. (2) Children are the least of all, and of these, those who by chance are of greater appetite than others of the same age.

Ḥ.

(1) المشائخ أحمل الناس للصوم ومن بعدهم الكهول والشبان أقلّ احتمالاً له (2) وأقلّ الناس احتمالاً للصوم الصبيان وما كان من الصبيان أقوى شهوة فهو أقل احتمالاً له.

(1) The elderly are the best of people to bear fasting, and after them the mature. Youths are less able to bear it. (2) The least able to bear fasting are children, and those children who are strongest of appetite are the least able to bear it.

The translations of this aphorism present a contrast between the Syriac translation on the one hand and the Arabic translations on the other. The Greek text is quite abbreviated. In the first sentence, the verbal phrase νηστείην φέρουσι 'they bear fasting' is modified by the comparative εὐφορώτατα 'best able to bear', which describes γέροντες 'the elderly'. The following phrases then compare the ability of people of different ages with this capacity of the elderly without restating any of the elements of the verb phrase. Instead, the adverbs δεύτερα 'second', ἥκιστα 'least', and πάντων δὲ μάλιστα 'least of all' refer the successive subjects back to the statement in the first clause.

The Syriac translation follows this approach closely. The main content of the aphorism is expressed in the phrase *ṭāḇ dalilā'iṯ msaybrin ṣawmā* 'very easily bear fasting', which modifies *sāḇē* 'the elderly'. As in the Greek, none of these elements are restated in the remainder of the text; rather, adverbs used as comparatives refer the subjects back to the first statement.

Both of the Arabic translations differ substantially from the Syriac version in their approaches to rendering this aphorism. In each of these texts, a form of the verb *iḥtamala* 'to bear' renders the Greek φέρουσι. Forms of this verb are then restated several times in the text that follows. In the early Arabic version, the verb is restated twice, and in Ḥunayn's version it is restated three times. Al-

Biṭrīq restated the noun *al-ṣawm* 'fasting' by means of pronouns like *dhālika*, and Ḥunayn's version departs even further from the Greek original by also repeating *al-ṣawm* itself in the second sentence.

Another example of the Syriac translator's greater concern for rendering literally each word of the Greek original may also be seen in these authors' approaches to translating the Greek τύχῃ 'by chance' in the second sentence of this aphorism. In fact, neither of the Arabic authors gave an equivalent for this word at all. The Syriac version, however, again translates it literally with *d-geḏšā* 'by chance'. Although the Arabic translators were not mistaken in regarding τύχῃ as a relatively insubstantial element of the Greek text, the presence of its equivalent in the Syriac version distinguishes the latter translation from the former two. Furthermore, a long, unattributed entry for the Syriac equivalent *geḏšā* in bar Bahlul's *Lexicon* helps further to emphasize the overtones of Aristotelian logic in the terminology of the Syriac *Aphorisms*:

453:19 **ܓܕܫܐ** عرض حتى العارض. **ܓܕ̈ܫܐ** ܕܒܢܝܢܫܐ **ܓܕ̈ܫܐ** ܠܡܣܟܢܘܬܐ ܗܘܘ܀ **ܓܕܫܐ** ܐܝܬܘܗ̄ ܗܘ ܡܐ
ܕܐܝܬܘܗ̄ ܒܡܕܡ. ܟܕ ܠܐ ܐܝܟ ܡܢܬܐ ܡܕܡ ܡܢܗ ܐܝܬܘܗ̄. ܘܠܐ ܡܨܐ ܕܢܗܘܐ ܡܦܪܫܐ ܠܒܪ ܗܘ ܡܐ
ܕܐܝܬܘܗ̄ ܒܗ. ܡܬܬܐܚܕ ܓܝܪ ܕܐܝܬܘܗ̄ ܒܡܕܡ. ܡܛܠ ܕܟܠ ܓܕܫܐ ܕܐܝܬ. ܒܡܕܡ ܐܝܬܘܗ̄ ܗ̄ ܒܟܝܢܐ
ܡܩܒܠܢܘܬܗ. ܗܘܝܢ ܐܝܟ ܕܠܐ ܡܬܬܐܚܕ ܡܢܗ ܐܝܬܘܗ̄. ܐܘ ܡܛܠ ܕܩܢܘܡܬܐ ܕܐܝܬܘܬܗ ܓܕܫܐ ܠܗ ܡܬܠܐ ܡܢ
ܠܡܥܒܕܐ ܡܩܒܠܢܘܬ ܐܝܬܘܬܗ. ܗܘܝܢ ܕܠܐ ܡܨܐ ܕܢܗܘܐ ܡܦܪܫܐ ܠܒܪ ܗܘ ܡܐ ܕܐܝܬܘܗ̄ ܒܗ. ܡܛܠ
ܕܩܢܘܡܬܐ ܠܗ ܡܢ ܗܝ ܕܬܗܘܐ ܠܒܪ ܠܡܥܒܕܐ ܡܩܒܠܢܘܬܗ. ܐܝܟ ܢܦܫܐ ܐܝܟ ܕܐܡܪ ܠܡܥܒܕܐ ܘܡܥܒܕܢܐ
ܐܝܟܐ ܕܗܘ ܒܐܬܪܐ ܦܐܝܡ. ܟܕ ܠܗ ܡܬܠܐ ܡܢܗ ܐܝܬܘܗ̄. ܘܠܐ ܡܨܐ ܕܢܗܘܐ ܡܦܪܫܐ ܠܒܪ ܡܢܗ̇, ܢܐܬ
ܕܠܐ ܒܗܝ ܕܒܥܠܐ ܦܐܝܡ ܠܡܥܒܕܐ ܒܐܬܪܐ. ܐܠܐ ܒܗܝ ܕܠܡܥܒܕܐ. ܒܗܝ ܕܠܐ ܒܥܠܐ ܐܝܬܘܗ̄ ܠܡܥܒܕܐ.
ܐܠܐ ܚܕ ܡܢ ܐܕ̈ܫܐ ܕܟܝ̈ܢܘܬܐ. ܡܬܬܐܡܪ ܕܝܢ ܐܦ ܓܕܫܐ ܗܘܝ. ܗܘ ܡܐ ܕܗܘܐ ܘܡܬܚܙܐ ܗܘܐ ܡܢ
ܣܘܟܠܐ ܕܗܘܐ ܒܗ ܗܘ ܡܐ ܕܗܘܐ ܘܡܬܚܙܐ. ܐܘܦ ܓܝܪ ܐܡܪ ܓܕ̈ܫܐ ܕܠܐ ܡܬܚܙܝܢ. ܐܝܟ ܐܘܪܟܢܘܬܐ
ܕܒܗܪ̈ܐ ܕܒܗܘܪ̈ܐ. ܐܠܐ ܒܬܪܥܝܬܐ ܡܬܬܚܙܝܢ ܐܦ ܗܠܝܢ. ܡܛܠ ܗܢܐ ܗܘ, ܓܝܪ ܕܝܕ̈ܝܥܝܢ, ܐܝܟ ܒܣܘܟܠܐ
ܠܒܗܪ̈ܐ ܝܗܘܒܐ ܘܠܢܦ̈ܫܬܐ ܐܘܟ̈ܡܬܐ. ܗܟܢܐ ܘܐܦ ܗܝ ܕܗܦܟ ܡܢ ܢܒܥܠܐ.[25] ܐܦ ܓܝܪ ܐܡܪ ܓܕ̈ܫܐ
ܕܡܬܝܕܥܝܢ ܠܡܕܡ ܕ̈ܓܕܫܝܢ ܒܗ̇. ܐܠܐ ܠܗ ܠܚܝܠܐ ܡܬܝܕܥܝܢ. ܐܠܐ ܠܡܚܙܐ ܓܒܐ ܐܘ ܠܓܫܝܫܘܬܐ ܐܘ
ܠܛܥܡܘܬܐ. ܐܘ ܠܣܪܝܐ ܡܢ ܐܝܠܝܢ ܕܝܬܒܝܢ ܠܥܝܢܐ. ܥܝܢܐ ܓܝܪ ܚܙܐ ܡܢ ܐܝܟ ܠܐ ܡܨܐ ܕܬܬܝܕܥ. ܡܬܬܐܡܪ
ܕܝܢ ܓܕܫܐ ܐܦ ܗܟܢܐ. ܗܘ ܕܠܐ ܩܝܡ ܒܩܢܘܡܗ ܕܢܦܫܗ. ܘܠܒܪ ܡܢܗ, ܡܩܒܠܢܐ ܕܡܕܡ. ܡܬܬܐܡܪ ܓܝܪ ܕܠܐ
ܦܐܝܡ ܠܢܦܫܗ ܘܠܐ ܡܩܒܠ ܠܡܕܡ ܕܢܬܦܪܫ ܡܢ ܚܝܠܐ ܕܦܐܝܡ ܠܢܦܫܗ ܘܡܩܒܠ ܠܡܕܡ ܕܡܬܬܚܫܒ ܠܗ
ܕܠܡܫܠܡܘܬ ܒܐܘܣܝܐ. ܐܟܚܕܐ ܕܡܬܦܪܫ ܠܗ ܕܠܡܫܠܡܘܬ ܒܬܪܥܝܬܐ. ܡܬܬܐܡܪ ܓܝܪ ܓܕܫܐ ܐܦ
ܗܟܢܐ. ܗܘ ܡܐ ܕܠܐ ܓܒܝܐ ܐܝܬܘܗ̄ ܘܠܐ ܐܕ̈ܫܐ ܘܠܐ ܦܘܪ̈ܫܢܐ ܘܠܐ ܕܝܠܝܬܐ. ܘܐܝܬܘܗ̄ ܡܩܒܠܢܐ ܒܟܠܗܝܢ
ܒܡܕܡ ܐܚܪܝܢ. ܘܡܬܦܠܓ ܕܝܢ ܠܬܫܥܐ ܦܘܪ̈ܫܢܐ. ܠܡܬܝܕ̈ܥܢܐ ܘܠܡܬܐ ܓܕ̈ܫܐ. ܠܥ̈ܠܬܐ ܘܠܫܘ̈ܚܠܦܐ.
ܘܠܐܘܚܕܢܐ ܘܠܕܠܐ ܡܚܝܠܐ. ܡܬܝܕ̈ܥܢܐ ܐܝܟ ܣܘܓܐܐ ܘܒܨܝܪܘܬܐ ܘܦܪܝܫܘܬܐ ܘܚܒܝܫܘܬܐ

25 Duval: ܢܒܥܠܐ.

ܘܣܟܠܘܬܐ ܘܟܠܗܘܢ ܐܝܠܝܢ ܕܒܢܦܫܐ ܐܝܬܝ̈ܗ ܩܘܝܡܗܘܢ ܕܝܠܗܘܢ. ܡܬܪ̈ܓܫܢܐ ܐܝܟ ܟܠ ܕܠܚܘܫܐ ܗ̈ ܓܫܐ
ܡܬܬܚܕܢ. ܓܘܢܐ ܐܘܡܪ ܐܝܟ ܘܩܠ̈ܐ ܘܪ̈ܝܚܐ ܘܛܥܡܐ ܘܡܓܫ̈ܐ ܟܠܗܘܢ ܀ ܕ ܓܒܬܐ. ܓܘ̈ܢܝܐ ܐܝܟ ܟܠܗ
ܐܢܫܘܬܐ ܘܟܠܗ̇ ܐܘܟܡܘܬܐ. ܡܢܬ̈ܢܝܐ ܐܝܟ ܐܢܫܘܬܐ ܕܦܠܛܘܢ. ܐܘ ܐܘܟܡܘܬܐ ܕܟܘܫܝܬܐ. ܕܡܫܬܚܠܦܢܐ
ܐܝܟ ܝܥܩ̈ܬܐ ܕܗܘܦܟܐ ܘܡܬܚܘܪܢܐ ܐܘ ܥܘܬܪ ܓܘܢܐ ܕܡܢ ܕܒܠܬܐ ܐܘ ܐܘܟܡܘܬܐ ܕܡܢ ܥܡܩܐ. ܕܠܐ
ܡܫܬܚܠܦܢܐ ܐܝܟ ܐܘܟܡܘܬܐ ܕܥܘܪ̈ܒܐ ܘܕܟܘ̈ܫܝܐ. ܗܠܝܢ ܕܐܦ ܒܢܝ̈ܐ ܡܫܬܡܗܝܢ ܐܘ ܥܘܫܬܐ ܕܡܬܦܪܫܢܐ
ܒܚܘܫܒܐ ܕܠܐ ܡܬܦܪܫܐ ܡܢܗ العَرَض܀

Geḏšā, *accident.* In a manuscript, *accidental.* Again, *gaḏšan* is masculine, and *gḏašen* is feminine. *Geḏšā* is that which is in a thing, but the form of that thing does not derive from it, and it is not possible that it subsist without the thing in which it is. It is thus restricted to being in some thing, for each accident that is, is in a thing which is receptive of it by nature, and whose form does not derive from it. It is thus, because whiteness, which is an accident, is not a part of the body containing it, and because it is not possible that it subsist without that in which it is. For it is not possible that whiteness subsist without a body to contain it. If someone says that a body or a substance, wherever it is, subsists in a place, when it is not part of (the place), and it is not possible that it subsist without (the place), he knows that that body does not subsist in that place by nature, but by virtue of that in the body which is not essential, and which is rather one of the types of quantity. Accident is thus defined in this way: That which may be thus separated without destruction of that in which it is, that which is and is separable. For though there are accidents that are not separable, like the blackness of ravens or of Cushites, they are (in fact) separable in the mind, as it is possible for people to imagine a white raven or black milk.[26] Thus this is without destruction. For if there were accidents (whose removal) would destroy the thing in which they occurred, but did not destroy the essence, but (only) the mixture or the embodiment or the surface, or one of the things that accompanies the essence, it is not possible that essence be destroyed in one of these ways. Accident is thus defined in this way: That which does not possess substance of itself, and is not the receptivity of the thing. For it is established that it does not exist of itself, nor does it receive the thing that is separate from the essence, which does exist of itself and does receive the thing of which it is stated to be receptive by definition, as it is so distinguished to be receptive by the judgment. Accident is thus defined in this way: That which is not a kind, nor a type, nor a form, nor a property, and which has its subsistence at all times in another thing. It is then separated into six types: The intelligibles and the sensibles, the generalities and the particulars, and the mutables and the immutables. The intelligibles (are things) like wisdom and ignorance, good and evil, righteousness and sinfulness, and all those things which properly have their

26 The white raven is a common example in Aristotelian logic, for example in the *Prior Analytics*, 27ᵇ5.

existence in the soul. The sensibles (are things) like all that stimulates the five senses, I say the colours, sound, smells, taste and all the varieties of touch. The generalities (are things) like all whiteness and all blackness. The particulars (are things) like the white which is in snow, or the black which is in ink. The mutables (are things) like a fever which is and is separable, or a change of colour due to fear, or the darkening of the Sun. The immutables (are things) like the blackness of a raven or of a Cushite, which are designated by nature, or a scar which is fixed upon the body, which does not change on account of it. *Accidents (*al-ʿaraḍ*).*

As King indicates in his glossary, *gedšā* was the Syriac equivalent for the Greek logical term συμβεβηκός 'accident' from an early stage.[27] While it clearly relies upon an Aristotelian conceptual framework and has Peripatetic overtones, the details of the entry do not readily appear to match exactly those found in any specific work of Aristotle. Furthermore, the presence of phrases like 'I say' (*āmar-nā*) indicate that this is an independent composition. Although due to its being unattributed to any author it is possible to attribute its authorship to Ḥunayn, comparison of the style and language to other of his Syriac works would be desirable for making a firm judgment on the question.

Aphorism iii. 1

(1) Αἱ μεταβολαὶ τῶν ὡρέων μάλιστα τίκτουσι νοσήματα (2) καὶ ἐν τῇσιν ὥρῃσιν αἱ μεγάλαι μεταλλαγαὶ ἢ ψύξιος ἢ θάλψιος (3) καὶ τὰ ἄλλα κατὰ λόγον οὕτως.

S.[28]

(1) ܫܘܚܠܦܝܗܘܢ ܕܙܒܢܐ ܕܫܢܬܐ ܠܚܕ ܝܬܝܪܐܝܬ ܡܘܠܕܝܢ ܟܘܪܗܢܐ. (2) ܘܗܟܘܢ ܒܙܒܢܐ ܕܫܢܬܐ

ܡܫܚܠܦܢܘܬܐ ܪܘܪܒܬܐ ܕܩܘܪܝܘܬܐ ܐܘ ܕܫܚܝܢܘܬܐ (3) ܘܗܢܝܢ ܕܫܪܟܐ ܦܚܡܐܝܬ.

(1) The alterations of the times of the year very often beget diseases, (2) and great variations of cold or heat in the times of the year, (3) and those of the others analogously.

Ḥ.

(1) إنّ انقلاب أوقات السنة ممّا يعمل في توليد الأمراض خاصّة، (2) وفي الوقت الواحد منها التغيّر الشديد في البرد أو في الحرّ، (3) وكذلك في سائر الحالات على هذا القياس.

(1) The alternation of the times of the year is one of the things that especially affects the generation of diseases, (2) and in one of these times severe changes in cold or heat, (3) and likewise for the remaining conditions in an analogous way.

---

27 King, *Earliest Syriac Translation*, 306.

28 Due to a lacuna in Houtsma's text of al-Biṭrīq's translation of this aphorism, I have placed the early Arabic translation last.

P.

(1) انقلاب الساعات [.........] (2) عن عظم البرد والحرّ (3) وغير ذلك ممّا يجرى مجراه أى انقلاب ساعات الزمان من اجزاء السنة.

(1) The alteration of the hours... (2) from the magnitude of cold, or hot, (3) or others of those that follow the same course (*yajrī majrāhu*), that is, the alteration of the hours of the time of the parts of the year.

The manuscript of the Arabic Palladius ends with aphorism ii. 19. For aphorisms that follow, then, our only source for al-Biṭrīq's translation is the *History* of al-Yaʿqūbī, as described in the Introduction. The text of the lemmas as found in Houtsma's edition has suffered some attrition, and they tend to be less reliable than those found in the Arabic Palladius. Despite this, it is still possible to draw interesting conclusions from them regarding the variety of approaches adopted in rendering the *Aphorisms* into Arabic.

When comparing the three versions of aphorism iii. 1 presented above, a picture that should be by now somewhat familiar emerges. Even considering the important lacuna in Houtsma's edition of the *History*, it is clear that al-Biṭrīq's translation of the aphorism suffers from a lack of clarity. The explanation of the sense of the aphorism found at the end of the translation, 'that is, the alteration of the hours of the time of the parts of the year', whether added by the translator, al- Yaʿqūbī, or some intermediary scribe, reflects nothing in the original Greek. It appears, however, that its addition was seen as a helpful supplement to the text of the translation itself.

Although the Syriac translation faithfully renders the Greek aphorism, it also reflects the source-text's quite concise character. This technique may be compared with the more expansive approach adopted by Ḥunayn in his Arabic version. For example, in the first clause of the aphorism, both the Greek and the Syriac version rather straightforwardly state the subject under discussion. First, each gives the subject 'the changes of the seasons' (Αἱ μεταβολαὶ τῶν ὡρέων, *šuḥlapayhon d-zabnē d-šattā*), then the verb 'beget' (τίκτουσι, *mwalldin*) modified by the adverb 'often' (μάλιστα, *ṭāb ittirāʾit*), and then the object 'diseases' (νοσήματα, *kurhānē*). The word order of the Syriac version thus follows the source-text exactly with barely anything added or removed.

This is not the case in Ḥunayn's Arabic translation, however. There, the single verb τίκτουσι is rendered with a more complex phrase *mimmā yaʿmal fī tawlīd (al-amrāḍ)* 'is one of the things that affect the generation (of diseases)'.

Furthermore, rather than adopting a similarly straightforward approach to translating μάλιστα to that of the Syriac version, Ḥunayn rendered this word with the adverb *khāṣṣatan* 'especially'. This type of distinction between the two versions is also evident in the translations of τὰ ἄλλα in the final clause. The Syriac version rendered this phrase literally with *hānēn d-šarkā* 'the others', while Ḥunayn explicated, using *fī sā'ir al-ḥālāt* 'for the remaining conditions'.

Beyond this, the phrase κατὰ λόγον in clause three of the aphorism affords the opportunity to consider the translations of the word λόγος in the context of these translations of the *Aphorisms* and their scholarly background.

λόγος/λόγια/λογισμός

947:9 ܠܘܓܘܣ ܡܐܡܪܐ قول كلام. ܠܘܓܘܣ ܗ̄ ܠܥܣܩ الغاية.❖

Logos, speech, *saying, speech*. *Logos*, this is 'with difficulty', *extremity.*

947:21 ܠܘܓܝܘܣ ܡ̈ܠܐ الكلام❖

Logios, words, *speech.*

948:10 ܠܘܓܘܣ ܘܠܘܓܝܐ ܐܝܟ ܝܘܢܝܐ ܡܠܬܐ ܡܬܦܫܩ ܐܝܟ ܣܘܪ̈ܝܝܐ. ܡܬܬܣܝܡܐ ܕܝܢ ܘܠܘ ܓܝܐ
ܒܝܘܢܝܐ ܒܙܢ̈ܝܐ ܣܓܝ̈ܐܐ. ܡܫܡܠܐ ܓܝܪ ܠܬܚܘܡܐ ܠܥܠܬܐ ܕܡܕܡ. ܘܠܡܠܬܐ ܢܦܘܩܬܐ ܕܡܢ ܦܘܡܐ
ܘܠܡܠܠܘܬܐ ܕܢܦܫܐ. ܘܠܗܝܡܢܘܬܐ ܕܝܗܒܝܢ ܒܢ̈ܝ ܐܢܫܐ ܠܚ̈ܕܕܐ. ܘܠܡܢܬܐ ܕܡܬܦܠܓܐ ܠܐܢܫ ܡܢ ܡܕܡ.
[ܘ]ܠܟܢܘܫܝܐ ܕܪ̈ܥܝܢܐ ܣܓܝ̈ܐܐ الكلام❖

Logos and *logia* in Greek are defined as is *mellṯā* 'word' in Syriac, for both it and *logia* in Greek are understood in many ways. It signifies the definition of the cause of a thing, the word uttered from the mouth, and the reasoning of the soul, as well as the trust men give to one another, the portion that divides a person from a thing, [and] the gathering of many minds, *speech (*al-kalām*).*

947:8 ܠܘܓܝܐ ܡܠܬܐ الكلام المنطق❖

Logya, word, *speech, logic (*al-manṭiq*).*

947:11 ܠܘܓܝܣܡܘܣ قياس المنطق فكرة ܚܘܫܒܐ قلب فكر❖

Logismos, *reason (*qiyās*), logic (*al-manṭiq*), thought,* thought, *heart, thinking.*

The Greek text of the *Aphorisms* contains approximately eight uses of forms of the word λόγος in various phrases and compounds, as well as one use of the related word λογισμός. The Syriac translation of the work uses three main approaches to rendering these nine instances, each of which has distinct treatment in bar Bahlul's *Lexicon*. I shall structure this discussion around these three translations and the relevant lexicographical material .

In aphorism ii. 27, the word λόγος occurs in the phrase τοῖσι μὴ κατὰ λόγον κουφίζουσιν 'those lightenings (of the disease) that are not usual (lit. not according to reason)'. The Syriac translation renders μὴ κατὰ λόγον with *law b-wālitā* 'not suitable', while Ḥunayn's Arabic translation gives *bi-khilāf al-qiyās* 'against reason'. In this case, the two translations differ significantly in their interpretation of the Greek source-text, with Ḥunayn's translation being somewhat more literal than the Syriac version. Two successive entries in bar Bahlul's *Lexicon* relevant to *wālitā* read like this:

665:17 **ܘܳܠܶܐ** ينبغي يجب ܡܬܚܫܒ ܙܳܕܶܩ ❖

*Wālē, to be appropriate (*yanbaghī*), to be necessary (*yajib*),* it is incumbent, it is necessary (*zādeq*).

665:18 **ܘܳܠܺܝܬܳܐ** واجبة. ܘܳܠܝܳܐܺܝܬ ܐܝܟ ܚܢܝܢ كما جاء به في موضع أجود و هو عندي الانفعال بالواجب ܒ
ܘܳܠܺܝܬܳܐ ܙܕܩܐ ❖

*Wālitā, necessary (*awjaba*). Wālyā'it* according to Ḥunayn *as he introduced in a certain place, better (*ajwad*), and for me it is 'being done of necessity'.* In a manuscript *wālitā*, right (*zedqā*).

What is especially important to note about these entries is the absence of Ḥunayn's translation in aphorism ii. 27 *al-qiyās*. This word is also absent in the lexicography for the second approach to translating λόγος in the Syriac *Aphorisms*. This approach involves *zedqā* 'necessity', a word that also figures in both of the above entries for *wālitā*.

Later in the same aphorism discussed above, ii. 27, for example, the compound word παραλόγως 'beyond reason' is employed in the Greek source-text. In place of this word, the Syriac version gives the phrase *lbar men zedqā* 'unduly', while Ḥunayn again followed much the same approach as above, writing *'alā ghayr al-qiyās* 'in (a way) other than reason'. Yet in other instances where the Syriac uses some form of *zedqā*, Ḥunayn adopted a different approach which aligns better with the Syriac lexicography given so far. For example, in aphorism ii. 28, the phrase μᾶλλον τοῦ κατὰ λόγον 'greater than that which is regular (lit. according to reason)' is translated in the Syriac *yattir men zedqā* 'more than is right', and similarly Ḥunayn's Arabic gives *akthar mimma yanbaghī* 'more than what is appropriate'. In aphorism v. 64, the Syriac again translates the phrase παρὰ λόγον with *lbar men zedqā* 'unduly', while in this place Ḥunayn uses the phrase *'alā ghayr mā tuwajjibuhu al-'illa* 'without the disease necessitating it'.

We have already seen the equivalence between *wālitā* and *zeḏqā* in bar Bahlul's entries for the former word. In these entries there also occur words related to two of the Arabic equivalents, *yanbaghī* 'to be appropriate' and *yajib* 'to be necessary', that Ḥunayn used to translate λόγος in the Arabic *Aphorisms*. An entry in bar Bahlul's *Lexicon* relevant to the Syriac *zeḏqā* also contains definitions related to Ḥunayn's approach to translating λόγος:

676:5 **ܙܕܝܩܐ** البارّ الصدّيق البرّ الصدق. **ܙܕܝܩܘܬܐ** صدّيقيّة برورة. **ܙܕܝܩܘܬܐ** ܗܝ ܡܝܬܪܘܬܐ ܕܝ ܨܒܝܢܐ ܡܠܝܠܐ ܕܪܕܦܐ ܒܙܕܝܩܘܬܐ. ܕܫܠܝܐ ܠܗ ܠܡܟܬܫܘ ܥܡ ܒܥܠܕܒܒܐ. ܡܬܐܡܪܐ ܗܟܝܠ ܙܕܝܩܘܬܐ ܥܠ ܐܠܗܐ. ܐܘ ܦܫܝܛܐܝܬ ܐܘ ܡܛܠ ܠܐ ܡܙܕܥܙܥܢܘܬܐ ܕܡܝܬܪܘܬܐ البرارة. **ܙܕܩܬܝܗ** أبررته ܐܝܟ ܒܪ ܣܪܘܫܘܝ أي جعلته برّاً. **ܙܕܩܬܢܝ** زكّيتني. **ܙܕܩܝܢ** زكّيني. **ܐܙܕܕܩ** تبرّر. **ܙܕܩܗ** ܒܕܘܟܐ ܕܦܪܕ̈ ܐܝܟ ܫܘܘܕܝܗ ܕܝܠܗ. **ܙܕܩ** ܗܘ ܙܕܩܐ ܐܝܟ ܗܿ ܕܒܗ ܗܘ ܙܕܩ ܗܘܐ ܕܢܬܦܣܩ܆ أوجَب. **ܙܕܩܐ** حَقّ واجب صَدَقة. **ܙܕ̈ܩܬܐ** صدقات. **ܙܕܩ** يجب. **ܙܕܩܢ** حقّنا واجبنا. **ܙܕܩ** ܗܘ ܝܐܐ ܘܦܐܐ܆ ܐܝܟ ܗܿ ܕܙܕܩ ܗܘܐ ܕܢܬܐܡܪ ܟܬܒܐ يجب وينبغي. **ܙܕܩ** ܗܘ ܡܢ ܙܕܝܩܐ ܘܟܐܢܘܬܐ أوجَبُوا وعَدَلوا. **ܙܕܩܐ** واجب. **ܙܕܩܐ** برّ صَدَقة. **ܙܕܩܢ** برّرنا. **ܙܕܩܢ** نصيبنا سهمنا. **ܙܕ̈ܩܐ** اقارب܀

Zaḏiqā, righteous, truthful, righteousness, truthfulness. Zaḏiquṯā, truthfulness, righteousness. Zaḏiquṯā, this is the excellence of rational will that pursues righteousness, which is fit to struggle against the enemy. *Zaḏiquṯā* is thus said of God, either simply or because He is unmoved in excellence, *righteousness. Zaddeqteh, you behaved righteously in it.* According to bar Serošway, *that is, you did it in a righteous way. Zaddeqṯān, you purified me. Zaddeqayn, purify me. Ezdaddaq, to do righteousness. Zaddeqeh* in a place in the Book of Paradise, 'according to his promise'. *Zaddeq*, this is necessity (*zeḏqā*), according to that which has been decided to be necessary, *to necessitate (*awjaba*). Zeḏqā, right, necessary, true. Zeḏqāṯā, alms. Zāḏeq, it is necessary (*yajib*). Zeḏqan, it is necessary for us, it is right for us. Zāḏeq*, this is to be seemly, to be fitting, according to that which is necessary to be said, a decree (*keṯbā*), *to be necessary (*yajib*), to be appropriate (*yanbaghī*). Zaddeq*, this is from righteousness and justice, *they adjudicated, they acted equitably. Zāḏqā, necessary. Zeḏqā, righteousness, truth. Zaḏqan, we acted righteously. Zeḏqan, our share, our portion. Zeḏqē, close acquaintances.*

Buried in this entry, we again find Ḥunayn's general equivalents for λόγος in the *Aphorisms*, *yanbaghī* and *yajib*. Thus far, then, these two Syriac equivalents have been shown to be more or less synonymous with one another. These accord both with certain approaches of Ḥunayn's in his Arabic version of the *Aphorisms* and with Arabic definitions of these words found in bar Bahlul's *Lexicon*. On the other hand, nothing related to Ḥunayn's third major equivalent for λόγος, *al-qiyās*, occurs in these contexts.

Forms of a third Syriac equivalent for λόγος, *peḥmā* 'analogous', occur in the aphorism under consideration here, iii. 1, and in aphorism iv. 71. In both of these places we find in Ḥunayn's Arabic version a form of *al-qiyās*, which is largely synonymous to this Syriac word. An entry for *peḥmā* in bar Bahlul's *Lexicon* reads like this:

> 1533:7 **ܦܚܡܐ** قال حنين ينتظم على معانٍ شَتّى فيقع على نظير مثل ندّ. ويقع على قياس بين شيئين ليعلم أيّما أفضل في جملة الأمر وظاهره. ويقع على النسبة وهي قياس بين شيئين متناسبين ليعلم بالحقيقة كم مقدار أحدهما من الآخر. شكل عدل كفو وآخرون نظير ܀
>
> *Peḥmā, Ḥunayn said: It is arranged according to six meanings. It is used for an equivalent, a like, (or) an equal. It is used for an analogy (*qiyās*) between two things in order to know which of them is more appropriate for the sum of an affair and its manifestness. It is used for the ratio, which is an analogy between two proportioned things making known the quantity of one to the other in reality. A shape, a balance, a match. Elsewhere, an equivalent.*

Although I have shown in several places above that the Syriac version of the *Aphorisms* and Ḥunayn's version are very often quite different in terms of the rate and types of variation in their respective translation techniques, the variations in these translations of λόγος are especially striking. The three approaches in the Syriac translation that I have described are all reflected both in Ḥunayn's Arabic translation and in glosses attributable to Ḥunayn in bar Bahlul's *Lexicon*. This is not the case, however, in the relevant Greek lexicography cited at the beginning of this discussion. Although these entries are important and interesting,[29] they only reflect Ḥunayn's translation choices in his Arabic version of the *Aphorisms* very partially. This is, again, emphatically not the case for the Syriac lexicography. Thus we may say that the scholarly background to Ḥunayn's Arabic translations of λόγος in the *Aphorisms* give strong evidence for the translator's use of a Syriac source-text in his production of this version of the Hippocratic work.

Yet, at the same time, these three interpretations of λόγος in the *Aphorisms* do not overlap in the Syriac *Aphorisms* and in Ḥunayn's Arabic version. In all of the cases where the Syriac version uses a form of the equivalent *peḥmā*, Ḥunayn employed the analogous Arabic equivalent *al-qiyās*. Yet in several places in the latter work *al-qiyās* is used where one of the other Syriac techniques (*zeḏqā* or *b-wāliṯā*) is used in the Syriac version. Again, these Syriac approaches are clearly distinct both in their meanings and in the approaches Ḥunayn used to carry them over into Arabic, as evidenced by the material in bar

29 In particular, the entry at 948:10 is very likely a fragment from Ḥunayn's lost glossary.

Bahlul's *Lexicon*. As such, while it is very likely that Ḥunayn used a Syriac exemplar at least in some capacity in his Arabic translation of the *Aphorisms*, it is almost equally as unlikely that the extant Syriac *Aphorisms* was in fact the Syriac exemplar employed by Ḥunayn. To say this is perforce to say that Ḥunayn was not the author of the extant Syriac translation of the Hippocratic *Aphorisms*.

To conclude this discussion, we may consider the two instances where translations of λόγος are found in al-Biṭrīq's early Arabic translation of the *Aphorisms*. In the aphorism directly under discussion here, iii. 1, al-Biṭrīq translated κατὰ λόγον with *yajrī majrāhu* 'following the same course' in the sense of 'analogous'. In aphorism v. 64, he translated παρὰ λόγον 'unusually' with the single word *jiddan* 'seriously'. Neither of these translations are represented anywhere in the lexicographical material presented above, nor do they resemble any of the translations presented from the other two works. Thus, despite what I believe to be the strong unlikelihood that Ḥunayn was the author of the Syriac *Aphorisms*, the contrast between al-Biṭrīq's translation and the two other translations under consideration is much stronger than that obtaining between the Syriac version of the *Aphorisms* and Ḥunayn's Arabic version. This may be explained at least in part because al-Biṭrīq did not have recourse to the Syriac medical tradition in producing this work, but instead translated directly from Greek to Arabic. The translations of λόγος thus provide clear insight into the part played by Syriac sources in the advancement in Arabic translation technique made by Ḥunayn ibn Isḥāq.

Aphorism v. 64

(1) Γάλα διδόναι κεφαλαλγέουσι κακόν· κακὸν δὲ καὶ πυρεταίνουσι καὶ οἷσιν ὑποχόνδρια μετέωρα καὶ διαβορβορύζοντα, καὶ τοῖσι διψώδεσι· (2) κακὸν δὲ καὶ οἷσι χολώδεις αἱ ὑποχωρήσιες ἐν τοῖσιν ὀξέσι πυρετοῖσιν ἐοῦσιν καὶ οἷσιν αἵματος πολλοῦ διαχώρησις γέγονεν· (3) ἁρμόζει δὲ φθινώδεσι μὴ λίην πολλῷ πυρέσσουσιν διδόναι καὶ ἐν πυρετοῖσι μακροῖσι βληχροῖσι, μηδενὸς τῶν προειρημένων σημείων παρεόντος, παρὰ λόγον δὲ ἐκτετηκότων.

E.

(1) أَعْطِ اللبن لمن يشتكي رأسه ولمن به عطش (2) وايضاً لمن به اختلاف من مرّة صفراء وحمّى حادّة ولمن اختلف دماً كثيراً (3) وهو موافق أن يعطى لمن به ضمر وقرح فى رئته اذا لم يكن محموما جدّا ويعطى لمن كانت حمّاه ليّنة فاترة مزمنة من غير أن يكون به شيءٌ من العلامات التى ذكرنا ويكون جسده ناحلا جدّاً.

(1) Give milk to one who complains of his head, or to one who has sneezes, (2) and again to one

who has diarrhoea due to yellow bile and an acute fever, or to one with extremely bloody diarrhoea. (3) It is appropriate that it be given to one with emaciation and ulceration in his lungs when he is not intensely feverish, and that it be given to one whose fever is gentle, weak, and chronic, without anything of the signs we mentioned, and whose body is seriously thin.

S.

(1) ܚܠܒܐ ܠܡܬܠ ܠܡܟܐܒܝ ܪܫܐ ܒܝܫܐ. ܒܝܫܐ ܕܝܢ ܕܢܬܝܗܒ ܘܠܐܝܠܝܢ ܕܐܚܝܕܝܢ ܒܐܫܬܐ. ܘܠܐܝܠܝܢ ܕܗܘܝܢ
ܐܬܪܘܬܐ ܕܬܚܝܬ ܣܚܘܣܩܘܬܐ ܕܐܠܥܝܗܘܢ. ܘܫܘܦܐ ܒܗܘܢ ܘܒܗ ܒܥܘܪܐ ܘܠܐܝܠܝܢ ܕܥܛܫܝܢ. (2) ܒܝܫ ܕܝܢ
ܘܠܐܝܠܝܢ ܕܡܪܬܐ ܡܬܚܠܛܐ ܒܡܦܩܬܗܘܢ ܘܐܝܬ ܠܗܘܢ ܐܫܬܐ ܚܪܝܦܬܐ. ܘܠܐܝܠܝܢ ܕܡܦܩܬܐ ܕܕܡܐ ܣܓܝܐܐ
ܡܦܩܬ ܠܗܘܢ. (3) ܢܦܫ ܕܝܢ ܕܢܬܝܗܒ ܠܡܫܥܠܢܐ ܡܢ ܕܠܐ ܐܫܬܐ ܐܚܝܕܝܢ ܒܐܫܬܐ ܕܠܒ ܪܒܐ[30]
ܘܒܐܫܬܘܬܐ ܘܒܐܫܬܘܬܐ ܢܓܝܪܬܐ ܒܕ ܠܝܬ ܡܢ ܡܕܡ ܡܢ ܐܝܠܝܢ ܕܐܬܩܕܡ ܐܬܐܡܪ. ܠܒܪ ܡܢ ܗܕܐ ܕܝܢ
ܡܕܝܒ ܦܓܪܐ.

(1) To give milk to those who suffer pain in the head is bad. It is also bad that it be given to those who suffer from fever, and to those with swelling and rumbling in the places beneath the cartilage of their ribs, and to those who sneeze. (2) It is also bad for those who have bile in their faeces while they have an acute fever, and for those who have very bloody faeces. (3) It is beneficial that it be given to consumptives who do not have a fever that is very great, and in fevers that are long and fine, when there is not anything of what was said previously, except what is fit for the wasting of the body.

Ḥ.

(1) اللبن لأصحاب الصداع رديء وهو أيضاً للمحمومين رديء ولمن كانت المواضع التي دون الشراسيف منه مشرفة وفيها قراقر ولمن به عطش (2) ولمن الغالب على برازه المرار ولمن هو في حمّى حادّة ولمن اختلف دماً كثيراً، (3) وينفع أصحاب السلّ إذا لم تكن بهم حمّى شديدة جدًّا ولأصحاب الحمّى الطويلة الضعيفة إذا لم يكن معها شيء ممّا تقدّمنا بوصفه وكانت أبدانهم تذوب على غير ما توجبه العلّة.

(1) Milk for the sufferers of headache is bad, and it is bad also for the feverish, and for the one whose area below the ribs is elevated and has rumblings, and for the one who has sneezes, (2) and for the one in whose faeces yellow bile predominates, and for the one with an acute fever, and for the one with very bloody diarrhoea. (3) But it benefits the sufferers of tuberculosis if they do not have a very severe fever, and the sufferers of long, weak fevers if there does not occur along with these anything of what we described previously, and whose bodies waste without the disease necessitating it.

The first matter which must be remarked upon when considering these translations is the corrupt state of al-Biṭrīq's translation as represented in

30 Pognon corrects to ܕܠܐ ܒܐܫܬܐ ܐܚܝܕܝܢ ܒܐܫܬܐ ܕܠܒ ܪܒܐ, but to me this appears unnecessary. See Pognon (ed.), *Une version syriaque des Aphorismes*, 39 n. 2.

Houtsma's edition of al-Yaʿqūbī's *History*. This is shown by the fact that the entire first part of the aphorism communicates precisely the opposite meaning as that which the Hippocratic author apparently intended; instead of milk being described as harmful for the sufferers of these illnesses, the text enjoins that it be given to them. Furthermore, certain elements of the text have dropped out, notably the mention of a disease of the diaphragm at the end of sentence (1).

Comparing the Syriac version with the Arabic version of Ḥunayn, the stronger adherence to the literal sense of the text of the former may be observed. For example, the two occurrences of *bīš* 'bad' in sentence (1) and the third occurrence at the beginning of sentence (3) mirror the repetition of κακόν in the original Greek in these places. This while Ḥunayn in his Arabic version only stated the equivalent *radī'* a single time to stand for all three.

A difference of interpretation in sentence (2) may also be observed amongst the different versions. Both the early Arabic version and the Syriac translation render the Greek phrase οἷσι χολώδεις αἱ ὑποχωρήσιες ἐν τοῖσιν ὀξέσι πυρετοῖσιν in ways that show their authors understood the prepositional phrase ἐν τοῖσιν ὀξέσι πυρετοῖσιν 'in acute fevers' to modify the clause οἷσι χολώδεις αἱ ὑποχωρήσιες 'for those whose faeces have bile'. The early Arabic version translates this phrase *li-man bih ikhtilāf min mirra ṣafrā' wa-ḥummā ḥādda* 'to one who has diarrhoea due to yellow bile and an acute fever', while the Syriac translation gives here *l-aylēn d-merṯā iṯeḇthon w-iṯ l-hon ešāṯā ḥarripṯā* 'for those who have bile in their faeces while they have an acute fever'. Ḥunayn's Arabic translation differs, however, in that the translator appears to have interpreted this clause to refer to two different cases rather than one. In translating this section, he wrote *li-man al-ghālib 'alā birāzih al-mirār wa-li-man huwa fī ḥummā ḥādda* 'for the one in whose faeces yellow bile predominates, and for the one with an acute fever'. In his commentary on this aphorism, Galen likewise differentiates slightly between the two.[31] Thus it appears that Ḥunayn translated the Hippocratic lemma to accord with Galen's interpretation, while the author of the Syriac translation preferred literally to render the original Greek of the aphorism.

Finally, I would like to consider the translations and lexicographical background of the anatomical term ὑποχόνδριον, which are of interest for the Syriac translation in particular:

31 Mimura (ed.), *Tafsīr Jālīnūs*, V 89.

ὑποχόνδριον

81:18 ܐܘܦܘܦܘܠܐܪܝܘܢ ܐܝܟ ܦܘ̈ܠܘܣ الشراسيف ܘܒܕܘܟ **ܐܦܘܟܝܕܪܝܐ** ܐܘܟܝܬ ܓܒ̈ܐ تحت الشراسيف
ܘܐܝܟ ܒܪ ܣܪܘ̈ تحت المراقّ؞

Upupularion according to Paul, *the epigastrium (*al-sharāsīf*)*, and in one place *apukidria*, meaning the sides (*gabbē*) *below the ribs*, and according to bar Serošway, *below the membranes (*taḥt al-marāqq*)*.

233:10 ܐܣܦܘܩܢܕܪܘܢ ܪܒܢ الشراسيف الأحد السُرّة وهو باليونانيّة وهو من مراق البطن؞

Aspukndrun (according to) our teacher, *one of the epigastria, the navel. It is in Greek, and it is one of the membranes of the stomach.*

254:6 **ܐܦܘܟܝܕܪܝܐ** ܒܪ ܣܪܘ̈ ܗܢܘ ܐܬܪܐ ܗܘ ܕܪ̈ܐܬܐ ܘܕܐܣܛܘܡܟܐ ܘܕܟܒܕܐ ܘܕܛܚܠܐ ܘܕܫܪܬܐ
ܥܙܐ الصدر والبطن؞

Apukidria (according to) bar Serošway, this is the place of the lungs, the stomach, the liver, the spleen, and the navel, *the breast and the stomach.*

Forms of the word ὑποχόνδριον occur some four times in the *Aphorisms*. In translating these instances, in something of an exception to the usual pattern I have observed over the course of this work, Ḥunayn's Arabic version follows a more regular pattern than does the text of the Syriac *Aphorisms*. In three of the four cases, the Arabic version translates this word with the phrase *mā dūn al-sharāsīf* 'that which is beneath the rib cartilage', while in aphorism v. 64 under consideration here, this varies slightly to *al-mawādi' allatī dūn al-sharāsīf* 'the places that are beneath the rib cartilage'. For its part the Syriac version adopts two very different approaches to this term. For the first two examples of ὑποχόνδριον in the *Aphorisms*, which occur in aphorisms iv. 64 and iv. 73, the Greek word is translated with a form of the word *gabbē* 'sides', which corresponds with the entry from bar Bahlul's *Lexicon* at 81:18 presented above. For the following two examples, a different translation is given, namely *a̱trawāṯā ḏa-ṯheyt ḥasḥusē ḏ-el'ē* 'the places that are beneath the cartilage of the ribs'. The sense of the latter translation is almost identical to Ḥunayn's preferred translations of all instances of ὑποχόνδριον in his Arabic version of the *Aphorisms*.

An entry in bar Bahlul's *Lexicon* relevant to the Syriac equivalent of ὑποχόνδριον, *gabbē*, reads like this:

445:10 **ܓܒܐ** الجانب ܘܐܝܟ ܒܪ ܣܪܘ̈ **ܓܒܐ** ܠܓܒܐ ܩܪܐ الخاصرة. ܓܒܗ ܗ̄ ܠܡܬܩܪܒܘܬܗ ܐܡܪ إلى جانبه؞

Gabbā, *the side,* and according to bar Serošway *gabbā*, for the side he read *the hip (*al-khāṣira*)*. *Gabbeh*, he says this for (someone's) being brought near, *to his side*.

This entry's irrelevance to the Arabic translations of the *Aphorisms* is clear. However, further resources regarding the Greek entries may be located in other places in the lexicons. First, an entry for ὑποχόνδριον in bar ʿAli's *Lexicon* reads in the following way:

ܐܘܦܘܩܘܢܕܪܝܘܢ. ܐܬܪܐ ܕܬܚܝܬ ܚܫܘܫܐ ܕܐܠܥܐ. الشراشيف.[32]

Upukundrion. The place below the cartilage of the ribs (*aṯrā ḏa-ṯḥeyt ḥashḥusā ḏ-elʿē*). *The rib cartilage (*al-sharāsīf*).*

This entry, likely attributable to Ḥunayn by virtue of bar ʿAli's stated reliance upon the translator's glossary, reproduces almost exactly the second of the two Syriac translations of ὑποχόνδριον in the *Aphorisms*. This constitutes evidence that Ḥunayn used this equivalent in his own Syriac translations. Yet again, the discrepancy between the Syriac and Arabic versions of the *Aphorisms* is remarkable, despite their convergence in the latter two instances of ὑποχόνδριον in the work. Given the strong agreement between these latter equivalents, the sense that the Syriac equivalent *gabbē* 'sides' is far less explicit than Ḥunayn's technique tended to be is only heightened. Yet on the other hand, the echo of Ḥunayn's technique in the latter two instances of the Syriac version must be admitted to be somewhat mysterious. The fact that the pairing ὑποχόνδριον/*gabbē* seems to be attributed to the translations of Paul in bar Bahlul's entry at 81:18 also adds another, albeit limited, example of the tendency for citations of the works of Ḥunayn and Paul in the *Lexicon* to be at variance with one another.

At any rate, it is quite clear that for the translations of ὑποχόνδριον the relevant Greek lexicography is of greater importance than is the directly relevant Syriac lexicography. This argument is further extended by the presence of a definition of this Greek word in an extended Greek-to-Arabic anatomical entry attributed to Ḥunayn in bar Bahlul's *Lexicon*, which reads as follows:

1160:26 ܡܪܘܩܐ ܐܝܟ ܣܘܡܩ مراقّ البطن يقال له باليونانية ܗܘܦܘܓܐܣܛܪܝܘܢ وهو يقسم ثلثة أقسام وله أسماء كثيرة باليونانية. فيقال لما دون الشراسيف الذي حذاء السُرّة ܐܘܦܘܟܘܢܕܪܝܘܢ[33] وما دون السُرّة الى العانة أمّا الموضع الأوسط منه فيقال له ܐܦܝ ܓܐܣܛܪܝܘܢ ويقال له ايضاً ܐܬܪܘܢ وبالعربية الثنّة. و أمّا ما عن جنبتيه يمينه ويساره الى الصُلب فيقال له باليونانية ܠܐܓܘܢܐ وتفسيره الخالي لأنّ تلك المواضع خالية من أجل الأحشاء وبالعربية الخاصرتان وما دون ذلك وهو القسم الثالث يقال الأوسط منه باليونانية

32 Hoffmann (ed.), *Syrische arabische Glossen*, 17:368.

33 Duval: ܐܘܦܘܟܘܢܕܪܝܘܢ.

ܗܦܝܒܐܘܢ ويقال له أيضاً ܗܦܣܝܘܢ ويقال لجنبتيه ܠܓܘܢܝܣ ويقال بالسريانية للموضع الاوسط منه ܡܚܨܢܐ ܘܐܙܒܐ ويقال لجنبتيه ܡܚܨܢܐ ܘܓܣܐ ܕܡܚܨܢܐ ويقال بالعربية للأوسط العانة. ܘܐܝܟ ܒܪ ܣܪܘܫܘܝ ܡܪܩܩܗ ܗܘ ܩܠܦܗ. ܡܪܩܩܐ غصون البطن. ܘܒܟܬܒܐ ܕܦܪܕܝܣܐ ܚܕܐ ܩܘܦ ܩܪܐ. ܢܝܠܒܐ ܢܝܠܒܗ ܐܝܟ ܗܘ ܕܫܦܛܐ. ܒܢ ܢܝܠܒܗ. ܘܐܘܣܦ ܒܪ ܣܪܘܫܘܝ ܟܪܣܗ المراقّ ثربه܀

*Marqāqā according to Ḥunayn, the membranes of the stomach (*maraqq al-baṭn*). It is called in Greek epigastron. It is divided into three parts, which have many names in Greek. That which is below the rib cartilage (*sharāsīf*) which is opposite the navel is called upokondrion. As for that which is below the navel up to the pubic region, the middle part of it called upogastrion, and it is also called itron, and in Arabic the abdomen (*thunna*). As for that which is from its two sides, the left and the right, to the backbone, it is called in Greek qênêon, the meaning of which is 'the empty' (*al-khālī*), because this part is empty on account of the bowels. In Arabic it is the haunches. That which is below this is divided into three sections. The middle of it is called in Greek êpibêon, and it is also called êpsion, and its sides are called lagunês. In Syriac the middle part is called maḥsānē w-ezbē* ('the loins and the genitals'), *and its sides are called maḥsānē w-gesē d-maḥsānē* ('the loins and the sides of the loins'). *In Arabic the middle is called* al-ʿāna *('the loins').* And according to bar Serošway *marqāqeh*, this is its membrane. *Marqāqā, the limbs of the stomach (*ghuṣūn al-baṭn*).* In the Book of Paradise, he reads a single *qop*. A hilt, its hilt, as it is in the Book of Judges.[34] In a manuscript, its hilt. Bar Serošway adds, its abdomen, *the membranes, its adipose membranes (*tharbuh*).*

34 Judg. 3:22.

Chapter 5

Conclusion

Ḥunayn ibn Isḥāq's Syriac Scholarship and the Study of Greek-to-Arabic Medical Translation

In surveying the material presented above, it is clear that the relationship obtaining amongst Ḥunayn ibn Isḥāq's Greek, Syriac and Arabic scholarly works was a complex one. It can only be assumed that small portions of Ḥunayn's Greek lexicographical work survive in the extant Syriac lexicons. However, certain examples presented above clarify the ways in which Greek and Syriac scholarship informed Ḥunayn's Arabic translation work as represented by his version of the Hippocratic *Aphorisms*.

The entries and translations of the Greek word αὐτόματον in Chapter One (1.1.3) and the long Arabic entry for ὑποχόνδριον (4., v. 64) both give strong evidence for significant Greek-to-Arabic lexicographical work on the part of Ḥunayn that informed his Arabic translation of the *Aphorisms* without any significant Syriac intermediary. Yet, the evidence for the very strong relationship that obtained between Ḥunayn's Syriac and Arabic philological work strongly outweighs these examples. In only a few cases has it proved difficult to discover parallels between Ḥunayn's Arabic translation of the *Aphorisms* on the one hand and entries in the Syriac lexicons on the other. This holds true even in spite of the evidence presented throughout the present work that Ḥunayn was not the author of the extant Syriac *Aphorisms*. This pattern is further strengthened by the existence in several cases of exact or nearly exact agreement between lengthy explicating translations in the Arabic *Aphorisms* and the definitions in the lexicons of Syriac equivalents of these words.[1]

To repeat, this pattern of agreement between the lexicons and Ḥunayn's Arabic translation of the *Aphorisms* is insufficient for the attribution of the authorship of the Syriac translation of the *Aphorisms* to Ḥunayn, due to the

1 Examples of this occur in the discussions of κιρσός (2.1.4) and λέπρα (3., iii. 20). The pattern of agreement mentioned has potential for (admittedly very tentative) reconstruction of Ḥunayn's lost Syriac translations in the event of the preparation of digitized versions of the lexicons of bar Bahlul and bar ʿAli.

strong pattern of divergent interpretations between the main Arabic and Syriac translations. Rather, the broad terminological agreement between the two translations and the contrasting interpretative and stylistic modes they adopt points to their having been composed by two different authors within the same scholarly milieu. This is consistent with Ḥunayn's account in the *Risāla* regarding his contemporaries' Syriac translations of Galen's *Commentary on the Aphorisms*. On this basis I believe it is very likely that the extant Syriac *Aphorisms* was composed by either Job of Edessa or Jibrīl ibn Bukhtīshūʿ.

This likelihood may be considered disappointing, given that it removes the best hope for the survival of a Syriac translation composed by Ḥunayn. However at the same time it would mean that in the extant translations of the *Aphorisms* we have a very good simulacrum of the state of both the Syriac and Arabic translation traditions prior to Ḥunayn's career. This allows for judgments about Ḥunayn's especial contribution to ʿAbbāsid-era Greek scholarship to proceed upon quite firm foundations.

The Characteristics of the Various Translations

Despite its being much less given to stylistic variation and creative adaptation than Ḥunayn's Arabic translation, the Syriac *Aphorisms* generally gives a reasonably good sense of the text. This is especially true when it is compared with al-Biṭrīq's early Arabic version, which can be quite awkward.[2] Again taking this version to represent the state of the art of Syriac medical translation prior to Ḥunayn, it is evident that the tradition by that time had reached what may be described as a tolerable degree of competency.

In contrast, as has been generally recognized for Ḥunayn's Arabic translations, the standard Arabic version of the *Aphorisms* is quite sophisticated. This may be observed both in its reader-oriented presentation of the sense of the Greek original and in its stylistic quality as a work of Arabic literature. On the basis of the evidence presented here, I hold that the high quality of Ḥunayn's Arabic translation owes a great deal to the translator's thorough familiarity with

---

2 The latter conforms to a pattern of relative inaccuracy and lack of sophistication noted for early Arabic medical and philosophical translation in previous studies. See for example J.M. Mattock, 'The Early Translations from Greek into Arabic: A Comparative Assessment' in *Symposium Graeco-Arabicum II* (Amsterdam 1987), 102, as well as Ullmann, *Wörterbuch zu den griechisch-arabischen Übersetzungen*, 47–8.

the methods of Syriac translation established by Sergius of Reš ʿAynā and his successors.[3]

At the same time, however, this does not mean that Ḥunayn's Arabic translation of the *Aphorisms* was in any sense a mechanical reproduction of his lost Syriac translation of the work. As may be seen for example in the discussion of the translations of ἄσθμα in Chapter One (1.2.10), there is evidence that Greek-to-Arabic and Syriac-to-Arabic lexicography were both involved in the production of Ḥunayn's translations. This points to a tri-lingual translation process that saw Ḥunayn first translate the Greek original into Syriac, and then use both the original and the Syriac translation in the production of his Arabic version.

Other evidence drawn from the lexicography and the comparison of the Syriac and Arabic versions also emphasizes the importance of Ḥunayn's knowledge of Arabic for the quality of his translations. Even in cases of clear Syriac influence such as the borrowing of the word *buḥrān* 'crisis' discussed in the treatment of κρίσις (4., i. 1), the exigency of clearly communicating the sense of the Greek original often prompted Ḥunayn to vary his approach or to rely on precedents established earlier in the Arabic medical tradition. In many places in the entries collected by bar Bahlul, furthermore, Ḥunayn displays a deep knowledge of the possibilities afforded by the Arabic lexicon.

In other examples, too, we see the limits of the influence of Syriac idiom on the Arabic translations. In the long entry for the Syriac word *pagrā* found in the discussion of the translations of σῶμα (3.1., ii. 9), for example, the non-existence of an exactly corresponding Arabic word prompted one of the lexicographers to suggest that the Syriac word should be taken over into Arabic. However, this borrowing does not appear to have been influential. Similarly in the discussion of κυνάγχη (3.2, iii. 20), there is evidence for an attempt at transferring the specific sense of the Syriac terminology into Arabic by means of calque translation. This adds a layer of complexity to an already extensive set of Arabic equivalents in the study of the lexicography, but again it does not appear to have been influential in the texts of the translations.

This evidence thus shows conclusively and in detail that the sophistication of Ḥunayn's Arabic translation techniques owed a great deal both to his own

3 A somewhat similar argument was put forward by Henri Hugonnard-Roche on the basis of a few examples in his article 'L'intermédiaire syriaque', 198–200, which is cited in the Introduction.

Syriac scholarship and that of his predecessors. Although the fact does not diminish the importance and value of Ḥunayn's Arabic scholarship, the complex interaction of Greek, Syriac, and Arabic in the scholarly background to his translations contrasts markedly with the simpler Greek-to-Arabic paradigm apparently underlying al-Biṭrīq's translation of the *Aphorisms*.[4] Perhaps somewhat counterintuitively, the existence of some form of a Syriac intermediary appears to have increased rather than to have decreased the quality of Ḥunayn's Arabic translation of the Hippocratic *Aphorisms*.

Evidence of Direct Syriac Influence upon Ḥunayn's Arabic Translations

This statement regarding the character of Syriac influence on the early Arabic translations of the Hippocratic *Aphorisms* may lead us to a broader consideration of the implications of the evidence presented herein. In several cases, such as for example the translations of παροξυσμός (3.2., iii. 19) and λέπρα (3.2., iii. 20), there is clear evidence that variations both in the general idiom and the specific medical terminology of Syriac came to be expressed in Ḥunayn's Arabic translation of the *Aphorisms*. If one were to read Ḥunayn's Arabic translation alongside the Greek original without reference to the Syriac translation, these variations would appear to be unexplainable anomalies. Furthermore, it is reasonable to expect that Syriac idiom likewise came to be expressed in other Arabic compositions of Ḥunayn's. This is so, since it is to be assumed that an even stronger relationship obtained between Ḥunayn's own Syriac works and his Arabic ones than that which I have shown to exist between the Arabic *Aphorisms* and the Syriac version now extant.

Perhaps more encouragingly, we may also expect that many of Ḥunayn's Arabic translations have a similar relationship to the Syriac lexicons of bar Bahlul and bar ʿAli as does his Arabic *Aphorisms*. Some understanding of Syriac medical and philosophical terminology is necessary for accessing this material. Yet as I have shown throughout the present work, interesting and at times enlightening discussions of Greek, Syriac, and Arabic terminology may be found in these lexicons. The foregoing research thus specifies the immense value

4 That is, at least as far as the preface to the Arabic Palladius may be trusted, where it is stated that the work was translated 'from Greek into Arabic'.

of these lexicons as tools for the study of the Greek-to-Arabic translation movement.

Implications for Arabic Translations Beyond the Field of Medicine

Although medicine and philosophy were certainly distinct disciplines for Greek, Syriac, and Arabic authors, at the same time the links between the two subjects were very strong. Even at the terminological level, the two fields were profoundly interwoven. The deep influence of Aristotelian terminology on the Syriac medical vocabulary shown in bar Bahlul's entries for *kyānā* (4., i. 3), and *gedšā* (4., i. 13) points to an interesting phenomenon whereby, in a sense, the long history of Greek thought comes to be compressed into a single idiom. The Hippocratic author's τύχη and the Aristotelian συμβεβηκός vary quite significantly both in tone and in conceptual weight, yet it is impossible to escape the impression that the two have been conflated in the Syriac translation of τύχη with *gedšā* in aphorism i. 13.

In this respect the study of Arabic medicine shares certain problems with that of Arabic philosophy considered more broadly. The types of variations in translation I have treated above pose similar or even greater problems for the latter study. As Gutas writes in his introduction to the study of Avicenna's philosophical works,

> By the fourth/tenth century... an Arabic speaking intellectual had to contend with three separate levels of Arabic: native and literary usage... the usage of the Islamic disciplines, and the usage of the translations, itself not uniform but varying according to different periods and complexes of translations.[5]

The evidence presented contributes to the process of delineating the types of effects produced by the interaction of Syriac with Arabic in one of these complexes of translation, the medical translations of Ḥunayn ibn Isḥāq. In doing so, it shows obliquely the types of benefit that may be expected to derive from

5 D. Gutas, *Avicenna and the Aristotelian Tradition* (Leiden 2014), 304. Although elements of this account should hold beyond the field of medicine, it bears repeating that the situation for a discipline like philosophy was a good deal more intricate, with various schools translating works of particular importance for their distinct intellectual or confessional positions. For a detailed account of some of these complexities, see A. Treiger, 'Palestinian Origenism and the Early History of the Maronites: In Search of the Origins of the Arabic *Theology of Aristotle*' in D. Janos (ed.), *Ideas in Motion in Baghdad and Beyond: Philosophical and Theological Exchanges between Christians and Muslims in the Third/Ninth and Fourth/Tenth Centuries* (Leiden 2016), 44–80.

the study of extant Syriac sources for other such complexes as well. In particular, the detailed study of bar Bahlul's *Lexicon* should provide significant insight into the philosophical translations of Ḥunayn and his successors in much the same way as I have shown it to do in regard to Ḥunayn's medical translations. Although the specific ways in which Syriac came to influence certain other bodies of Arabic translation beyond this one will differ according to context, the types of relationships I have observed herein I hope will prove to be useful models.

Syriac Scholarship in the Social and Intellectual History of Islamicate Societies

These findings are also of importance for areas of research beyond the relationship between Syriac and Arabic translations of Greek texts. The examples of longer entries I have provided above point to the value of bar Bahlul's *Lexicon* as a window into the intellectual life of Ḥunayn and his successors. This is especially true in entries for words like *ḥešokā* (1.3.14) and *ā'ar* (2.3.1), which display a certain tension between theological and philosophical conceptions. These entries along with many others in the *Lexicon* that I have not treated in the present work provide valuable material for the study of Syriac philosophy.

Other material cited herein from the Syriac lexicons is of importance for the history of Greek-to-Arabic translation without particular reference to Syriac exemplars. Most prominently, there is significant evidence against the traditional ascription to Ḥunayn of the Arabic translation of Paul of Aegina's *Pragmateia*. This evidence is found primarily in the discussion of τέτανος (2.2.6). There, an entry from bar Bahlul's *Lexicon* very likely written by Ḥunayn refers to the translator as someone other than himself, and in other entries the later compilers bar Bahlul and bar ʿAli explicitly state that Ḥunayn did not use an Arabic equivalent for τέτανος, *al-kuzāz*, that occurs frequently in the Arabic version of the *Pragmateia*. Furthermore, in other places it appears that Pauline material appears in bar Bahlul's *Lexicon* without attribution. This may be observed for example in the discussion of the translations of ἀπόστημα (1.3.8).

Finally, I would like to say a few words about the relationships of these findings to debates concerning the broader social and cultural history of Arabic and Syriac intellectual life. Regarding the former, an ongoing debate concerning the character of the impulse that drove the classical Arabic engagement with

Greek philosophy and science has tended to divide into two camps. One of these, centred around the work of George Saliba, has tended to focus on the interactions between Greeks and Arabs in the late Umayyad caliphate, when certain Byzantine administrative literature came to be rendered into Arabic.[6] The other, whose position has been articulated forcefully by Dimitri Gutas, favours a later date for the beginnings of serious engagement with Greek literature on the part of Arabic speakers. Gutas argues that rationalism and scientific inquiry played a key part in early ʿAbbāsid political propaganda, and that political dynamics should be considered the fundamental impulse behind the institutionalization of the Arabic sciences.[7]

Certain elements of this material arguably support each of these perspectives. For example, the very existence in any form of an early Arabic translation of the rather obscure Alexandrian physician Palladius' *Commentary on the Aphorisms*, performed directly from Greek into Arabic, would seem to support at least to a certain extent the idea of an early, western stratum of translation. Furthermore, the clear evidence against Ḥunayn's authorship of the Arabic translation of Paul's *Pragmateia* discussed above is accompanied by certain examples of convergences between the Greek-Syriac-Arabic lexicography attributed to Paul in bar Bahlul's *Lexicon* and al-Biṭrīq's early Arabic version of the work.[8] These convergences perhaps suggest a heavier reliance on late-Hellenic Alexandrian works in the early period of the translation movement. On the other hand, the definite inferiority of al-Biṭrīq's translations compared with Ḥunayn's tends to amplify somewhat the nuances of Gutas' position.

Gutas' work has also figured prominently in debates concerning the character of the Syriac contribution to the establishment and development of Arabic philosophy and the relative merits of these two traditions considered separately from one another. Neatly summarized in Siam Bhayro and Sebastian Brock's article 'The Syriac Galen Palimpsest and the Role of Syriac in the Transmission of Greek Medicine in the Orient',[9] this discussion has likewise

6 Saliba, *Islamic Science*, passim.

7 Gutas, *Greek Thought*, 29.

8 Notably in the discussions of τέτανος (2.2.6), again, as well as those of λέπρα (3., iii. 20), κίνδυνος (2.1.4), ἀποπληξία (2.2.2), and φρενός (2.2.8).

9 S. Bhayro and S. Brock, 'The Syriac Galen Palimpsest and the Role of Syriac in the Transmission of Greek Medicine in the Orient', *Bulletin of the John Rylands Library* 89:1 (2013), 25–43.

seen different voices adopt two opposing perspectives. Gutas' position, as characterized by Bhayro and Brock, has been decisively to favour the work of the ʿAbbāsid-era Greek-to-Arabic translation movement over that of earlier exponents such as Sergius of Reš ʿAynā. Whatever their quality and importance, from this perspective it is possible to view the ʿAbbāsid-era Syriac medical works of Ḥunayn and others as mere extensions of the same processes that underlay the Greek-to-Arabic translation movement, and thus to relegate the Syriac element to the background of the historical account.[10] In countering this view, Bhayro and Brock point to the inchoate scholarly understanding of much of the Syriac medical tradition while again emphasizing the independent value Ḥunayn accords to his Syriac translations in the *Risāla*.[11]

Although the somewhat narrow focus of the material presented in this work makes difficult the drawing of sweeping conclusions, it may be said that the evidence presented herein tends to favour the latter account of Bhayro and Brock. This may be seen first of all in the varying quality of the Syriac and Arabic translations of the *Aphorisms* that directly preceded Ḥunayn's career, represented above by the Syriac *Aphorisms* and al-Biṭrīq's early Arabic translation. Although neither of these translations reaches the standard of Ḥunayn's nuanced Arabic translation of the *Aphorisms*, the Syriac *Aphorisms* is also very much superior to al-Biṭrīq's version. This suggests that the Syriac translation tradition, in its development between Sergius' career and the early years of the ʿAbbāsid dynasty, had much more to contribute to Ḥunayn's project than did the nascent Arabic tradition of the time.

Again assuming that the extant Syriac *Aphorisms* is not the work of Ḥunayn, the comparisons in Chapter Three that show development in Syriac translation technique take on greater importance. In the discussions of words like σῶμα (3.1., ii. 9), γνώμη (3.2., ii. 6) and λέπρα (3.2., iii. 20) it appears that the later Syriac version of the *Aphorisms* is more precise than the earlier version found in the Syriac *Epidemics*. Furthermore, in the discussions of σῶμα and λέπρα, I presented strong evidence from bar Bahlul's *Lexicon* that these specific developments in Syriac translation technique had implications for the Arabic translation techniques of Ḥunayn and his school. Even if these developments were not as dramatic as the advances in translation technique associated with

10 Ibid., 41.

11 Ibid., 42.

Ḥunayn's work, they still represent important contributions on the part of the medical translation tradition initiated by Sergius to Arabic medical translation.

Both of these lines of argumentation support Bhayro and Brock's call for the addition of the word 'Syriac' to the usual phrase 'Greek-to-Arabic translation movement'. Furthermore, this evidence sits alongside numerous examples of less individual import that demonstrate that Ḥunayn's Syriac lexicography was a very important locus for the establishment of the Arabic terminology the translator used in his rendering of works like the Hippocratic *Aphorisms*. Yet in this way to consider Ḥunayn's translation techniques without reference to their broader historical context is to enter significantly murkier waters.

Even in the absence of Ḥunayn's own Syriac translation of the *Aphorisms*, it is possible with the aid of bar Bahlul's *Lexicon* to observe some of the ways in which Ḥunayn's work must have differed from the extant Syriac version. In the discussion of the scholarly background to the translations of the Greek word κατάστασις in the *Aphorisms* (4., i. 12), I observed the Syriac translation to render this word in an entirely regular fashion, whereas Ḥunayn used different Arabic equivalents for the term according to context. In particular, the use of κατάστασις with reference to the atmosphere prompted Ḥunayn to adopt a dramatically different approach. In one of bar Bahlul's entries for this Greek word, a definition of κατάστασις attributable to Ḥunayn provides in Syriac an atmospheric sense broadly analogous to that Ḥunayn used in his Arabic translation. Given the strong evidence that Ḥunayn used a Syriac version in preparing his Arabic translation of the *Aphorisms*, it is quite likely that he employed this or a similar Syriac phrase in his Syriac version.

It seems reasonable to suggest that Ḥunayn's greater attention to detail as manifested in his Arabic translations should also have figured in his Syriac translations. This kind of phenomenon points away from the influence of the tradition of Sergius upon Ḥunayn's translations, and tends to lend weight to the otherwise polemical remarks in the *Risāla* concerning Ḥunayn's fellow translators into Syriac. Furthermore, as I mentioned in the Introduction, there is important evidence that Ḥunayn's trial at the court of al-Mutawakkil represents a signal break between the Syriac court physicians and the translator.

For these reasons, I would suggest that personality was a key factor in these historical developments alongside language and religion, and that recognition of this may help the organization of historical research. This may be expressed in the following way: Prior to the accession of the ʿAbbāsids, there existed a

Sergian tradition of Greek-Syriac medical translation. This tradition continued to be pre-eminent in eastern Mesopotamia up to the time of Ḥunayn. Although Ḥunayn originally undertook his medical translations as an extension unto Arabic of this Syriac tradition, the historian should judge his translations as the beginning of a distinct 'Ḥunaynī' tradition of translation.[12] This tradition in effect, if not in intent, used Syriac as an intermediary between Greek and Arabic.

Effectively, the two debates concerning Arabic and Syriac that I have discussed each reflects the same fundamental parodox in the writing of history. Any event or complex of events may be approached by considering the ways in which that event displays continuity with the historical events that preceded it. However, at the same time no historical phenomenon may be reduced to a mechanical reproduction of its material causes. That is to say, every historical event is, in some sense, new and irreducibly unique.

The Syriac medical literature practiced by Ḥunayn's contemporaries was advanced enough to be mistaken for the work of the famous translator. Yet Ḥunayn did not content himself with reference to these standards of Syriac translation. Rather, he consistently strove to bring the older Greek and Syriac intellectual traditions into contact with the newly emergent standards of Arabic literature. It thus appears that the standards, styles and referents of Arabic literature considered as a whole represent an important element of the new in the Greek-Syriac-Arabic translation movement as represented by Ḥunayn.

Despite this, it is clear that the findings I have presented strongly emphasize the importance of what might be called the broader Aramaic culture of translation. As is generally well-known, many of the central works of Aramaic literature were translations, the main example of this in Syriac being of course the numerous detailed translations of the Bible.[13] Ḥunayn's extensive

---

12 In terms of translation technique, Ḥunayn's Arabic translations represent an important advance over the earlier Syriac tradition that he inherited. However, in other respects, such as for example the general body of texts with which he worked, Ḥunayn stands closer to the Sergian tradition than he does to other schools of translation. See the discussion of Ḥunayn's relationship to the Syriac tradition in J.W. Watt, ' The Syriac Aristotelian Tradition and the Syro-Arabic Baghdad Philosophers' in D. Janos (ed.), *Ideas in Motion in Baghdad and Beyond: Philosophical and Theological Exchanges between Christians and Muslims in the Third/Ninth and Fourth/Tenth Centuries* (Leiden 2016), 27.

13 Brock relies extensively on this literature in his study of the Syriac *Aphorisms* 'Syriac Background', *passim*. For a more detailed exposition, see idem., *The Bible in the Syriac Tradition* (Piscataway 2006).

employment of Syriac sources in his translation of the Hippocratic *Aphorisms* strongly emphasizes the importance of this long tradition for these Arabic translations. This highlights the kinds of organic processes that influenced Greek-to-Arabic translation alongside the more intentional institutional efforts emphasized by Gutas. In this reading, the political interests of the ʿAbbāsid elites provided the impetus for sustained contact and competition between the Syriac and Arabic intellectual traditions, each of which however had its own life apart from the machinations of princes.

While it is impossible to disregard the importance of religious and political management for the translation movement, the integrity of the various intellectual traditions that in effect served as its material cannot be ignored either. By dividing this history into two, the identity and contributions of the Sergian Graeco-Syriac tradition on the one hand and the Ḥunaynī Graeco/Syriac-Arabic tradition on the other may be more easily distinguished. Given their quite different historical, social and political contexts and aims, it makes sense to study these two as discrete yet related phenomena. This may be accomplished without denigrating the intellectual value or historical importance of either one.

In sum, the figure of Ḥunayn ibn Isḥāq represents the point of confluence between two traditions, that of ancient Aramaic and that of blossoming Arabic. No matter the various translators' knowledge of Greek sources, and no matter the desire of the ʿAbbāsid intellectual elites to see works of classical Greek literature rendered both elegantly and accurately into Arabic, it was ultimately by recourse to the praxis of translation maintained in the Syriac tradition that a satisfactory Arabic translation of the Hippocratic *Aphorisms* was performed. Certainly the extent to which this characterizes Ḥunayn's other translations and the broader work of Greek-to-Arabic translation will admit of further specification. However, the evidence I have presented here clearly demonstrates the great potential of Syriac sources for enriching scholarly understanding of both the details and the general character of these profoundly important historical subjects.

Bibliography

Barnes, J. (ed.). 1984. *The Complete Works of Aristotle.* Two volumes (Princeton)

Bergsträsser, G. (ed.). 1925. *Ḥunain ibn Isḥāq über die syrischen und arabischen Galen-Übersetzungen.* (Leipzig)

—— (ed.) 1932. *Neue Materialien zu Ḥunain ibn Isḥāq's Galen-Bibliographie* (Abhandlungen für die Kunde des Morgenlandes 19:2. Leipzig)

Bhayro, S. and S. Brock. 2013. 'The Syriac Galen Palimpsest and the Role of Syriac in the Transmission of Greek Medicine in the Orient'. *Bulletin of the John Rylands Library*, 89:1, 25–43.

Biesterfeldt, H. 2007. 'Palladius on the Hippocratic Aphorisms', in C. d'Ancona, *Libraries of the Neoplatonists* (Leiden). 385–98

—— (ed.). *Sharḥ Kitāb al-Tafṣīl l-Aflidhus.* Personal copy. ARABCOMMAPH/ Hinrich Biesterfeldt Palladius Transcription/Palladius.pdf.

Boudon-Millot, V. 2012. *Galien de Pergame: Médecin et Philosophe* (Paris 2012)

—— 2000. 'Galien de Pergame', in R. Goulet (ed.), *Dictionnaire des philosophes antiques, III: d'Eccélos à Juvenal* (Paris). 400–66

Brock, S. 2006. *The Bible in the Syriac Tradition.* (Piscataway, NJ)

—— 2015. 'Charting the Hellenization of a Literary Culture: The Case of Syriac', *Intellectual History of the Islamicate World* 3:1–2, 98–124

—— 1980. 'From Antagonism to Assimilation: Syriac Attitudes to Greek Learning', in N. Garsoïan, T. Mathews and R. Thompson (eds), *East of Byzantium: Syria and Armenia in the Formative Period* (Washington, D.C.). 17–34

—— 1991(1993). 'The Syriac Background to Ḥunayn's Translation Techniques', *ARAM* 3, 139–62

—— 1984. *Syriac Perspectives on Late Antiquity.* (London)

Brockelmann, C. 1895. *Lexicon Syriacum.* (Edinburgh). Reprint 1928 (Halle) http://www.dukhrana.com/lexicon/Brockelmann/index.php.

Butts, A.M. 2009. 'The Biography of the Lexicographer Isho' bar 'Ali', *Oriens Christianus* 93, 60–71

—— 2016. *Language Change in the Wake of Empire: Syriac in its Greco-Roman Context.* (Winona Lake, IN)

Carpentieri, N., K. Karimullah, T. Mimura and E. Selove (eds). *Sharḥ al-Kitāb al-Fuṣūl li-Aḥmad ibn Muḥammad Al-Kīlānī.* ARABCOMMAPH/editions/al-Kīlānī/al-Kīlānī bk. i.– iv. 72

—— *Al-Uṣūl fī Sharḥ al-Fuṣūl li-Abī al-Faraj ibn al-Quff.* ARABCOMMAPH/editions/QUF book 6

Cooper, G. 2011. *Galen, de Diebus Decretoriis, from Greek into Arabic.* (Surrey)

Cooperson, M. 2001. 'Two 'Abbāsid Trials: Aḥmad ibn Ḥanbal and Ḥunayn ibn Isḥāq', *Al-Qantara. Revista de estudios árabes,* 22:2, 375–93

Degen, R. 1981. 'Galen im Syrischen. Eine Übersicht über die syrische Überlieferung der Werke Galens', in V. Nutton (ed.), *Galen: Problems and Prospects* (London). 131–66

—— 1978. 'Zur syrischen Übersetzung der Aphorismen des Hippokrates', *Oriens Christianus* 62, 36–52

Dunlop, D.M. 1959. 'The Translations of al-Biṭrīq and Yaḥyā (Yuḥannā) b. al-Biṭrīq', *Journal of the Royal Asiatic Society* 91:3–4, 140–50

Duval, R. (ed.). 1901. *Lexicon Syriacum auctore Hassano Bar-Bahlule.* (Paris). Reprint 1979 (Amsterdam) http://www.dukhrana.com/lexicon/BarBahlul/index.php.

Endress, G. 1987–92. 'Die wissenschaftliche Literatur', in W. Fischer (ed.), *Grundriss der Arabischen Philologie*, Vol. 2, 400–506 and Vol. 3 (supplement), 3–152. (Wiesbaden)

Freytag, G.W. 1830–7. *Lexicon Arabico-Latinum.* 4 Vols. (Halle)

Gottheil, R. (ed). *The Syriac-Arabic Glosses of Isho' bar 'Ali.* 2 Vols, (Rome 1908–28)

de Groot, J. 1991. *Aristotle and Philoponus on Light*. (London)

Gutas, D. 2014. *Avicenna and the Aristotelian Tradition*. (Leiden)

—— 1998. *Greek Thought, Arabic Culture*. (London)

Hankinson, J. (ed.). 2008. *The Cambridge Companion to Galen*. (Cambridge)

Hoffmann G. (ed.). 1874. *Syrische-arabische Glossen: Autograph einer Gothaischen Handschrift enthaltend Bar 'Ali's Lexicon von Alif bis Mim*. (Kiel)

Horn, P. 1893. *Grundriss der neupersischen Etymologie*. (Strassburg)

Hugonnard-Roche, H. 1989. 'Aux origines de l'exégèse orientale de la logique d'Aristote: Sergius de Reshʿayna (d. 536), médecin et philosophe', *Journal Asiatique* 277, 1–17

—— 2004. *La logique d'Aristote du grec au syriaque: études sur la transmission des textes de l'Organon et leur interpretation philosophique*. (Paris)

—— 1991. 'L'intermédiaire syriaque dans la transmission de la philosophie grecque à l'arabe: le cas de l'Organon d'Aristote', *Arabic Sciences and Philosophy* 1:2, 187–209

Houtsma, M.T. (ed.). 1883. *Ta'rīkh ibn abī Ya'qūb*. (Leiden)

Iskandar, A.Z. 1976. 'An Attempted Reconstruction of the Late Alexandrian Medical Curriculum', *Medical History* 20:3, 235–58

Jones, W.H.S. (ed. and trans.). 1998. 'The Aphorisms of Hippocrates'. (Loeb Classical Library 150, Hippocrates IV, Heraclitus, 98–221. 9th ed. Cambridge)

Joose, N.P. and P.E. Pormann. 2012. 'Commentaries on the Hippocratic Aphorisms in the Arabic Tradition: The Example of Melancholy', in P.E. Pormann (ed.), *Epidemics in Context* (Berlin). 211–50

Jouanna, J. 1992. *Hippocrate*. (Paris)

Jouanna, J. and C. Magdelaine. 2000. 'Hippocrate de Cos', in R. Goulet (ed.), *Dictionnaire des philosophes antiques, III: d'Eccélos à Juvenal* (Paris). 771–90

Jourdain, A. 1843. *Recherches critiques du l'age et l'origines des traductions d'Aristote et sur des commentaires grecs ou arabes employés par les docteurs scolastiques*. (Paris)

Käs, F. 2010–11. 'Eine neue Handschrift von Ḥunayn ibn Isḥāqs Galenbibliographie', *Zeitschrift für Geschichte der arabisch-islamischen Wissenschaften* 19, 135–93

Kessel, G. 2012. 'The Syriac Epidemics and the Problem of its Identification' in P.E. Pormann, *Epidemics in Context* (Berlin). 93–124

—— 2014. 'Sergius ar-Ra'sī has Translated it into Syriac, but Poorly'. Paper presented at the conference 'Medical Translators at Work', Berlin, March 20–1

King, D. 2010. *The Earliest Syriac Translation of Aristotle's* Categories. (Leiden)

Klamroth, M. 1886. 'Über die Auszüge aus griechischen Schriftstellern bei al-Jaʿqūbī'. *Zeitschrift der deutschen morgenländischen Gesellschaft* 40, 189–233

Lamoreaux, J. 2015. *Ḥunayn ibn Isḥāq on His Galen Translations*. (Provo, UT)

Lewis, G. 1999. *The Turkish Language Reform: A Catastrophic Success*. (Oxford)

Liddell, H.G., H.S. Jones and R. Scott. 1940. *A Greek-English Lexicon*[9]. (Oxford) http://www.perseus.tufts.edu/hoppertext?doc=Perseus:text:1999.04.0057.

Löw, I. 1893. 'Review of R. Payne Smith, *Thesaurus Syriacus*'. *Zeitschrift der deutschen morgenländischen Gesellschaft* 47, 514–37

Magdelaine, C. 2003. 'Le commentaire de Palladius aux *Aphorismes* d'Hippocrate et les citations d'al-Yaʿqūbī', in J. Jouanna and A. Garzya (eds), *Storia e Ecdotica dei testi medici* (Naples). 321–34

—— 1988 'Histoire du texte et édition critique, traduite et commenté, des *Aphorismes* d'Hippocrate'. PhD diss., Université de Paris-Sorbonne

Mattock, J.M. 1987. 'The Early Translations from Greek into Arabic: A Comparative Assessment', in G. Endress (ed.), *Symposium Graeco-Arabicum II* (Amsterdam). 73–102

Mimura, T. 2016. 'Comparing Interpretative Notes in the Syriac and Arabic Translations of the Hippocratic *Aphorisms*', *Aramaic Studies* 14

—— (ed.) *Tafsīr Jālīnūs li-Fuṣūl Abuqrāṭ*. Translated by Ḥunayn ibn Isḥāq. ARABCOMMAPH/editions/Ḥunayn ibn Isḥāq (tr. Galen)/Galen commentaries books 1–7

Mingana, A. (ed.). 1935. *Book of Treasures by Job of Edessa*. (Cambridge)

—— (ed.) 1932. *Commentary of Theodore of Mopsuestia on the Nicene Creed*. (Cambridge) tp://www.tertullian.org/fathers/theodore_of_mopsuestia_nicene_01_intro.htm

Nöldeke, T. 1904. *Compendious Syriac Grammar*. (London). Reprint 2003 (Eugene)

Overwien, O. 2012. 'The Art of the Translator, or: How did Ḥunayn ibn Isḥāq and his School Translate?' in P.E. Pormann, *Epidemics in Context. Greek Commentaries on Hippocrates in the Arabic Tradition* (Berlin). 151–70

—— 2015. 'The Paradigmatic Translator and His Method: Ḥunayn ibn Isḥāq's Translation of the Hippocratic *Aphorisms* from Greek via Syriac into Arabic', *Intellectual History of the Islamicate World* 3, 158–87

Pietruschka, U. 1997. '"Puššāq šmāhē' und 'sullam": Mehrsprachige Wörterbücher bei Syrern und Kopten im arabischen Mittelalter', *Das Mittelalter* 2, 119–33

Pognon, H. (ed.). 1903. *Une version syriaque des Aphorismes d'Hippocrate*. (Leipzig)

Pormann, P.E. 2010. 'Arabic Astronomy and the Making of the European Renaissance'. Review of *Islamic Science and the Making of the European Renaissance*, by George Saliba. *Annals of Science* 67, 243–8

—— 2012. 'The Development of Translation Techniques from Greek into Syriac and Arabic: The Case of Galen's *On the Faculties and Powers of Simple Drugs, Book Six*', in R. Hansberger, M. Afifi al-Akiti and C. Burnett (eds), *Medieval Arabic Thought: Essays in Honour of Fritz Zimmermann* (London). 143–62

—— 2011. 'The Formation of the Arabic Pharmacology: Between Tradition and Innovation', *Annals of Science* 68:4, 493–515

Pormann, P.E. and E. Savage-Smith. 2007. *Medieval Islamic Medicine*. (Washington)

—— 2004. *The Oriental Tradition of Paul of Aegina's* Pragmateia. (Leiden)

—— 2003. 'Theory and Practice in the Early Hospitals in Baghdad: Al-Kaškarī on Rabies and Melancholy', *Zeitschrift für Geschichte der Arabische-Islamischen Wissenschaften* 15, 197–248

Richter-Bernburg, L. 2002. 'Gondēšāpur'. *Encyclopedia Iranica* 11:2, 131–5. Article updated online in 2012. http://www.iranicaonline.org/articles/gondesapur.

Rosenthal, F. 1966. 'Life is Short, the Art is Long: Arabic Commentaries on the First Hippocratic Aphorism', *Bulletin of the History of Medicine* 40:3, 226–45

Sachau, E. (ed.). 1870. *Inedita Syrica*. (Vienna)

Saliba, G. 2007. *Islamic Science and the Making of the European Renaissance*. (Cambridge, MA)

Smith, J. Payne. 1903. *A Compendious Syriac Dictionary*. (Oxford) http://dukhrana.com/lexicon/PayneSmith/

Smith, R. Payne. 1879. *Thesaurus Syriacus*. (Oxford) http://dukhrana.com/lexicon/RPayneSmith/

Strohmaier, G. 1991 (1993). 'Ḥunain ibn Isḥāq- an Arab Scholar Translating into Syriac', *ARAM* 3, 163–70

—— 1974. 'Ḥunayn b. Isḥāk as Philologist', in *Ephrem-Ḥunayn Festival* (Baghdad). 529–44.

Takahashi, H. 2010. 'The Sciences in Syriac from Serverus Sebokht to Barhebraeus', in H. Kobyashi and M. Koto (eds), *Transmission of Sciences: Greek, Syriac, Arabic, and Latin* (Tokyo). 16–32

Tannous, J. 2010. 'Syria Between Byzantium and Islam: Making Incommensurables Speak'. PhD diss., Princeton University

Thackston, W.M. 1999. *Introduction to Syriac*. (Bethesda)

Treiger, A. 2016. 'Palestinian Origenism and the Early History of the Maronites: In Search of the Origins of the Arabic Theology of Aristotle', in D. Janos (ed.), *Ideas in Motion in Baghdad and Beyond: Philosophical and Theological Exchanges between Christians and Muslims in the Third/Ninth and Fourth/Tenth Centuries* (Leiden). 44–80

Tytler, J. (ed.). 1832. *Kitāb al-Fuṣūl li-Abuqrāṭ*. (Calcutta)

Ullmann, M. 1978. *Islamic Medicine*. (Edinburgh)

—— 2011–12. *Die Nikomachische Ethik des Aristoteles in arabischer Überlieferung*. 2 Vols. (Wiesbaden)

—— 1977. 'Die Tadhkira des ibn as-Suwaidi, eine wichtige Quelle zur Geschichte der griechisch-arabischen Medizin und Magie', *Der Islam* 54, 33–65

—— 2002–7.*Wörterbuch zu den griechisch-arabischen Übersetzungen des 9. Jahrhunderts*. With 2 supplementary Vols. (Wiesbaden)

—— 2009. *Untersuchungen zur arabischen Überlieferung der Materia medica des Dioskurides*. (Wiesbaden)

Vagelpohl, U. 2011. 'In the Translator's Workshop', *Arabic Sciences and Philosophy* 21:2, 249–88

Watt, J. 2016. ' The Syriac Aristotelian Tradition and the Syro-Arabic Baghdad Philosophers' in D. Janos (ed.), *Ideas in Motion in Baghdad and Beyond: Philosophical and Theological Exchanges between Christians and Muslims in the Third/Ninth and Fourth/Tenth Centuries* (Leiden). 7–44

Wehr, H. 1994. *A Dictionary of Modern Written Arabic*. Edited by J.M. Cowan. (Wiesbaden). 1979. Reprint 1979 (Urbana)

APPENDIX

An Alphabetized Version of Duval's Greek Index to Bar Bahlul's *Syriac Lexicon*

As discussed at the beginning of Chapter One, Rubens Duval, the editor of Bar Bahlul's *Syriac Lexicon*, prepared an extensive index of Greek terms that he had identified as present in the latter work. However, this index has until now remained ordered according to the terms' column and line numbers rather than alphabetically, making it very difficult to consult systematically.

The following represents an alphabetically-ordered list of the Greek and Latin terms identified by Duval as present in Bar Bahlul's *Lexicon*. Although I provide it here with the intention of facilitating reference to the *Lexicon* for all interested scholars, I hasten to add that it should not be taken to replace Duval's index entirely. The original index includes important references that I have not included in this list. Furthermore, in numerous cases several Greek terms occur in the context of thematically-ordered entries, as may be seen in the entry for the word *marqāqā* in the discussion of ὑποχόνδριον at the end of Chapter Four above. This and like phenomena are emphasized by Duval's approach but suppressed here. Thus cross-reference between this list and Duval's index is generally recommended.

Finally, another slight problem in the original edition may be noted. For the intial pages of the sections in the *Lexicon* for the letters *ālep* to *pē*, the line-numbers given in Duval's index differ from those added in the Philo Press edition due to the editor's including the lines occupied by the section titles in his count. This approach was not adopted, however, in the Greek index for the letters following *pē* nor in any of the other indices. For this reason, the references in the index to columns 5, 6, 349, 350, 441, 442, 525, 526, 599, 600, 663, 664, 671, 672, 708, 709, 783, 784, 833, 834, 858, 859, 931, 932, 985, 986, 1207, 1208, 1291, 1292, 1471, and 1472 will differ from the Philo edition's line numbering.

Greek Words

A

ἀάατος 106:23

ἄατον 106:23

ἄβατος 10:13

ἀββᾶς 18:7

ἀβέλτερος 10:15

ἀβής 15:25

ἀβιληνή 15:4

ἀβραμίς= ἄγνος, τὸ δένδρον τοῦ Ἀβραάμ 20:3–4

ἀβραμίς (ἰχθύς) 20:3–4

ἀβροτόνινον 20:19

ἀβρότονον 20:21–4, 422:27, 594:8

 κεκαυμένον 20:21–4

ἀβρύνων 20:17

ἄβυσσος 14:19, 160:17

ἀγαθά 22:26, see ἀγάθων

ἀγαθός 22:27, 33:17

 ἄνθρωπος 26:17

ἀγαθοῦ 24:8

ἀγαθυνεῖς 22:22

ἀγαθυνθήσεται 33:19

ἀγάθων 33:16, see ἀγαθά

ἀγαλλιᾶσθε 22:11

ἀγαλλιάσομαι 22:9

ἀγάλλοχον 22:3, 28:25

ἀγάπη 26:20, 30:24, 156:12

ἀγαπητός 23:11, 31:1

ἀγαρικόν 22:16, 32:16, 445:3

ἀγαστός 23:1

ἀγγείδιον? 198:11

ἀγγελία 198:15

ἄγγελος 23:12, 198:12

ἀγένητος 30:16

ἀγέρωχος 22:28

ἄγη (ἡ)? 33:15

ἀγήρατον 27:15

ἀγήρατος (λίθος) 27:12, 864:14

ἅγιον πνεῦμα 27:10

ἅγιος 7:8, 26:19, 28:4

ἁγιώτατος 28:2

ἀγκύλη 145:24?, 276:8, 851:1

ἀγκύλιον 275:21

ἀγκύλωσις 214:3

ἀγκών 273:16

ἀγλαοφῶτις 26:4, 29:10–12,13

ἄγλωσσος 29:7

ἄγνοια 28:6, 30:6, 30:7, see ἄνοια

ἄγνος 27:25, 30:12, 948:18

ἀγορά 25:14

ἀγρία

 ἐλαία 22:20, 23:25–6, 32:20

 κάνναβις 32:12, see κάνναβις

 κνίκος 22:13, 32:24–5

 κράμβη 22:18, 32:14?, see κράμβη ἀγρία

ἀγριορίγανος 32:21

(ἐρέβινθος) ἄγριος 32:11, see ἐρέβινθος (ἄγριος)

ἄγριος 26:12

ἄγριος (τόπος) 32:10, 51:7

 σίκυς 33:7, 200:1–2, 518:5, see σίκυς ἄγριος

Ἀγρίππας 33:5

ἀγρός 25:24

ἄγρωστις 28:12

 ἄλλα ἐν Παρνασσῷ 31:24

ἀγύρτης 25:15

ἀγχίλωπα (ἀγχίλωψ) 211:6

ἀγχίλωπας (ἀγχίλωψ) 211:2

ἀγχίλωψ 253:24, 606:8

ἄγχουσα 126:22–6, 202:25, 210:22–3

ἑτέρα 126:22–6

τρίτη 126:22–6

ἀγωγάς 24:12–20

ἀγωγή 24:12–20

ἀγωγός 24:12–20

ἀγών 24:25

ἀγωνιστής 25:1

ἀδαμαντικὸς (λίθος) 33:28, 39:19–22, 39:23, 297:3–4?, 297:7, 331:27

ἀδάμαντος (λίθος) 565:17

ἀδάμας 34:10, 36:7, 39:14, 39:24, 135:20, 179:4 (-αντος), 331:27, 863:2, 1987:9

ἀδάρκης 33:25, 41:26, 43:7, 43:11, 99:15, 704:10, 718:22

ἀδάρκιον 718:22

ἀδελφύς 38:8

ἀδένες (ἀδήν) 34:21

ἄδηλον 37:2

ἀδήν 37:10, 1500:5, see ἀδένες

ἅδης 37:13

ἀδηφαγία 36:9, 53:8

ἀδίαντον 33:27, 37:4, 826:4

ἀδικία 37:15

ἄδικον 37:17

ἄδικος 37:17

ἄδιψον? 37:12

ἀδολεσχία 35:7

Ἀδονίς 35:21

Ἀδραμυττηνός 43:2

Ἀδρίας 42:17, 610:8

ἀεὶ ὤν 125:5, 137:17, 140:14, 210:13, 211:12

ἀείζων 122:6, 122:7, 148:3

ἕτερον τρίτον 6:23–6, 46:1

μικρόν 6:23–6, 46:1

ἀέρας 8:19, 9:8

ἀερία 9:4

ἀέρινον 344:6

ἀέριον 7:4, 7:12, 8:23

Ἀέτιος 6:17, 9:1

ἀέτιος 6:18

ἀέτος 107:2, 207:22

ἀετός 6:20

Ἄζωτος 100:14, 305:24

ἀηδών 7:2, 45:21, 212:25

ἄηπτον 17:12?

ἀήρ 8:14–16, 147:6

ἀθανασία 317:8

Ἀθανάσιος 317:6, 333:24

ἀθάνατος 7:9–10, 333:25

ἀθετῶν 321:18

Ἀθῆναι 327:20–7, 333:23, 662:7

ἀθήρα 37:21, 216:10, 328:4, 592:17?, 603:20, 676:1

ἀθηρώματα 321:24

ἀθληταί 330:22–8

ἀθλητής 330:22–8

ἄθλιος 331:4

ἀθυμία 326:28

ἀθῶος 322:5

αἴγειρος 27:23, 51:4, 111:3, 606:15

αἰγιαλός 26:21

αἰγίδιον 111:6

αἰγίλωψ 28:11, 28:21, 29:8, 98:10?, 111:26, 198:20, 605:25, 867:8

αἰγοθήλης 731:2

αἰγόκερως 111:22, 472:18, 605:16

αἰγύπτια 31:4

Αἰγυπτία (ἄκανθα) 198:17, see ἄκανθα Αἰγυπτία

αἰγύπτιον (ἐλένιον) 31:5

Αἴγυπτος 23:8, 30:26, 115:20

αἰδοῖον 602:12
αἰθάλη 331:6
αἰθήρ 8:14–16, 327:28, 662:5
αἰθιοπικός 233:15
Αἰθοπίς 933:13?
Αἰλώμ 127:23
αἷμα 132:10, 135:14, 636:27 (-ατος),
αἱματίτης (λίθος) 185:8, 637:7, 758:11, 865:5, 1837:7 (confused with κρύσταλλος), see λίθος (αἱματίτης)
αἱμορροΐδες 67:21, 616:7, 637:5
αἴνεσις 137:6
αἶνος 137:8
Αἰολίς 5:20
αἶρα 8:21, 147:20, 147:26, 655:27
αἱρεῖ 284:22
αἴρειν 149:21
αἵρεσις 299:12, 659:13
αἱρεσιῶται (αἱρεσιώτης) 280:3, 283:24
αἱρετικοί 658:1
αἴρω 149:10
πέντε αἰσθήσεις 1555:10, 1580:4
ἡ αἰτιατική? 124:19
Αἴτνη 108:19
αἰχμαλωσία 126:20, 158:16
αἰών 118:7, 599:11
Ἀκαδημαϊκοί 272:13
Ἀκαδημία 272:13
ἀκαδημία 1713:8
ἀκακαλίς 271:4
ἀκακία 272:3, 277:14, 1479:23
ἄκακος 272:1
ἀκαλύφη 271:16, 276:1
ἄκανθα 59:13, 271:11–17
Αἰγυπτία 59:13, 271:22, see Αἰγυπτία (ἄκανθα)
Ἀραβική 215:6, 590:16
λευκή 213:21, 248:14, 271:20, see λευκὴ ἄκανθα
ἀκάνθιον 272:4
ἀκανθίς 271:8
ἄκαρπος 278:11, 13
ἀκατέργαστοι 271:18
ἄκαυστον 75:28
ἀκέφαλος 240:20?, 242:17?, 277:12
ἀκηδιάσειν 275:15
ἄκινος 275:18
ἀκίντον 7:6
ἀκίντος 7:6
ἀκμή 276:13
ἄκμων 179:22
ἀκοή 272:22
ἀκολουθία 273:12, 273:21, 276:3
ἀκόνη 276:17, 25
ἀκονημένα 145:27
ἀκόνιτον 272:23–8, 273:4, 277:4, 828:19, 1740:3
λυκοκτόνον 272:23–8
κυνοκτόνον 272:23–8
ἄκοπα 273:25
ἄκοπον 274:4
ἄκορον 85:19, 85:24, 275:13, 278:9, 667:7
ἀκούβιτον 272:9, 273:13, 274:13
ἀκουσταί 276:21–2
ἀκουστή 276:21–2
ἀκούστιζέ με 276:24
ἄκρατον 274:25?, 277:19?, 1839:14?
ἀκρατῶς 145:6
ἀκρίβεια 278:1, 19
ἀκριβῶν (ἀκριβής) 277:25
ἀκρίς 278:16
ἀκρίδες 278:21
ἀκροβυστία 274:12

ἀκροστόλιον 1839:18?

ἀκρότομος 278:17

ἀκροχορδόνες 277:20?, 278:5, 942:20?

ἀκροχορδών 278:7, 278:14

ἀκτή 274:18

ἀλάβαστρος 165:26

ἀλάβαστρον 352:7

ἀλαλαγμός 165:19

ἄλαλος 165:16

ἀλγηδών 166:1–2

ἄλγος 166:1–2

ἄλειμμα 171:4–6, 1169:11

ἀλεκτορίς 167:23?

ἀλέκτορος (ἀλέκτωρ) 167:23?

Ἀλεξανδρία 176:15–16

Ἀλέξανδρος 176:6

ἄλευρον 171:19

ἀλήθεια 174:10

ἀληθινὸν ἐλατήριον 173:21, 180:20, see ἐλατήριον

ἀλθαία 181:3, 936:4, 983:1

ἁλικάκαβον 174:4

ἢ στρύχνον ἄλλο 174:16

ἄλιμος 172:7

ἄλιξ 173:14, 174:7, 174:8, 632:29, 633:20, 1393:6

χόνδρος 817:25–6

ἄλισμα 174:14

ἀλιστὸς (λίθος) 863:28?

ἀλκέα 180:4

ἀλκυόνια? 180:8

ἀλκυόνιον 63:8, 179:18

ἀλκύων 175:10, 180:9

ἀλλ᾽ἤ 176:21

ἀλλαγή 166:3

ἀλλαχθήσονται 176:22

ἄλλη? 625:4

ἀλληγορία σχηματική 174:20

ἄλλο κύφι 1744:11–14

ἀλλοίωσις 176:19

ἀλλότριος 176:18, 183:19?

ἀλλόφυλος 184:22

ἁλμάδες 177:6

ἅλμη 177:7

ἄλογοι 65:15

ἀλόη 165:1–2, 168:1, 168:9, cf. 28:25

Σοκοτορία 1382:27

ἁλός (ὁ ἅλς) 165:18, 166:19, 168:28, see ἁλῶν

ἄνθος 169:4, 170:5

ἄχνη 169:6, 170:3

ἅλς 177:19 see ἁλῶν

ἀλσίνη 177:15

ἀλυπίας (ἄλυπον) 169:17

ἄλυπον (σπέρμα.... ὡς ἐπιθύμου)169:26

ἁλυσίδια 169:19

ἁλυσίδιον 169:3, 170:24

ἄλυσσον (ἀσπίδιον) 168:8, 170:13

ἀλύσσων? 168:29

ἄλφα 178:24

ἀλφοί 178:17

ἁλῶν (ὁ ἅλς) 168:15, cf. 165:18, 166:19, 177:19, see ἁλός (ὁ ἅλς), ἅλς

ἁλώνια 169:20

ἀλωπεκία 169:25

ἀλώπεκος 169:24, cf.169:10

ἀλώπηξ 169:10, 164:24

ἅμα 181:17

ἀμαράκινον 187:12–14, 193:16

ἀμάρακον 181:14, 193:8, 215:15, 986:13, 1721:12, cf. 1155:1, 1477:10, 1485:2, 1811:6, see παρθένιον ἀμάρακον

ἀμάραντον 193:8–12, 1721:11

ἀμάραντος 634:12
ἀμάρας (ἀμάρα) 182:3, 193:13
ἁμαρτάνετε 181:18
ἁμαρτία 181:19
ἁματωλός 182:4, 193:18
ἀμαύρωσις 67:16, 181:21
ἀμβλυωπία 182:19, 190:24
ἀμβροσία 182:6, 182:18, 366:10–11
ἀμβρόσιος 182:21
ἄμη 181:13
ἀμίαντον 2077:17
ἀμίαντον (λίθον) 186:1, 1074:25
ἀμίαντον (ὑφάσμα) 185:25
ἀμίαντος 17:12?, 186:21
ἀμίαντος (λίθος) 136:6, see λίθος (ἀμίαντος)
ἀμίδα (ἀμίς)? 185:12
ἀμίς 185:13, 188:5, 188:7, 211:10
ἄμμεως 181:16, cf. 185:10
ἄμμι 181:16, 986:15 (-εως), 993:12 (-εως)
  τὸ κοπτικόν 185:10
ἄμμος 187:15
ἀμμωνιακόν 183:11–12, 297:1, 1090:5
ἀμμωνιακόν (θυμίαμα) 409:7
ἀμνός 133:14
ἀμόργη 184:1
ἀμπελόκαρπος 272:6
ἀμπελόπρασον 188:12, 189:20–2?
ἄμπελος 188:19–20
  ἀγρία 188:23, 191:8, 1146:10
  ἥμερος 188:21
  λευκή 188:15–18
  μέλαινα 183:3, 189:1, 191:13
  οἰνοφόρος 191:18
ἀμπώτινος 190:18
ἄμπωτις 190:18, 639:1
ἀμυγδαλέων (ἀμυγδαλή) 182:22
ἀμυγδαλή 184:11
ἀμυγδάλινον (ἔλαιον) 184:16
ἀμύδρωσις? 42:18
ἄμυλον 65:25, 184:26, 186:24, 1974:8
ἀμύνομοι 133:24
ἄμυρον 49:7
ἀμφῆλιξ 189:14
ἀμφίβληστρον 191:5
ἀμφιθαλής 191:3
ἀμφίκοπος 189:4
ἀμφίκυρτος 189:9
Ἀμφίπολις 189:16
ἀμφίσβαινα 1380:17
ἀμφόδοντα 934:4
ἀμφόδους 189:3
ἀμφοῖν 191:7
ἀμφορεύς 84:14, 144:1, 191:20
ἀμφότερα 183:19?, 191:24?
ἀμφότεροι 183:19?
ἀμωμίτης 977:1
ἄμωμον 184:13
ἄμωμος 184:24
ἀνάβα χύριε 22:24
ἀνάβασις 194:11
ἀναβιβάζων 194:17–21
ἀναγαλλίδος 197:21
ἀναγαλλίς 195:17, 197:11, 1453:5
ἀναγγέλετε 194:9
ἀναγκαῖον 211:15
ἀνάγκας 211:14
ἀνάγκε 211:13
ἀναγκεφαλαιωθέντα 214:9
ἀναγνώστης 28:8, 30:15, 76:13, 111:8, 199:1
ἀνάγυρις 198:21
ἀνάγυρος 197:13
ἀναδενδράδες 196:22

ἀνακαινιθήσεται 196:25
ἀνακάρδια (ἀνακάρδιον) 214:1
ἀνακολλήματα 196:14
ἀνακύκλησις 145:24
ἀναλαβεῖν 197:9
ἀνάληψις 195:25
ἀνάλλακτος 29:5, 195:7
ἀναλογία 194:26
ἀναλογική 203:1
ἀναλογιστικός 196:16
ἀνάλογον 195:3
ἀνάλογος 201:27
ἀνάλυσις 195:6, 197:7
ἀναλυτική 195:9, 203:25
ἀναλώματα 195:4
ἀνανέωσις 197:1
ἄναρχος 196:11, 214:18
ἀνάρρινον 110:17–19, 124:20, see ἀντίρρινον
ἀνάστα 195:22–3
ἀνάσταθι 195:22–3
ἀναστάς 211:25
ἀναστασία (ἀνάστασις) 154:5, 177:18, 195:19, 211:26
ἀναστήσονται 196:1
ἀναστροφή 195:24
ἀνατέλλουσα 205:12
ἀνατολή 195:14, 205:1
ἀναφορά 142:25, 196:3–7, 683:11?
ἀναφοράς 141:23, 213:9
ἀναφορικόν 196:8
ἀναφορῶν 213:8–9
ἀναψύξω 197:3
ἄνδρα (ἀνήρ) 199:6, see ἀνήρ
ἀνδράποδα 42:25
ἀνδράχνη 114:22, 199:4
ἀνδρεία 197:5
ἀνδριάς (-άντα) 18:8–9, 42:22, 121:20, 200:6, 932:13, 956:3
ἀνδρίζεσθε 197:16
ἀνδρόσαιμον 113:9, 200:3, 200:16
ἀνδρόσακες 115:3, 199:24
ἀνδροφονεῖς 200:23
Ἀνδρώνιος (τροχίσκος) 891:19, see τροχίσκος Ἀνδρώνιος
ἀνεβάλλετο 194:15
ἀνέβη 201:16
ἀνέθαλλεν 201:17
ἀνεθέμην 198:3
ἀνεκαινίσθη 201:18
ἀνεκαλύφθη 201:20
ἀνελόμενον 195:15
ἀνελπιστία 215:11
ἄνεμος 201:19, 209:8, 211:10
ἀνεμώνη 115:22, 132:12, 201:6, 209:20, 899:20
ἀνεξέλεγκτος 210:14
ἀνερώτησις 214:14?
ἄνεσις 211:23
ἀνέσκαψεν 201:21
ἀνεστηκώς 216:13
ἀνετράπην 201:5
ἀνεύρυσμα 71:5, 203:21
ἀνευρύσματα 201:11
ἀνεψιός 198:6
ἀνέψυχέ με 201:23
ἀνεῳγμένος 201:3
ἀνήγαγεν 198:18
ἀνήθινον 209:4
ἄνηθον 208:16, 214:27
ἀνήρ 210:8, see ἄνδρα
ἀνήφθησαν pro ἀνήφτην? 209:10
ἀνθεμίς 215:13, 15
ἀνθερίκη 214:25, 754:17

ἀνθερικός 210:3
ἄνθος 152:14, 214:23, 216:3
  χαλκοῦ 153:24
ἄνθρακες (ἄνθραξ) 216:15, 426:19
ἀνθρωπάρεσκος 216:18
ἄνθρωπος 71:7–8, 152:10, 215:8, 216:20
ἀνθύλλιον 214:23
ἀνθυλλίς 217:10–13
ἀνθύπατος 215:9
ἀνία 208:23
ἀνίκητον (ἀνίκητος) 209:9
ἀνίκητος 213:18
ἄνισον 139:4–8, 208:24, 209:1?
ἀνισοταχεῖς 209:16
ἀννώνα 118:5, 118:9, 202:2, 202:23, 680:28
ἀννώνας, 202:24, 203:20, 680:28
ἀνόητος 203:7
ἄνοια 201:24, 203:9, see ἄγνοια
ἀνοίγων 203:10
ἀνοίσω 203:11
ἀνομία 201:26
ἄνους 209:11
ἀνταείρατο 206:22
ἀντάλλαγμα 207:18
ἀντάμειψις 206:20
ἀνταπέδωκα 206:24
ἀνταποδιδούς 206:26
ἀνταπόδοσις 207:1
ἀνταρσία 206:9
ἀντάρτης 206:7
ἀντελάβετο 207:2
ἀντιγείτονας 206:13?
ἀντίδοτοι (ἀντίδοτος) 205:3
ἀντίδοτος 216:4, 677:23
  διουρητικός 1740:1
ἀντίθεσις 205:17
ἀντικειμένων (ἀντικείμενος) 207:16
ἀντικλείδων (ἀντικλείς) 204:8
ἀντικνήμιον 205:23
ἀντικυρικόν 1344:19
ἀντιλήπτωρ 207:4
ἀντιλήψεται 207:6
ἀντιλογία 207:7
Ἀντιόχεια 999:13
Ἀντιόχου (θηριακή) 208:12?
ἀντιπαθές 207:23
Ἀντιπατρίς 207:25
ἀντίρρινον 110:17–19, 124:20–1, 207:26
ἀντιστήριγμα 207:9
ἀντιστροφή 205:14
ἀντίτυπος 205:8
ἀντίφασις 204:12, 205:4, 208:11
ἀντιφατικάς (ἀντιφατικός) 206:16
ἀντιφατική 206:18
ἀντίφορος 205:10?
ἀντίχθωνας (ἀντίχθων) 206:13?
Ἀντίχριστος 205:27
Ἀντώνιος 204:6
ἀντωνυμία 204:24, 207:13, 220:13
ἀντωνυμιῶν 207:11
ἄνυδρος 209:12
ἀνυπόστατον (ὕδωρ) 209:14
ἄνω 203:12
ἀνωνίς 69:14, 202:19
ἀνώρθωσεν 203:16
ἄξαις 28:14
ἀξία 163:7, 202:1, see ἀναξία
ἀξιάς (ἀξία) 160:12
ἀξίδα 156:13?
ἀξίνας (ἀξίνη) 159:1, 160:7?, 160:21, 161:4
ἄξιοι 163:6
ἀξιόλογοι 163:3, 163:12, 628:26

ἀξιόπιστος 161:23

ἀξίωμα 161:6, 162:11?

ἀξιώματα 809:11

ἀξούγγιον 60:7, 140:16, 159:21, 159:26

ἀόρατος 5:15, 1305:2

ἀπαγωγή 248:19

ἀπαθής 84:29

ἀπαθητῶς 247:10

ἀπαλλοτριώμενος 264:11

Ἀπάμεια 263:23

ἀπάξει 247:27

ἀπαράλλακτος 268:24

ἀπαρίνη 247:15, 272:6, 443:23, 909:1

ἀπαρκτίας 247:7, 268:12, 373:20

ἀπαρχή 248:1

ἀπεδοκίμασαν 249:5

ἀπέδων 249:8

ἀπειθῶν 249:9

ἀπεκρίθη 249:10

ἀπέναντι 249:3

ἀπενεχθήσονται 249:12, see ἀχθήσονται

ἀπέπεσον 256:16

ἀπέρρηγμαι 249:14

ἀπέστησας 249:21

ἀπέστρεψεν 249:15

ἀπέτινον 249:16

ἀπεψία 265:23

ἀπῆλθον 249:11

ἀπηλιώτης 260:18, 649:24

ἀπηνήνατο 264:13

ἀπῆρεν 262:1

ἀπηχήματα 141:7, 259:26, 261:22

ἄπιον 260:3–5

ἄπιος 260:3–5

  τὸ φυτόν 262:4

ἀπιστοσύνη? 261:19

ἀπίτης οἶνος 83:16

ἁπλῆ ὠνή 1829:18

ἁπλοῦν 263:5

  μέν 263:18

ἁπλῶς 652:4

ἀπό 255:22

ἀποβλέπει 255:23

ἀπογεγαλακτισμένος 255:24

ἀπογονή? 255:1

ἀπογραφή 248:23

ἀποδεικτική 143:26–7, 250:14, 258:3, 1186:3

ἀπόδειξις 38:11, 143:25, 250:13, 251:20, 258:10

ἀπόδος 255:26

ἀποιήτως 247:10

ἀποκαθίσταθι? 256:3

ἀποκαθιστῶν 255:27

ἀποκαλύψει 256:1

ἀποκατάστασις 257:4

ἀποκομήτων 254:17, 257:9

ἀποκόψει 256:4

ἀπόκρισις 142:18?, 266:5

ἀπόκρουσις 253:8

ἀποκρυβήσεται 256:6

ἀποκρύπτεσθαι 256:6

ἀποκρυφή 256:8

ἀπόκρυφοι 80:12

ἀποκτείνειν 255:6, 256:9

ἀπόκυνον 252:16, 257:17

ἀπολεῖς 255:8

ἀπολεῖται 256:10–11

ἀπόλειψις 254:14

ἀπολελυμένον 255:20

ἀπόληψις 253:14?

Ἀπολινάριος 250:24

Ἀπόλλων 257:11, 258:13, 263:4, 350:15?

Ἀπολλωνία 257:15, 258:12

ἀπολογία 250:26, 257:27, 264:20
ἀπόλοιντο 256:10–11
ἀπόλοιτο 256:10–11
ἀπολοῦνται 256:10–11
ἀπολωλώς 256:13
ἀπόμελι 251:12, 254:9, 257:6, 1022:14
ἀπόπατος 257:16
ἀποπεσοῦνται 256:14
ἀποπληξία 251:6, 253:25, 263:8, 265:12
ἀπορία 374:4
ἄπορος 374:5
ἀπορρεύσεται 256:19
ἀπορρίψει 256:17
ἀποσκορακίσεις 255:9
ἀποστάντες 256:20
ἀπόστημα 251:23, 251:24, 253:21, 264:26,
    1586:17?
ἀποστήματα 251:24
ἀποστῆτε 256:22
ἀποστολήν (ἀποστολή)142:8
ἀποστολικοί 251:10
τρισκαίδεκα ἀπόστολοι 827:12
ἀπόστολος 251:9
ἀποστραφείησαν 256:24
ἀποσύρματα? 81:3
ἀποσφαγή 255:18
ἀποτελεσματικός 257:28, 264:21
ἀπουσία 251:13
ἀποφαίνεσθαι 252:14, 253:19, 265:28
ἀποφάναι 1576:14
ἀπόφανσις 252:12, 254:22–4
ἀποφαντικαί 252:18
ἀποφαντικός 252:13, 254:22–4
ἀπόφασις 252:4, 253:10, 1477:21, 1557:15, 1689:5
ἀποφατικός 254:20, 1320:20
ἀποφῆσαι 255:12
ἀποφθέγματα 546:16
ἀποφθέγξονται 256:26
ἄπυρον 261:15, 267:20, 2058:14
ἀπώμοτος 251:19
ἀπώσω με 256:28
ἄρα 278:25
    Πορφύριος 279:22
ἆρα 278:25
ἀρά 33:22, 279:2, 24
Ἀραβία 279:9, 280:9, 280:26
ἀραβικός (λίθος) 864:1, see λίθος (ἀραβικός)
ἄρακος 280:2
ἄρατε 279:27
ἀρατωματικά? 287:28
ἀράχνη 279:11, 293:25
ἄραχος 280:2
ἄργεμον 34:12, 15, 281:26, 291:24?
ἀργέστης 283:12
ἀργημώνη 149:19, 209:20–2, 282:3
ἀργυροπράκτης 283:19
ἄργυρος 283:8
    ἄργυροι 283:10
Ἀρειομανίτης 292:14
Ἄρειος 289:7
    παγός 291:25
ἀρέσει 284:21
Ἀρέτας 289:2
ἀρετάς (ἀρετή) 288:16, 288:28
ἀρετή 279:20, 287:22
ἄρηξις 289:4, 291:20
Ἄρης 291:6
ἄρθρα 304:25, see ἄρθρον
ἀρθρῖτις 98:25
ἄρθρον 304:18, 622:10, 1668:9, see ἄρθρα
ἀριθμητική 304:22
ἀριθμητικόν 291:23

ἀριθμητικός 291:22
ἀριθμοί 291:21
ἀριθμός 305:1
ἀρίσαρον 292:1
ἀριστερά 299:22
ἀριστήϊος 291:16
ἀριστητής 291:13–15
Ἀριστόβουλος 291:13, 299:3
(ἀριστό)δημος 565:9
ἀριστολοχία 290:16, 299:18
ἄριστον 291:13–15, 299:7
ἄριστος 291:16, 299:8
Ἀριστοτέλης 289:23, 299:13, 299:20
Ἀριστοχράτης 1476:6?
ἀριώθ 292:10, 1889:13
ἄρκειον 1356:13
ἀρκευθίδες 1705:4
ἀρκευθίδος 302:18–22
ἄρκευθος 302:18–22
ἄρκτιον 37:21?, 302:23?, 302:25, 303:6–11
ἄλλο 303:6–11
ἡ Ἄρκτος μεγάλη? 38:14, 42:15
Ἀρκτοῦρος 302:15–17
Ἀρκτοφυλάξ 302:15–17
ἄρκυς 41:1
ἅρμα 297:15
ἁρμάτιον 297:11
ἀρμενιακά? 135:15
ἀρμενιακόν 295:26, 297:1
ἀρμενιακός (λιθός)? 114:14, 296:28, 297:18
ἀρμενιακῶν (ἀρμενιακὰ μῆλα) 296:24
ἄρμενον 296:15, 670:6
ἁρμονία 295:28, 297:16, 297:20, 1036:8
ἁρμόνιον 295:27
ἀρνόγλωσσον 284:6?, 284:23?, 292:12, 298:18, 298:22?
ἀρωματοθήκη 287:28
ἄρον 9:3, 89:17, 95:24, 285:9, 548:22, 955:17
ἀροτραῖος? 216:23
ἄροτρον 206:12
ἁρπάζειν 302:3, 302:10
ἅρπαξ 302:1
ἁρπᾶσαι 302:10
ἀρρενικός 284:19–20
ἄρρην 303:12
ἀρσενικόν 284:19–20, 298:25, 299:15, 303:5
ἄρσις 299:12
ἀρτάβας (ἀρτάβη) 288:27
ἀρτάμη (ἄρταμος) 288:29?
ἀρτάρια 91:17
Ἄρτεμις 287:20
ἀρτεμισία 287:17
Ἀρτεμίσιος 1074:21
ἀρτηρία 288:1, 288:4, 288:6, see ἀρτηριῶν
ἀρτηρίας 289:1
ἀρτηριακάς 284:7, 287:25
ἀρτηριακή? 571:25
ἀρτηριακόν 288:4
ἀρτηριῶν 288:25, see ἀρτηρία
ἀρτοκόπος 199:3, 284:1, 288:9
ἄρτος 284:17–18, 287:23, 288:18, 288:23
ἀρχάγγελος 294:5
ἀρχαῖα 303:27
ἀρχαιολογία 293:8, 295:10
ἀρχαῖον 294:7, 388:6
ἀρχάς 281:7, 293:15, see ἀρχή
ἀρχέζωστις 295:13
Ἀρχέλαος 293:21
ἀρχέτυπον 295:9
ἀρχή 293:5–7, 293:19, 304:1, see ἀρχάς
τῆς ὥρας? 294:13
ἀρχίατρος 293:27, 554:7, 571:25?

Ἀρχιγένης 293:14, 295:12
ἀρχιδιάκονος 200:11, 294:1
ἀρχιερέων? 561:18
ἀρχιμανδρίτης 294:6, 295:16
Ἀρχιμήδης 294:25
Ἄρχιππος 295:17
ἀρχιταχύτερος? 295:4
ἀρχιτέκτονος 294:12
ἀρχιτέκτων 294:14
ἄρχοντα 294:10, see ἄρχων
ἄρχοντας 280:19, 293:17, see ἄρχων
ἄρχοντες 295:8, see ἄρχων
ἀρχός 304:2
ἄρχων 293:5–7, 293:12, see ἄρχοντα
ἄρωμα 657:15
ἀρωματικόν (φάρμακον) 297:11?
ἀρωματικόν κολλύριον 1601:17?
Ἀσαμωναῖοι 139:1
ἄσαρον 243:10, 1277:10, 1931:1
ἄσβεστος 99:6?
ἀσβόλη 217:20
ἀσθένεια? 245:17
ἀσθενής 245:20
ἀσθματικοί 227:13
ἀσίδα 229:16
ἀσίκητον 2077:10?
ἀσκάλαβος 192:8
ἀσκαλαβώτης 241:7
Ἀσκάλωνα 241:24
ἀσκαρίδες 241:3, 1378:26
ἀσκαρίς 241:3
ἀσκητικόν= ἀσκητήριον 241:23
ἀσκίδιον 160:7?
Ἀσκληπιάδης 240:6, 240:17, 1457:4
ἀσκληπιάς 240:11
Ἀσκληπιός 223:19, 239:24
ἀσκός 242:3
ἀσκυροειδές 239:11
ἄσκυρον 239:11, 242:12
ἀσόκιτον 2077:10?
ἀσπάλαθος 233:12
ἀσπάλακος (ἀσπάλαξ) 234:17
ἀσπάραγος 233:17, 237:19, 238:12, 239:18–20, 1371:10, 1459:5
ἀσπίς 237:11, 636:7
ἄσπληνον 236:26–237:1
ἀσσάριον 130:9, 217:18, 242:22–3
ἄσσιος (λίθος) 865:16, see λίθος (ἄσσιος)
ἀστεργής? 223:17
ἀστερίσκος? 228:21
ἀστέρος 224:13
δὶα ἀστέρων 567:20?
ἀστήρ 224:13
ἀστὴρ Ἀττικός 223:8, 228:6
ἀστράγαλος 224:20, 227:21, cf. 283:7
ἀστραπή 226:20
ἀστρόλαβον 226:21
ἀστρολογία 224:7
ἀστρολόγος 224:9
ἄστρον 224:12
ἀστρονομία 223:25
Ἀστυάγης 223:5, 228:22
ἀσύκητον 2077:10?
ἀσύνετος 230:4
ἀσύφη 1701:26
ἀσφάλεια 235:10, 239:21
ἄσφαλτος 233:6, 236:20, 236:22, 238:23, 260:1, 263:6, 1587:12
Ἰουδαϊκή 233:6
ἀσφόδελος 131:17–18, 218:18, 234:12, 238:7, 1150:20, 1372:22, 1432:1, 1493:25
ᾆσω 139:19

ἀσώματα 1311:26
ἀσωτία 76:9, 218:8
ἄσωτος 218:11
ἀτάραχος 110:2
ἀτελής 107:10, 208:6
ἀτέραμνος 106:16
Ἀτθίς 345:27
Ἀτλαντική 322:4?, 332:4?
Ἀτλαντικόν 108:1, 123:14, 208:4
Ἀτλαντικός 108:3
Ἄτλας 107:23, 28
ἄτομα 106:24, 124:7
ἄτομος 107:6–7, 194:25, 207:14
ἀτρακτυλίς 109:7, 227:17
ἀτράφαξις 109:21, 199:7
ἀτριβής 110:2
ἀτταγήν 124:11
Ἀττική 107:9, 107:22, 327:20–7
αὐγουστάλιος 26:8, 50:25
Αὔγουστος 25:6, 9, 50:23, 1303:29
αὐθάδεις 98:17
αὐθέντης 98:2
αὐθεντία 97:24, 98:15
αὐθεντική 98:1
αὖλαξ 117:26
αὐλείας 169:5?
αὐλή 62:18, 64:7, 117:19
αὐλητρίδος (αὐλητρίς) 64:17, 950:7
αὔλιον 64:12
αὐλισθήσεται 117:22
αὐλύ? 57:16, 64:9
αὐλών 62:25, 168:17
ἄυρα 116:3
αὐτή 117:9
αὐτοί 117:12
αὐτοκράτωρ 57:2, 58:8, 207:20
αὐτοματισταί 58:2
αὐτόματον 57:19, 58:1, 58:5, 106:18
αὐτοπτικός 57:23
αὐτοσχεδίως 57:6, 57:7, 57:27, 58:13, 1171:3
αὐτοῦ 47:28, 117:11
αὐτοφυῆ (τερμὰ ὕδατα) 57:14
αὐτόφυσις? 208:14
αὐτοψία 57:25
ἡ μὲν αὐτῶν 132:26
αὐχήν 59:24, 117:21
ἀφαιρούμενος 247:23
ἀφάκη 247:20, 248:18?
ἀφανίσει 247:25
ἀφείθησαν 249:17
ἄφες 249:19
ἀφῆκαν 262:3
ἄφθαρτος 269:19
ἀφόρητον 21:7
ἀφοριεῖς 255:11, 257:1
ἀφορισμοί 252:24, 924:1
Ἀφροδίτη 244:8, 266:23, 383:7, 599:17, 1608:21
ἀφρόνιτρον 251:3, 264:2, 267:11, 965:14, 1289:20
ἀφροσέληνος (λίθος) 267:23, 1631:1
ἀφρώδης 268:26
ἄφρων 268:19
ἀφχάγγελος 198:12
Ἀχαΐα 154:8
Ἀχαϊκὰς (μνας) 154:10
ἀχάτης 156:10
ἀχθήσονται 164:24, see ἀπενεχθήσονται
ἀχίλλειος 156:18–19, 172:5 ((ἀχί)λλειος)
ἄχιλος 62:11 (vel Ἀχιλλεύς), 156:20
ἀχλύς 157:16
ἀχράς 164:12

ἀχρειώθησαν 127:1

ἄχυ 1701:25

ἄχυρον 156:27

ἀχυρών 155:10

ἀχῶρος (ἀχώρ) 155:5, 1914:4

ἀχώρων (ἀχώρ) 60:10

ἀψίδα (ἀψίς) 163:1

ἀψίνθιον 265:1

θαλάσσιον 1349:1

ἀψινθίτης οἶνος 265:7

ἀωρία 5:17, 92:11

B

βαβαί 349:5, 354:3

βάθεα 353:15, 382:5

βαθεῖα 353:15, 382:5

βάθος 382:5, 995:10

βάκλος 373:9

βακτηρία 352:15

βάκχαρις 352:12

βαλανεῖον 394:22, 399:18

βαλανευτικός? 396:10

βαλάνινον (ἔλαιον) 351:20, cf. 351:1–3

βάλανοι δρυός? 383:15, 397:21

βάλανος μυρεψική 351:1–3, see μυροβάλανος

βαλαύστιον 351:5–10, 395:26

βάλλοντες 351:24

βαλλωτή 351:22

βάλσαμον 351:11–12, 369:23, 399:23

βάμβαξ 1576:11, cf. μπόμβυξ

βαναυσία 352:2

βάναυσοι 352:2

βάπτισμα 418:24

βαπτισμός 1129:6

Βαραββᾶς 423:10

βάραθρον 427:11

Βαρθολομαῖος 438:28

βάρις 353:1

Βαρνάβας 432:17

βαρύγυιον 352:22

βαρυκάρδιος 353:2

βαρύς 353:4

βάρυτον 427:12

Βασάν 409:22, cf. 386:12

βάσανος 408:17

ἐπί τῇ βασικῇ ὁδῷ 1540:7?

βασιλεία 408:10

βασιλείας 408:11

βασιλεύς 352:6, 408:11

βασιλική 408:23

βασιλικόν 408:21, 789:4

βασιλικός 408:20

Βασιλικῶν? 598:6

βασιλίσκος 352:5, 823:11, 20

βάσις 409:24

βάτος 349:9 (βάδος), 349:13, 380:14

βάτου φύλλον? 380:15

βατράχιον 350:7, 381:27

βάτραχος 349:15

βαττόλογος? 381:3

βαφή 352:10

βδέλλιον 357:26

βεβηλοῦνται 361:9

βέλεα 383:10, see βέλος

Βελίαρ 397:23

βέλος 361:10, see. βέλεα

βελόστασις 398:17

βελουάκος 2068:18

βέλτερα? 351:14

βέλτερος 352:1

Βένετοι καὶ Πρασινοί 413:20, see Veneti et

Albati, πράσινος
βερενίκιον 362:5 (νίτρον), 375:4, 1289:22 (νίτρον)
βετονίκη 1816:5, 2058:17
Βηθφαγή 391:16
Βήλ 350:19
βηλός 367:9, cf. 12:1
βῆμα 384:5
Βηρσαβεέ 432:22
βήχιον 383:3, 393:11
ὦ βία 49:24, 50:1, 60:6, 286:1
βιβλιοθήκας 382:13
βιβλιοθήκη 354:16, 383:12
βιβλιοθήκην 396:9
βιβλιοθηκῶν 354:14
βιβλίον 354:12
βιβλίων 354:12
βίβλος 382:7
Βιθυνία 387:20
βίκος 373:1
βλαστός 1701:25
βλασφημία 384:3–4
βλάσφημος 384:3–4
βλέπειν 395:10
βλεφαρόξυστον 395:5
βλέφαρον 395:12
βλῆτον 397:16, 398:12, 430:20
βόες 364:16
βοήθεια 370:11
βοηθός 366:20
βόθριον 376:18
βόθρος 376:25, 376:27
βοιδάρια (βοιδάριον) 374:23
βοίδια (βοίδιον) 364:7
βολαῖς (βολή) 370:1
βόλβοι? 33:23
βολβός 48:25, 394:26, see βάλιοι
ἐδώδιμος 367:15
ἐμετικός 367:15
βολή 368:22, 369:1
βομβυλιός 2044:22
βολχόν 63:10
βορέας 373:20, 373:24, 375:17
βοτάνη 191:8
βότρυς 366:10–11, 873:6
βου- 362:10
βούβαλοι 362:21, 367:14
βούβαλος 362:21
βουβῶνες (βουβών) 362:16
βουγάϊος 363:14
βούγλωσσον 363:7, 368:14, 2040:3
Βουκέφαλος 92:23, 1823:19
βουκέφαλος 176:15–16
βούκινα 373:2, 373:10, 1380:7, see βυκάνη
βουκινάτορ 373:2, 373:10
βουλευτήριον 369:3
βουλευτής 368:16
βουλή 367:11, 368:22, 369:25, 388:18, 637:1
βούλιμος 369:9, 896:8
βουνιάδος 362:7 (βουνιάς), 376:23
βουνιάς 370:12, 376:23
βούνιον 303:6–11, 370:12
βουνοί 371:26
βούπαις 371:26
βούπρηστις 372:4
βούτυρον 366:3
βούφθαλμον 362:14, 372:1, 843:6
βράκαι 422:15, 431:25?
βραχίων 422:19
βραχύ 422:18
βρέξας μικρός 421:17, 431:4
βρεταννική 422:16?, 425:18
Βριάρεως 430:9

βρογχία 426:24, 432:15
βρόμος 426:22
βροντή 428:5
βροῦχος 428:6
βροχή 428:7
βρόχος 427:22?
βρυγμὸς τῶν ὀδόντων 920:8
βρύον 421:22, 425:19, 425:25, 426:8, 427:15, 543:5, 1341:5
  θαλάσσιον 427:5?, 427:18
βρυωνία 86:5–7, 178:21, 188:15–18, 191:13–17, 422:26–8, 427:1, 472:4, 1296:1, 1296:3, 1573:20
βρυωνίς 427:25?, cf. 22:19
βρῶσις 428:8
βύας 362:9
βυζαντία 364:26
βυκάνη 373:2, 373:10, see βούκινα
βυκανίστης 373:2
βύνης (βύνη) 370:9
βυούσης 382:23
βυρσεύς 375:9
βωλώδης? 369:6, 369:18
βωμός 370:3

Γ

γαγάτης 441:8
γαγάτης (λίθος) 863:14, see λίθος (γαγάτης)
γάγγλια 441:6
γαγγλία 198:16
γάγγλιον 503:1
γάγγραινα 444:8–12
Γαδάρων? 487:10
Γάδειρα 441:12
Γάδηρα 453:15
Γάζα 442:12
γαζοφύλαξ 478:24
γαῖα 441:4
Γάϊος 442:20
γαλακτίτης (λίθος) 859:2, 865:7, see λίθος (γαλακτίτης)
γάλακτος (γάλα) 443:13
γαλαξίας 1930:4
γαλάριον 443:13, 490:11
Γαλατίας (ῥητίνη) 495:10?
γαλεώτης 443:8
γαλῆ 443:16
γαληνός 443:12, 498:3
γάλιον 443:22, 858:9
γαλίοψις 443:20
γαλλικόν 443:26
γάμος 499:26
γαμψάς 444:6
γαμψός 444:6
γάρος 366:7?, 445:4, 518:17
γαστήρ 444:14, 508:9
γαστριμαργία 508:15
γαυρίασις? 442:8
γέα 441:4
γεγέννηκα 456:9
Γέεννα 457:5, 487:8
Γεθσημανεῖ 453:8
γείτων 455:26
Γελασία 498:24
Γελάσιος 444:1
γέμει 456:27
γένεσθε 487:15
γενέσια 507:14
γένη 457:4
γενητόν 504:18

γεννήματα 457:1
Γεννησάρ 505:19
γεννήσεως (γέννησις) 457:15?
γεννική 457:12
γένος 457:3
γένου 457:2
γεντιανή 457:10, 504:13
γεραίος 444:28
γεράνιον 458:9
Γερμανική 520:3
Γερόντιος 445:1
γεύσασθε 457:14
γεῦσις 485:19, 504:6
γεωγραφία 607:3
γεώδης (λίθος) 864:5, see λίθος (γεώδης)
γεώμετραι 442:4, 485:17
γεωμέτρης 561:3
γεωμετρία 442:6, 456:1, 465:17–18
γεωμετρικόν 465:17–18
γεωπονική 457:12
γεωργία 456:6
γεωργίας 442:9
γεωργικόν 474:2, 933:2
γεωργικός 456:8, 482:5, see γεωργικόν, γεωργός
γεωργός 484:27
γῆ 22:2, 111:25, 441:4, 482:3, 487:5, see κρητικὴ γῆ, λημνία γῆ, χία γῆ
  ἀμπελῖτις 484:23
  ἐρετριάς 484:21
  κιμωλία 489:3, see κιμωλία, 1378:24
  μηλία 487:6
  πνιγῖτις 489:1
  σαμία 29:13, 488:15, 508:22, 890:15, see σαμία (γῆ)
  χῖα 486:5
γηγενεῖς 483:1
ἐπὶ γῆν ὄντα 1032:8
γῆρας 489:13
  ὄφεως 489:15, 891:9
γηροκομεῖον 67:4, 517:21
γῆς 1812:10 (καὶ ἐπὶ γῆς)
  ἀστήρ 508:22, 971:13
  ἔντερα 487:16, 498:1, 890:19
γίγαντες 483:4, see γίγας
γίγαρτον 482:26
γίγας 482:24, see γίγαντες
γιγγίδιον 50:22, 487:12, 905:15
γίζιρ 1701:24
γίνεσθαι? 488:18
γινώσκει 487:14
γλαύκιον 490:15, 494:7
γλαῦκος? 494:14
γλαυκός (γλαύξ) 491:10
γλαύκωμα 491:4
τὰ Γλαφυρά 403:10, 494:18
γλεύκινον 492:27
γλήχων 490:13, 497:22, 897:10
γλοῖος 493:12
γλυκίας? 464:14, 493:2, 493:4, 493:7, 493:9, 493:15
γλυκύ 496:6, see γλυκύτερος
γλυκύρριζα 494:4, 494:16
γλυκύτερος 496:18, see γλυκύ
γλυκυσίδη 29:10–12, 472:20, 1580:11
  Παιονία 493:22
γλυπτόν 496:20
γλυφή? 488:24
γλῶσσα 493:14
γλωσσόκομον 493:20
γναφάλιον 482:7, 502:10, 905:13
γναφεύς 507:15
γνῶμα 503:4, 17, 504:5, see γνωμικόν

γνώμη 504:3

γνωμικόν 465:19?, 500:2, see γνῶμα

γνώμων 184:14, 468:10, 503:10, 905:25

γνῶσις 484:25, 503:16

γνωστικός 493:19, 503:22

γνωστός 504:2

γνώστωσαν 503:25

γνῶτε 504:1

γογγύλη 468:7

γογγύλις 468:7

γογγυλίς 871:6

γογγύσουσι 460:3

γόμφιος 469:14

γόνασι 431:8

γονή 468:19–20

γόνος 485:20

γόνυ 468:9

γονυκλισία 431:8

γραικός? 32:17

γράμμα 512:5, 518:26, 567:3, 1207:14?

γραμματεύς 512:13

γραμματική 512:3, 8

γραμματικόν 1968:1

γραφεῖα 517:8

γραφείδιον? 517:6

γραφεῖον 517:11, 518:18?, 701:18?

γραφή 512:4

γραφήτωσαν 512:14

Γρηγόριος 518:19

γυμνάζων 612:16

γυμνάσια 465:21

γυμνάσιον 388:25, 465:23, 466:14, 500:1

γυμνάσμενος 612:16

γυμναστική 503:20

γύργαθος 473:24?

γύριν 474:9

ἡ γύρις 111:23, 198:24

γύψος 459:9, 471:24

γωνία (ἀμβλεῖα, ὀρθή, ὀξεῖα) 469:2–3

γωνίας (γωνία) 468:22

Δ

δᾳδίον 525:14

δαιμο...(?) 561:17

δαίμων 525:21

δάκρυα 303:4

δάκρυος (δάκρυ) 528:12

δάκτυλοι τρεῖς 528:7

δάκτυλος 528:10

δάμαλις 526:17, 692:14 (-εως)

δαμασκηνά 579:20, 582:19, 679:11, 1862:1

δαμασώνιον 526:11

δαμασώριον 11:22

δανείζεσται? 526:18

δανειστής 527:1

δάνος 526:21

Δανούβιος 1559:24

δαπάνη 247:22, 527:12, 586:10, 586:21, 586:23, 586:24

δασύτης 525:16, 527:2

δαῦκοι 547:23

δαῦκος 528:13, 546:27, 547:6, 1479:3, 1495:2

δαφνή 527:3, 586:10, 587:14, 932:19, 1511:6, see δαφνίς

Ἀλεξανδρίνη 527:15

δάφνης τῆς ποάς 527:13

δάφνινον (μύρον) 527:5

δαφνίς 527:3, 587:4, see δαφνή

δαφνοειδές 527:8, 527:19, 1789:17

δαφνός 587:5?

δεδωρῆσθαι 534:21?, see δωρεῖσθαι

δέησις 535:25

δείκτης 36:20, 536:4, 562:8
δείξει 534:23
δειλιάσω 535:20
δειμός 566:9
δεῖπνον 1900:7
δέκα 528:5
δεκανοί 527:11, 589:7
δέκανος 528:5
δέκαρχος 570:24
δεκάχορδα 536:6
δεκάχορδος 587:25
δέλφιν 542:25, 578:6
Δελφοί 578:5
δεξία 535:22, 541:5, 562:13, 574:21
Δέρβη 591:7
δέρμα 526:15, 536:11
δέρματα 536:13
δέρρος 536:12
δεσμός 536:2
δεσπόζει 536:1
δεσποτεία 536:3
δεῦτε 534:22
δευτέριον 36:26
δηλητήρια (φάρμακα) 564:9
δηλητηριώδης 564:20
δηλοῖ 564:21
δῆλος 564:8
Δημᾶς 565:13?, 566:4
δημηγορία 561:8
Δημήτριος 566:1
δημοκρατικοί 543:24
Δημόκρατος 560:15, 565:7
δῆμος 565:11
δημοσία 526:16 (ὁδός), 560:13
δημόσιον 543:15, 565:19, 680:4
δημόσιος 566:3, 579:24
δηνάριον 567:3
διαβαίνειν 555:4
διαβήματα 555:5
διαβήτης 525:12, 552:11, 552:18, 554:1, 554:20, 558:10, 558:16
διάβολος 555:6, 558:1, 558:18
διαγέομαι 555:8
διάγνωσις 561:23
διαγνωστική 556:22, 556:26
διάθεσις 162:1, 554:11
διαθήκη 37:20?, 555:9, 573:14
διαιρετική 559:7
δίαιτα, -ης 559:16
διακενῆς 555:11
διακονία 556:12, 571:17
διακονικόν 571:9, 572:8
διακόνιον 114:16, 389:5, 570:8
διακόνισσα 571:18
διάκονοι 571:19
διάκονος 571:16, see δικαιοκρίτης
διακόπτων 555:12
διάκρισις 553:24
(ξηρὸν) διάκροκον 554:2
διακύσιοι 554:8
διαλείπων 553:7
διαλεκτική 564:11, 564:12
διαλεκτικός 564:11, 564:12
διάλληλος 556:14
διαλογή 555:14
διαλογική 556:17
διάλυσις 559:25, 562:1
διαμαρτυρία 553:10, 565:24, 566:11
διαμαρτύρομαί σοι 555:16
διαμενεῖ 555:19
διαμενοῦσι 555:18
διαμέρισον 555:20

διαμέτρησον 555:21

διάμετρον 553:13, 559:5, 565:21–2

διάμετρος 553:5, 553:11, 553:16, 565:26, 565:28

σύμμετρος 1898:2

ἐκ διαμέτρου 272:18?

ἐκ διαμέτρων 272:16?

διανεύοντες 556:1

διανόημα 555:7

διαπορευόμενα 555:25

διαρρηξάμενος 556:3

διάρροια? 561:16

διασκεδάζει 556:4

διασκόρπισον 556:5

διαστρέψεις 556:6

διάταξις 552:25

διαταραχή? 570:23

Διατεσσάρων 552:19

διατηρήσεις 553:3

διατητής 552:23

διατρέψεις 555:10

διαφορά 553:21

διάφραγμα 553:23, 569:10, 749:5

διόφυτος 245:3

διάχρυσος 556:10

διάχυλον 553:6

διάψαλμα 557:8

δίγλωσσος 349:7

διδάξει 558:25

δίδαξον 558:23

Διδασκαλία 558:21

διδασκαλία 559:3, 1602:11

διδασκαλοί 556:18, 558:20, 558:26, 559:3

διδάσκαλος 558:19–22, 568:14, 568:20, 1254:6, 1257:13

Δίδυμος 2023:14

δίδυμος 558:24, 559:1

διέκυψεν 559:6

διελεύσομαι 559:8

διελογίζοντο 555:13

διεμέρισαν 559:9

διέξοδος 559:10

διεπετάσαμεν 559:11

διεπέτασεν 559:12

διερμενευτής 572:20

διέστειλαν 559:13

διεσχίθησαν 559:14

διήγαγεν 556:24

διηγέσομαι 556:25

δικαιοκρίτης 571:15, 571:16, 572:10, see διάκονος

δίκαιος 570:9, 570:12, 571:5

δικαιοσύνη 570:10, 571:7, 572:11

δικαίως 570:14

δικαστήριον 560:21, 571:21, 572:6

δικάστης 560:24

δικαστής 571:20

δίκελλα 547:5, 570:26

δίκη, -ας 572:2

κατά δίκην 1760:16?

δίκροτος 571:3

δίκταμνος 570:16, 571:10, 2068:19

δικτάτωρ 570:21

δικτυβόλος 571:13

διόβολον 558:3, see ὀβόλος

Διογενής 559:21

δίοδος? 561:16

Διόδωρος 559:18

διονυσίας 1038:7

Διονύσιος 567:5

Διοπετοῦς 562:2

δίοπτρα 561:9

διόρισμος 553:27

Διοσκορίδης 559:22
Διόσπολις 560:1, 560:25
Διοσπολίτης 560:1
Διοσπολιτοῦς (φάρμακον) 561:5, 568:12
διότι 556:8
διουρητική 554:9
διπλοΐς 569:6
δίπλωσις 569:4
δίπους, -οδος 561:1
δίπτυχα 568:27
δίπτυχον 560:7
δίσκοι 567:14
δίστομα (πνεύματα) 568:19?
δίστομος 567:22
δίφρος 546:11, 546:14, 569:14
διφρυγές 569:8, 569:17
διφυής 561:21?, 568:23
διχοτομῶν 556:16
δίχρωμος (ἔμπλαστρος) 562:14
δίψα 568:25
διψακός 553:25, 554:20, 557:1, 569:1, 569:23
διψάς 567:25
διώκων 561:20
διώξω 561:22
δόγμα 538:14
δόγματα 538:17
δογματική 538:15
δογματικοί 538:12
δοθιῆνες 684:23
δοκιμάζων? 546:25
δοκιμασία? 543:12
δοκίμιον 547:3
δόκιον? 574:12
δόλιος 542:11, 542:18
δολιότατος? 542:10
δολιχοί 542:14, 542:24
δόλος 542:9
δόμα 543:26
δομεστικόν 543:16, 582:16
δομεστικός 543:19, 553:19, 582:16
δόμος 543:8
δόξα 541:1, 574:15
δόρατα (δόρυ) 547:16
δορύκνιον 56:26, 548:11, 548:12
δός 544:16
δουλεύσατε 543:3
δοῦλος 542:9
δούξ 535:11, 540:24, 541:6
δοχεῖον? 574:12
δράβη? 590:6
δράγματα 591:14
δρακόντειον 132:19, 548:22
δρακοντία 591:5
δρακόντιον 590:17
δράκων 590:4, 595:19, 821:17
δραμεῖν 590:5
δράξασθε? 590:7
δραχμάς 590:21, 594:25
δραχμή 590:21, 594:25
δρέπανον πετόμενον 594:10
δρόμος 43:14
Δρουσίλλη 593:11
δρύϊνος 592:12, 1881:7
δρυμός 593:22
δρυοπτερίς 592:14, 593:8, 593:12
δρύος 548:1
δρυπετής 621:1
δρῦς 548:1, 593:1
Δρώπακος 593:9
δρῶπαξ 593:3, 593:7
δύναμις, (-εως) 560:6, 566:17
δυναστεία 560:16

δυνατός 560:20
δύο 536:18, 562:4
χίλια 572:19?
δὶα δύο 556:20
δυσεντερία 544:13
δύσις 567:15, 567:21
δυσκολία 562:3, 568:6
δυσμός 560:22
δυσουρία 567:17, 617:23?
δύσπνοια 568:1
δωδεκάθεον 538:26
δῶμα 544:1
δωρακινά 547:17, 548:21, 549:25
δωρεά 547:7, 549:3, 572:16
δωρεάν 549:10
δωρεῖσθαι? 548:5, see δεδωρῆσθαι
δώρημα 548:6
δωρήματα 548:4
δῶρον 549:15
δώσω 544:16

E

ἔαρ 599:10
ἔβαλον 602:27
ἐβαρύνθη 602:29
ἐβδελύχθησαν 603:30
ἑβδομάδα 11:11, 198:9, 1211:13
ἑβδομήκοντα 11:13, 21:5
ἐβεβαίωσας 604:1
ἔβενος 18:3–4, 86:18, 604:27
αἰθιοπική 18:3–4
ἐβουλεύσαντο 604:4
ἔβρυξαν 604:28
ἐγγίζειν? 605:7
ἐγγίζεταί σου 111:17
ἔγγιστα 605:8
ἔγγραπτον 605:9
ἐγγυραῖος 198:25?
ἐγγύς 605:10
ἐγένετο 605:11
ἐγήρασα 606:4
ἐγκαίνια 146:1, 213:15
ἐγκαίνισμα 352:17
ἐγκαίνισον 607:1
ἐγκανθίδες 621:17, 626:26, 642:17
ἐγκάρδιον 1523:3
ἔγκατα 606:23
ἐγκατάλειμμα 605:3
ἐγκατέλιπες 606:24
ἐγκέφαλος 146:16, 214:13, 275:9
ἐγκράτεια 121:14, 655:21?, see Ἐγκρατίται
ἐγκρατής? 33:1
Ἐγκρατίται 146:27
ἐγκρίς 214:2
ἐγκύκλια 146:11, 214:10
ἐγκύκλιον 214:5
ἐγκύκλιος 1748:11
ἐγλύκανας 606:6
ἐγνώρισας 606:22
ἐγόγγυσαν 606:5
ἐγχείριον 210:26, 1592:19
ἐκγελάσεταί σε 653:14 (ad ἐκδίκησις glossa pertinente)
ἐγχελύδια (ἐγχελύδιον) 211:1
ἔγχελυς 211:5
ἐγχυμώματα 653:12
ἐγχύμωσις? 156:22
ἐδαφιεῖ 607:13
ἔδαφος 607:15
ἐδειλίασαν 607:18
ἐδέσματα 607:19
ἐδίψησεν 608:21

ἐδοκίμασας 607:20

ἐδολιοῦσαν 607:21

ἕδος 53:24

ἐδούλευσαν 607:22

ἕδρα? 572:24

ἔδραμον 610:13

ἔδωκας 607:24

ἐθαυμάστωσε 661:8

ἐθεμελίωσας 662:1

ἐθίζων? 327:1

ἐθιστά (ἐθιστός)? 326:31

ἔθυσα 662:9

εἰ 599:20

εἶ 599:20

εἶδεν 599:19

εἴδη 602:9

εἶδος 112:25, 113:24

εἰδωλολατρία 542:5

εἴδωλον 600:4

εἰκῆ 145:18

εἴκοσι 274:16

εἰκών 145:10–11?, 600:6

τοῦ θεοῦ τοῦ ἀοράτου 213:16, 850:9

εἰλεός 128:17, 167:25–7, 869:2, 872:6

εἰλίξεις 600:8

εἰμί 133:20, 600:10?

εἶπεν 600:11

Εἰρηναῖος 298:24

εἰρήνη 291:19, 600:12

εἰρηνικάς (εἰρηνική) 148:26

εἰρωνικὸν μέτρον 259:14–15

εἷς 600:14

εἰς 600:13?

τέλος 601:5

εἰσαγωγή 138:15

εἰσάκουε 600:15

εἰσελεύσομαι 600:16

εἰσελθέτω 600:18

εἰσεπορεύετο 600:19

εἰσήγαγεν 600:21

εἰσήκουσεν 601:1

εἰσῆλθοσαν 601:3

εἰσόδια 233:3

εἰσόδιον 217:17?

εἴσοδος 138:18

εἶτα 123:1, 123:5 (confused with αἴτει), 123:9, 623:22

εἴτω 123:25

ἐκάθισας 653:5

ἐκαθίσω 653:4

ἐκάλυψεν 653:6

ἐκάστη 653:7, see ἕκαστος

ἑκατόμβη 653:9?

ἑκατὸν χίλια 572:19

ἕκαστος 653:11, see ἐκάστη

ἑκατοστός 653:28

ἐκαύθη 653:8

ἐκβαλόντες 655:15

ἐκδικητής 653:16

ἔκδικος 23:21, 266:20?

ἐκεῖ 654:6?

ἐκέκραξα 653:17

ἐκέραννυν 654:8?

ἐκζητήσει 655:19

ἐκζητῶν 655:20

ἔκθεσις 655:25

ἐκθλίψω 655:26

ἐκίνησαν 654:19

ἐκίσσησεν 654:20

ἐκκένωσις 275:12

ἐκκλησία 275:26, 655:16, 1790:13

ἐκκ(λησιασ)τικά 653:27?, 654:4

ἐκκλησιαστική 1791:4, 1794:12
ἐκκλῖναι 655:18
ἔκκλινον 655:1, 655:17
ἔκλαιον 654:26
ἔκλειγμα 131:3
ἐκλείπωσι 654:25
ἔκλειψις 29:15, 321:23, 330:16, 605:1, 606:18, 635:4, 655:5, 1796:16
ἐκλεκτός 654:27, 655:2
ἐκληροδότησε 654:28
ἐκλογή 276:5
ἐκμυκτηριεῖ 655:9
ἐκοιμήθην 653:19
ἐκόπασεν 653:20
ἐκοπίασα 653:22
ἑκουσίως 653:23
ἐκπιεσμός 655:13
ἐκπορευόμενος 655:12
ἔκρυψαν 655:24
ἔκρυψάς μοι 655:22
ἐκσκέπτωρες 1129:14?
ἔκσπασας 655:10
ἔκτασις 655:1
ἐκτήσατο 654:10
ἐκτήσω 654:11
ἑκτικά 623:24?, 653:24?, 654:3?
ἑκτική 146:9?
ἑκτικοί 654:3
ἑκτικός (πυρετός) 228:16, 653:24, 1496:26
ἐκτιλεῖ σε 654:7
ἔκτομον 654:17
ἐκτρόπιον 613:11, 642:27, 654:12, 655:3
ἐκφανείς 528:16
ἔκχεον 654:24
ἔλαβεν 631:1
ἐλάθετο 631:2
ἐλαία 165:11, 631:19, 635:24
ἐλαιόμελι 632:10
ἔλαιον 631:20, see ἀμυγδάλινον (ἔλαιον), βαλάνινον (ἔλαιον), Ἰστρικόν ἔλαιον, κίκινον (ἔλαιον), κνίδινον (ἔλαιον), κομμωτικὸν (ἔλαιον), κρόκινον (ἔλαιον), κύπρινον (ἔλαιον), μολόχινον (ἔλαιον), μύρσινον (ἔλαιον), οἰνάνθινον (ἔλαιον), ὀμφάκινον (ἔλαιον), ῥόδινον (ἔλαιον), σαβῖνον (ἔλαιον), σαμψύχινον (ἔλαιον), σούσινον (ἔλαιον), σχίνινον (ἔλαιον), ὑοσκυάμινον (ἔλαιον), ὠμοτριβές (ἔλαιον)
ἐλάλησεν 631:3
ἐλάτη 165:20, 171:12, 630:24, 1358:18, see ἐλάτος, ἰτέα
ἐλατήριον 171:10, 200:1–2, 1347:3, see ἀληθινὸν ἐλατήριον, σάρδιον
  ἕτερον 171:26, 518:6
ἐλατίνη 631:8
ἐλάτινον (μύρον) 631:17
ἐλάτος 631:4, see ἐλάτη
ἐλαττωθήσονται 631:5
ἐλαφοβόσκον 631:12, 23
ἔλαφος 130:2, 165:25?, 169:18?, 631:7, 1899:17?
ἐλέγξεις 632:1
ἔλεγξις? 349:10
ἐλεγμός 631:29
ἐλεημοσύνη 127:27, 632:2
ἐλεήμων 128:1
ἐλέησον 129:26, 632:3
  ἡμεῖς 172:19
ἔλειον 177:12 (ἀσπάραγον), 633:22
ἐλειοσέλινον 967:27?
ἐλειτίς? 398:26
ἐλελίσφακον 172:21, 632:13, 633:15, 634:14

ἐλελίσφακος 968:3
ἐλελίσφασκον 526:8
ἐλένιον 130:24, 173:23, 189:20, 291:4, 633:14, 634:1
αἰγύπτιον 632:8
ἔλεος 165:12, 632:4
ἐλευθερία 169:1
ἐλευθεροπρεπής 128:3
ἐλεύθερος 128:11?, 128:16, 211:9?, 632:5
Ἐλευσῖνα 168:29?
Ἐλυσίς 168:29?
ἐλεφάντινος 632:6
ἐλέφας 631:27, 1899:17?
ἐλθέτω 636:25
ἑλίκη 633:25, 636:9, 636:15, 636:20, cf. 396:26
Ἑλικωνιάς? 633:17
ἕλιξ 633:25, 636:9, 636:15, 636:20, cf. 396:26
ἐλίπανας 634:8
ἑλίχρυσον 634:11
ἀμαράντινον 633:9
ἑλκύσαι 636:12
ἕλκυσμα 526:5, 636:23
ἕλκω 633:24
Ἑλλάδα 327:20–7, 361:11
Ἑλλάς 327:20–7, 635:27
ἐλλέβορος 165:23, 635:6, 1073:13
λευκός 635:21
μέγας 635:22
Ἕλλην 175:4–8
ἕλληνες 764:16
ἑλληνικά 635:25
Ἑλληνισμός 175:4–8
ἑλληνισμός 635:26
ἑλξίνη 176:10, 177:10, 632:16, 634:17, 635:1, 910:7?, 926:19, 1485:1, 1499:8
Ἑλπίδιος 179:3
ἐλπίζει 634:9
ἐλπίς 178:12, 636:2
ἐλπίσατε 636:1
ἐλύδριον (pro χελιδόνιον) 168:10, 1455:19, see χελιδόνιον
ἔλυμος 632:23
ἐλυπήθη 634:10
ἐμάκρυνα 636:26
ἐμάταζον 1062:28?
ἔμβλεψις 132:1–2
ἔμβροχος 182:11
ἐμελέτησαν 637:2
ἐμίαναν 638:1
ἐμίγησαν 638:2
ἐμίσησας 638:3
ἐμμέλεια 187:8
ἔμμορθος 214:16?
ἐμός 135:13, 17
ἐμπαγῆναι 639:16
ἔμπαιγμα 639:5
ἐμπειρίας 252:21
ἐμπειρική 190:20, see ἐμπερικοί, ἐμπερική
ἐμπειρότατος 209:3
ἐμπερική 640:7, see ἐμπειρική
ἐμπερικοί 639:3, see ἐμπειρική
ἐμπεσεῖται? 639:18
ἔμπετρον 639:10, 640:4, 645:13
ἔμπλαστρος, see δίχρωμος (ἔμπλαστρος), λειχηνικόν (ἔμπλαστρον), μικτόν ἔμπλαστρον
ἐμπλησθήσῃ 639:12
ἔμπνευσις 639:19
ἐμπύημα 190:16, 640:1
ἐμπυρίζεται 639:14
ἐμφανῶς 639:24
ἐμφράξει 639:25

ἐμφύσημα 620:11, 626:6, 639:8, 639:26
ἔμφωμα 189:23, 190:22?, 1104:20, 1643:22
ἔνδειξις 535:26
ἔνδημα 640:14, 640:25
ἐνδιαβάλλοντες 640:18
ἐνδιέβαλλόν με 640:20
ἔνδοξος 136:22, 200:22, 214:16?
ἔνδυμα 640:22
ἐνδύομαι 640:24
ἐνεγράφη 641:14
ἐνέδρα 641:4
ἐνεδρεύει 640:23
ἕνεκα 641:5
ἕνεκεν 641:6
ἐνεκότουν 641:7
ἐνενήκοντα 121:17
ἐνεπάγησαν 641:9
ἐνέργεια 196:13, 209:19, 214:17?
ἐνέργημα 196:23–4
ἐνεργήματα 196:23–4
ἐνεσκαμμένη 200:13
ἐνετείλω 641:10
ἐνέτεινον 641:11
ἐνευλογεῖται 641:12
ἐνθέους (πράξεις) 216:16?
ἐνθουσιασμός 154:3, 217:8
ἐνιαυτόν (ἐνιαυτός) 208:20
ἐνιαυτός 117:10
ἐννακόσιοι 214:12
Ἔννατον 624:25
ἐννενήκοντα 203:26
ἔνοπτρον 1229:9?
ἐντελέχεια 123:3, 204:2, 205:7
ἐντεροκήλη 206:10, 642:1
ἔντερον 84:18
ἐντολή 641:23
ἐντολικόν 58:17, 115:1, 124:3, 203:27, 205:25
ἐντραπείησαν 641:24, see ἐπισημασία
ἔντρομος 641:26
ἐντυβία 103:1, 204:25
ἔντυβον 641:28
ἐν τῷ 641:27
ἐνύδριον (ἐνυδρίς) 115:7, 200:7
ἔνυδρον? 68:7
ἐνύπνιον 642:3
ἐνύσταξαν 641:17
ἐνσφράγισμα 141:1
ἐνώπιον 641:18
ἐνωτικόν 200:21
ἐνώτισαι 641:19
ἐξαγγελῶ 628:8
ἐξαγορεύσω 628:10
ἑξάγωνος 160:3, 160:15, 628:9
ἑξακόσιοι 156:28, 163:5
ἐξάλειψον 629:4, see ἐξήλειψας
ἐξανθήματα 628:18
ἐξαπέστειλε 629:6
ἐξάπινα 629:7
ἐξέβαλεν 629:10
ἐξεβιάσαντο 629:11
ἐξεγέρθητε 628:12
ἐξεδείξατε 629:8
ἐξέδρα 158:18, 158:25
ἐξέθρεψε? 629:12
ἐξειργάσατο 628:14
ἐξειργάσω 628:13
ἐξείρπυσεν 630:7
ἐξεκενώθη 629:14
ἐξέκλινον 629:13
ἐξελέξατο 629:18
ἐξέλθοι 629:19
ἐξέλιπεν 629:15

ἐξέλιπον 629:16

ἐξέλοι 629:19

ἐξέλου 629:20

ἐξεναντίας 629:21

ἐξεπορεύετο 629:22

ἐξερευγόμενα 629:24

ἐξέρκητον 159:14, 163:19

ἐξετάζει 629:26

ἐξετεινάχθην= ἐξετινάχθην 630:1

ἐξέτηξας 629:27

ἐξεχύθη 629:28

ἕξεως (ἕξις) 161:25

ἐξήγαγε 628:6

ἐξήγαγεν 628:16

ἐξήγγειλα 628:17

ἐξηγέρθη 630:5

ἐξηγητής 158:22

ἐξηγητικόν 242:14

ἐξήλειψας 630:3, see ἐξάλειψον

ἐξηράνθη 630:4

ἐξηρίθμησαν 630:6

ἐξίλασμα 630:8

ἕξις 162:3, 628:24, 629:1, 630:10, see ἕξεως

ἐξισωτής 163:8

ἐξιτήριον 163:13

ἐξιχνιασάμην 630:12

ἔξοδος (ἐξοδίασις) 159:20, 628:20

ἐξοίσει 628:23

ἐξολοθρεύσει 630:14

ἐξομολογήσεται 630:17

ἐξορία 159:6, 159:11

ἐξορῖσαι 159:11

ἐξορισθέν 159:8

ἐχορισθῆναι 159:8, 159:10, 159:12

ἐξόριστος 163:17

ἐξουδενώθη vel ἐξουδενώθεις 630:20

ἐξουδένωμα 155:9

ἐξουδένωσις 630:19

ἐξουσία 630:21

ἐξοχάδες 628:22

ἔξω 630:16

ἐξωμοσία 162:11

ἔξωσον 630:22

ἑορτάζων 599:12

ἑορταστική 844:4

ἑορτή 599:14

ἐπαγγελία 644:3

ἐπαγωγή 620:13, 644:19

ἐπάγων 644:4

ἐπᾴδων 644:5

ἐπαίδευσαν 644:26

ἐπαινεῖται (ἐπενεῖτε) 645:18

ἔπαινος 645:19

ἐπάκουσόν μου 644:7

ἐπαλαιώθη 644:6

ἐπαλαιώθησαν 644:8

ἐπανιστάμενοι 644:9

ἐπανίσταντο ἐπ᾽ἐμέ 644:11

ἐπάρθητε 644:13

ἐπάρκης? 268:14

ἐπάρκιος 268:14

ἔπαρον 644:14

ὑπὸ ἐπάρχων 79:27?

χώρα 79:21?

ἐπάταξας 644:15

Ἐπαφρίδιτος 266:1

ἐπέβη 644:23

ἐπεβίβασας 644:24

ἐπεῖδον 645:10

ἐπείνασαν 644:27

ἐπεκαλύφθησαν 645:2

ἐπελήσθην 645:1

ἐπενεῖτε (ἐπαινεῖται) 645:18
ἐπενθήθησαν 645:3
ἐπεξεργασία? 617:24
ἐπερρίφην 645:4
ἐπετάσθη 645:6
ἐπετίμησας αὐτοῖς 645:7
ἐπετίμησεν? 604:2
ἐπευθύνειν 257:26
ἔπη 259:2, 259:14–15
ἐπήγαγεν, -γες 646:17
ἐπήκουσεν 646:18
ἐπήρθη 648:15
ἐπῃτήσαντο 644:21
ἐπιβρέξει 648:16
ἐπιγάστριον 648:7, 1160:24, 1486:25
ἐπίγαστρον 648:7, see ὑπογάστριον
ἐπιγραφή 142:22
ἐπίδημα (νοσήματα) 651:27
ἐπιδημία 646:19
ἐπιεικής 648:17
ἐπιθετικοί? 144:18
ἐπιθρόνιοι 262:26
ἐπιθρονίων 262:26
ἐπιθυμητός 648:18
ἐπιθυμία 645:9
ἐπιθύμιον 261:17
ἐπίθυμον 269:12, 653:2
ἐπικαλεῖσθαι 648:19
ἐπικάρσιος 266:6
ἐπίκαυμα 647:26, 648:3, 652:1
Ἐπίκουρος 261:27
ἐπίκυκλοι 261:26
ἐπιλάβον 648:23
ἐπιλανθανόμενα 648:24
ἐπιλήσεται 648:26?
ἐπιλησμοσύνη 647:13
ἐπιληψία 143:11, 144:20, 646:22, 647:21
ἐπιλογισμός 649:26
ἐπίλογος 260:25, 647:9
ἐπιμελητής 260:22
ἐπιμήδιον 646:14
ἐπι(νε)νευκώς 650:9
ἐπίνευσις 646:26
ἐπινυκτίδες 647:3
ἐπιπακτίς 651:21
ἐπίπεδον 647:5
ἐπιπεφυκώς 1534:9
χιτών 79:5, 254:13, 260:17, 262:11, 534:3, 647:17, 651:15
ἐπιπλεῖον 648:27
ἐπίπλοος 647:6
ἐπιποθεῖ 649:1
ἐπιπολῆς 143:17
ἐπίρρημα 648:4, 649:20
ἐπίσειον 652:3?, 1161:7
ἐπίσεισμος 144:22
ἐπίσειστος 144:22
ἐπισημασία 648:12, 651:24, see ἐντραπείησαν
ἐπισιτισμός 645:21
ἐπισκέπτῃ 649:2
ἐπίσκοπος 141:11, 260:11, 261:24, 650:16
ἐπίσπαστρον 1378:6
ἐπιστάτα 15:26, 259:16, 259:27
μου 259:16
ἐπιστολεύς 261:1
ἐπιστολήν 213:7
ἐπιστόλιον 213:7, 264:19–20
ἐπιστραφῆτε 649:7
ἐπίστρεψον 649:8
ἐπιτήδευμα 649:19
ἐπὶ τί 649:9
ἐπὶ τοσοῦτον 649:15?

ἐπιτίμησις 649:13

ἐπιτίμησον 649:17

ἐπιτόνια 650:13?

ἐπίτριψις 650:17

ἐπίτροπος 258:22, 258:23

ἐπιφάνεια 260:7, 527:7?

Ἐπιφάνιος 261:2

ἐπίφανον 649:12

ἐπιφανῶν πόλις 650:14

ἐπιχαρείησάν μοι 649:18

ἐπιχείρημα 142:20, 259:19, 650:11

ὑπὸ ἐπιχείρων 79:23?

ἐπίχυσις 1543:21

ἐπιχώρια 640:14, 640:25 (νοσήματα)

ἐπιχώριον 79:21?

ἐπλανήθησαν 647:7

ἐπλατύνας 652:7

ἐπληθύνθησαν 652:9

ἐπλήσθη 647:12

ἐποίησα 650:7

ἐποίησας 650:8

ἐπολιόρκησεν 261:18

ἐπολυώρησας 645:22

ἐπομένη σοί? 626:28

ἔποπος (ἔποξ) 262:15

ἐποπτική 250:17, 254:18

ἐπορεύθη 645:20

ἐπόρθουν 258:6

ἐπορούων? 627:3

ἐπόρωευσαν 645:24

ἐπότισάν με 645:25

ἐπόψωμαι (ἐποφθήσομαι) 645:26

ἐπτά 646:10

ἐπτάγωνα, -ων 569:16

ἐπτάκις 646:9

ἐπτακόσια 145:5

ἐπταπλάσιον 646:11

ἐπτάπλευρον 298:18–22?, 1570:5?, 1570:8?, 1722:18?

ἐπῳδή 250:4

ἐπῴδια (ἐπῴδιον) 250:11

ἐπωμίδιον? 161:3, 21

ἐπώνυμος 1516:21

ἐραγαστήρια 147:18

ἐργαζόμενος 657:24

ἔργον 656:15

ἐρέβινθος 15:18, 280:15, 656:2

ἐρέβινθος (ἄγριος) 26:12, 32:11

ἐρεγμός 656:17

ἐρείκη 21:10, 149:25, 658:13, 1479:19

ἐρεῖτε 656:25

ἔρειψις 660:22

ἐρεύξεται 656:27

ἔρημος 289:22, 658:15

ἔρινος 604:15

ἔριον 658:9

ἔρις 658:10

ἐρισύβη 658:11

ἑρμηνεία 296:19

περὶ ἑρμηνείας 1311:18, 1496:11, 1625:7

Ἑρμῆς 658:19, 686:16, 1211:23

Ἑρμῆς Τρισμέγιστος 296:20, 658:25

Ἑρμογένης 298:9

ἑρμοδάκτυλος 296:4, 659:1, cf. 33.25

ἑρπετά 660:3

ἕρπης 660:9

ἕρπυλλον 291:4

ἕρπυλλος 189:20–2, 302:8, 617:15, 660:6, 1345:12

Ἐρυθρά θάλασσα 659:3

ἐρυθραῖος 292:16

ἐρυθρόδανον 285:18–19, 304:28, 622:19,

657:13, 647:14
ἐρυθροείδης (χίτων) 632:20
ἐρύσιμον 657:18, 752:7
ἐρυσίπελας 657:1, 1295:3?
ἐρχομένη 658:18
ἐρωδιός 89:16, 96:10, 212:26, 657:7
ἔρως 525:11?
ἐρώτησις 214:14?
ἐσάπησαν 642:22
ἐσείσθη 642:23
ἐσεμειώθη 643:11
ἔσεται 642:26
ἔση 643:10
ἐσίγησα 643:13
ἐσκαλεύθην 1293:1?
ἔσκαλλον 140:1
ἐσκίρτησαν 644:1
ἐσμίκρυνε 643:18
ἔσπασαν 643:26
ἑσπέρα 217:24
Ἐσσηνοί 232:26
ἔσταξεν 643:1
ἐστέρησας 643:2
ἐστεριγμένη 643:6
ἐστεφάνωσας 643:3
ἔστη 643:4
ἐστιητεόν? 123:12
ἔστιν 226:10, 643:4
οὐκ ἔστιν 48:4, 48:29
ἐσχάρα 643:15, 643:19, 1349:28, 1943:17, 1958:11
ἐσχάρας 643:22, 1349:19, 1352:4
ἔσχατος 643:14
ἔσωθεν 642:25
ἐσώθησαν 642:24
ἐτάζων 623:3
ἐτάκησαν 623:4
ἐταπεινοφρόνουν 623:5
ἐταράχθη 623:7
ἐτάχυναν 623:8
ἔτεκον 623:9
ἐτέκταινον 623:10
ἐτελέσθησαν 623:11
ἑτερο... 822:26
ἑτερώνυμος 109:25, 623:12
ἐτησίας (ἐτησίαι) 57:9
ἔτι 623:22
ἔτνος 623:25
ἑτοιμασία 623:17
ἔτος 623:18
ἐτυμολογία 57:12, 107:3, 124:25, 613:10, 623:15
ἐτυρώθη 623:23
εὐαγγέλια 68:19–25
εὐαγγέλιον 68:19–25, 1017:16
εὐαγγελισταί 68:19–25, 69:1
Εὐάγριος 51:6
Εὔβουολον 49:2
Εὔβουλος 49:2
Εὐγενής 50:17
Εὐγένιοι 50:14–15
Εὐγένιος 50:14–15
εὐδαίμων 54:1
εὐδόκητος 54:9
εὐδοκία 54:7, 601:6, 613:4
εὐεξία 613:5
εὐεργήτεσας 601:7
εὐεργέτης 33:1
εὐηγγελισάμην 601:9
εὐηρέστουν σοι 601:11
εὔζωμον 53:25, 55:19, 613:8
εὔθετον 97:22

εὔθετος 601:15
εὐθηνία 601:16
εὐθύς 601:18
εὐθύτης 98:3, 601:19
εὐίλατος 601:20
εὐκαιρία 601:21
εὔκηλος 63:20
Εὐκλειδής 561:3
εὐλάβεια 117:16, 131:27
εὐλαβέστατος 117:18
εὐλαβής 117:17
εὐλογεῖτε 169:21
εὐλογήσεις 601:23
εὐλογία 601:22
Εὐνίκη 75:16
εὐνοῦχος 70:11, 203:13, 276:16?
Εὔξεινος (πόντος) 160:14
Εὐοδία 55:9
εὐόδωσον 602:8
εὐπαθοῦντες 601:24
εὐπατώριον 10:21, 617:11, 620:15, 1455:24
εὐπειθής 261:1?
εὐπρέπεια 601:26
εὑρέθη 602:20
εὐρίζων 89:27, 91:26
Εὔριπος 92:21, 96:20, 302:5
Εὐρυκλύδων 1837:16
εὐρόνοτος 89:14, 622:15
εὖρος 90:23, 621:25, 1883:13
εὔροτος? 622:14
εὐρύς? 601:28
εὐρύχωροι? 601:27
Εὐρώπα 95:25
Εὐσέβιος 76:15, 78:26
εὔσημος 602:1
εὔτονος 601:13
Εὐτύχιος 58:16
εὐτύχιος (λίθος) 124:1
Εὔτυχος 58:14
εὐφάρμακος 843:1
Εὐφρατησία 84:10
εὐφόρβιον 84:25, 521:10?, 620:25
εὐφράνθησαν 602:4
εὐφρανθήσομαι 602:3
Εὐφράτιος (ἰχθύς) 268:6?
εὐφροσύνη 84:22, 602:6
εὐχαριστία 62:3
εὐχάριστος 62:1
εὐχή 117:13, 121:22, 602:7
Εὐχῖται 59:18
εὔψυχος 85:7
ἐφάνθη 639:23?
ἐφείσατο 645:11
ἐφεκτική 250:17?, 254:18?
Ἐφεκτικοί 250:19, 264:9, 266:21
ἐφέλκυσμα 1572:12?
Ἔφεσος 264:15
ἐφηβαῖον 1161:7
ἐφηβείας 110:26
ἔφηλις 649:23
ἐφημερινός 189:18, see ἐφήμερος (πυρετός)
ἐφήμερον 150:5–6, 647:15, 647:24, 648:6, 651:17, 651:19, 656:18
ἐφήμερος (πυρετός) 647:11, see ἐφημερινός
ἐφιάλτης 650:5, 652:10
ἔφοδος 217:17?, 250:6
ἐφόδια 527:12
ἐφόνευσαν 646:2, 3
ἐφονοκτονήθη 646:1
ἐφορεία? 252:21
ἐφρύαξαν 652:24
ἔφυγον 649:22

ἐχενηΐς 211:8
ἔχθρα 164:26, 210:6
ἔχιδνα 154:18, 627:6
ἐχῖνοι 627:22
ἐχῖνος 15:15, 110:23, 627:5 (τοῦ στομάχου), 628:2, 643:8
  θαλάσσιος 627:24
  τὸ φυτόν 627:18
  χέρσαιος 627:26
ἔχιον 627:7
ἐχόμενος 627:1
ἐχορτάσθησαν 627:2
ἐχώλαναν 627:4
ἐψεύσαντο 652:18
ἐψιθύριζον 652:15
ἕως 599:15
ἑωσφόρος 599:16

Z

ζάλεια 526:9, 527:26
ζάλη 689:2
ζέα 671:4, 676:24, 687:6, 967:14
ζεία 676:24
Ζεῦγμα 678:21
ζεῦγος 677:5
Ζεύξιππος 525:18?, 680:4
Ζεύς 677:24, 681:6, 686:22
ζέφυρος 1890:20
ζῇ 686:7
ζῆλος 687:7
ζημία 566:12, 687:8
ζῆν καλῶς 695:17
Ζηνοβία 687:12
ζήτημα 671:14
ζητήματα 686:4
ζίβυναι 1305:15
ζιγγίβερις, -ιν 1315:22
ζοῦρα 684:11, 1140:7
ζυγομαχία 680:18
ζυγός 686:8, 686:10, 686:24, 686:26
ζυγοστάτης 560:18, 1129:14, 1299:19, 1350:8, 1741:16, 1815:17
ζύγωμα 99:12, 99:19, 217:25, 678:19
ζύθος 684:22, 688:4
ζυμάρυστρον 64:23?
ζύμη 680:23, 1887:4
ζωγρεῖα 678:17
ζώδια 678:24
ζωδιακός 679:3, 679:4
ζώδιον 589:7, 679:1
ζωή 525:19, 671:12, 677:25
ζωμὸς ἰχθύων 679:12
ζώνας (ζώνη) 427:22?, 681:1, 681:3
ζώνη 680:27
ζώπισσα 683:13
Ζωροάστρης 684:17

H

ἡ 110:3
ἠγάπηκα 111:4
ἤγγισαν 111:13
ἡγεμονική 24:5, 29:25, 111:10, 111:12
ἡγεμονικοί 111:14
ἡγεμών 112:1, 606:17, 606:20
ἠδολέσχουν 114:3
ἡδύ
  μου 114:12
  σοι 114:12
ἡδυοσμόν 568:16?
ἡδύοσμος 51:27, 113:16, 612:23, 836:6

ἡδύσαρον 113:18–22, 113:26, 114:7–8

ἥδυσμα? 568:18

ἡδύχρουν 115:8–13

ἡδύχρουν (μύρον) 115:8–13

ἠθικοί 327:13

ἠθικόν 154:6, 216:8, 327:18

ἠθικός 327:17

ἠλάττωσες 133:3

ἠλειμμένος 171:4–6, 176:13, 1169:10

ἤλεκτρον 131:16, 179:14, 180:3, 565:17, 634:3, 1373:18

ἦλθον 130:23

ἡλιακάς (ἀκτῖνας) 128:15?

ἡλικία 174:11

Ἡλιόπολις 38:6, 128:13, 131:25, 171:17, 633:11, 635:8 (confused with Ἑλλήσποντος?)

ἥλιος 128:8, 129:24, 171:16

Τιτάν 802:19, see Τιτάν

ἡλιοστασία 129:24

ἡλιοστάσιον 129:24

ἡλιοτρόπιον τὸ μέγα, τὸ μικρόν 131:6–12

ἠλλοιώθης 130:6

ἧλος 63:7, 128:5, 128:7, 130:27

ἠλύσιον (πεδίον) 131:17–18

ἠλύσιος 128:15?

ἡμᾶς 135:17

ἡμεῖς 133:18

ἡμέρα 133:6

ὅλη 133:9 note 4

(ἀφ᾽) ἡμέρας 133:8

(δι᾽) ἡμέρας 133:9

Ἡμεροβατισταί 618:18

ἡμερόκαλλις 132:3, 132:15, 134:1–2

ἡμεροκατάλλακτος 134:1–2

ἡμίθεος 640:9

ἡμικρανία 133:11, 638:21

ἡμῖν 133:19

ἡμίνα 135:18

ἡμιονῖτις 132:17–22

ἡμίονος 132:23, 846:26

ἡμιπληγία 133:13, 1562:9?

ἡμισεύσουσι 133:22

ἡμιστάτηρ 64:23?

ἥμισυ 133:21, see ἥμισυν

ἥμισυν 638:11, see ἥμισυ

ἡμιτριταῖος 133:15–16, 638:13

ἡμῶν 133:25

ἦν 136:7

ἠνέγκατε 641:3

ἤνεγκε 137:1

ἠνέμιον? 209:20–2

ἡνίοχος 642:8

ἤνοιξαν 137:2

ἠντιασάμην 206:15

ἥξει 127:3

ἧπαρ 143:15, 602:14, 644:17

ὄνειον 849:1

ἠπατήθην 144:10

ἡπατικοί 618:3

ἡπατικόν (πάθος) 652:6

ἡπατικός 619:11 , 621:16?

ἡπατῖτις 165:1–2

ἥπατος 141:6

ἠπίαλος 143:20, 648:10

ἦρα 149:10

Ἡράκλεια 148:15–16, 297:3–4

ἡρακλεία 660:17, 863:6, 1315:11, 1362:5

Ἡράκλειος 150:11

Ἡρακλῆς 660:10

ἠρετισάμην 149:11

ἠριγέρων 147:24, 149:13, 149:24

ἠρξάμην 149:16

ἦρος 1790:11

ἠρύγγιον 89:21, 148:7, 657:21

Ἡρώδης 657:8, 954:23

Ἡρωδιανοί 150:12

Ἡρωδιάς 657:3

ἡρῶον 259:7

ἡρώτων 149:18

ᾗσαν 139:23

ἧσθα 139:24

ἡσύχασε 139:26

ἡσυχία 1315:4?

ἥσυχος 141:3

ἤσχαλεν 140:1

ᾐσχύνθησαν 140:6

ἦτα 125:4

ᾐτησάμην 206:15

ᾔτησε 125:3, 208:3

ἦτρον 124:13

Ἥφαιστος 142:21

ἤχησα 154:11

ἤχησαν 125:24

ἦχος 126:1, 1261:4

ἠχώδεις 1261:8?

Θ

θάλασσα 2027:23, 2065:4, 2068:16

θαλάσσης ῥόδον 2027:16?

θαλάσσιος 1577:5

θαλασσόμελι 2027:11

θαλάττιον

οἶνος 2027:13

ὕδωρ 2027:9

θαλεία 2066:4?

θάλικτρον 2027:20

θαλλία 2028:1

θαλλίας 828:18

θάμνος 2028:10, 2072:15

θάνατος 2029:2

θάπτει 2029:20

θάπτων 2029:20

Θάσος 2077:5

θαυμάσιον 2021:1

θαυμαστόν 2021:3

θαυμαστός 2025:17

θαυματουργός 2025:16

θαψία 621:20, 2029:7, 2081:4, see ἐρυθρόδανον, herba rubia

θεατρίσαι 2026:18

θέατρον 260:21, 2023:1, 2026:14, 2036:17

θεῖον 2029:1, 2037:26, 2057:19, 2058:12

Θέκλα 2083:10

θέλημα 2038:2

θέλων 2038:3

θεμέλια 2038:7

Θεοδοσιόπολις 2037:14

Θεόδοσιος 2022:2, 2036:1

Θεόδοτος 2025:15

θεόδουλαι 2036:10

Θεόδουλος 2022:4, 2036:4

Θεόδωρε 2022:13

Θεοδωρῖτα 2022:11, 15

Θεοδωρίτης 2022:9

Θεόδωρος 2022:6, 2035:25

θεολογία 2026:10, 2036:7

θεολόγος 2023:10, 2027:7, 2036:8

θεοπασχῖται 2024:19, 2035:20

θεοπασχίτης 2025:11

Θεόπολις 2037:7

θεός 98:20, 316:28, 317:1, 2025:12, 2036:5, 2037:17

θεοσέβαστοι 2025:7

θεοσέβαστος 2025:7
θεοτίμητος 2025:9
θεοτόκος 2027:3, 2037:1
βοήθει 2027:1
θεοφανία 2025:2
Θεόφιλε 2024:4
Θεόφιλος 2037:9
Θεοφόρε 2024:2
θεοφόροι 2023:24
Θεοφόρος 2024:23, 2026:20
θεοφόρος 2037:3
Θεόφραστος 2025:1, 2037:5
Θεοφύλακτος 2024:24
θεραπευτής 817:20
θερίσουσιν 2038:15
θέρμη 799:26?, 826:6?, 826:25?, 2038:17
θέρμος 2038:19, 2050:5, 2060:13
ἄγριος 2060:14
θέρος 2038:18
θεσαυροί 139:16?
Θερσίτης 2030:5
Θεσσαλονίκη 2038:12, 2077:8
Θεσσαλός 2038:9
θεωρετής 2035:24
θεώρημα 2025:19
θεωρῆσαι 2023:11, 2030:1
θεωρηταί 2037:18
θεωρητική 2026:4
θεωρητικός 2027:5, 2036:11
θεωρητικῶν 2026:1
θεωρία 1181:6, 2023:4, 2026:12, 2030:2, 2035:18
ἰατρός 2025:5?, 2026:8
Θῆβαι, -ας 2021:10
θηβαϊκόν 2021:7, 2031:4
Θηβαῖοι 2021:9
θήβαϊς 783:4?, 2030:19
θήκη 2029:21, 2082:1
θηλάζων 2059:8
θῆλυ 2059:6
θηλύκον 2059:7
θηλυπτερίς 2059:9
θῆξις 127:4, 2058:21
θήρα 2060:8
θηρατής 2060:10
θηρία 806:17, 2060:5, 2060:11
θηριακή 2050:3, 2060:6, see Ἀντιόχου (θηριακή)
θηριακοί (ἅλες) 1090:7
θηριώδης 2060:15
θησαυρός 218:25, 2059:17, 2059:21
θῆσθαι 2038:11
θήσομαι 2059:19
θλάσματα 2027:18
θλασπέως 183:21?, 399:26, 2068:20
θλάσπι 570:17, 2068:20
θλιμμός 2067:14
θλίψις 2067:15
θνησιμαῖα 2076:13
θολός 2045:5
θρακίας 2083:22, see λίθος θρακίας
θρασκίας 2084:8, 2084:15, 2089:13
θραῦσις 2084:10
θρησκεία 2088:3, 2089:9
θρίδαξ 1389:22, 2087:2
θριχές 303:26
θρονίον 2086:3
θρόνος 1859:7, 2086:1
θρύψις 2084:10
θυγάτηρ 2058:15
θυλάκιον 2045:17
θυλακῖτις 1276:20, 1809:12

θύμαλον 1358:13, 2046:3
θύμβρα 2046:11
θυμέλαια 1355:22?, 2046:14?, 2046:15?, 2046:16
θυμίαμα 2058:3, see ἀμμωνιακόν (θυμίαμα)
θυμοξάλμη 2046:6
θύμος 2045:20, 2045:22?, 2046:8, 2058:5
θύρα 2058:6
θυρεός 2058:7, 2060:7
θυρσίνη 375:13–15
θύσατε 2058:8
θυσία 1009:14, 2058:9
θυσιαστήριον 140:24, 1009:13, 2058:10, 2059:20
Θωμᾶς 2023:12
θώραξ, -ακος 2050:15

I

Ἰακωβίτης (Ἰακώβ) 848:19
ἴαμβος 259:14–15
Ἰαννῆς καὶ Ἰαμβρῆς 847:19
Ἰανουάριος 110:4
ἶᾶσαι 110:11
ἰάσπεως (ἴασπις λίθος) 864:6, see λίθος (ἰάσπις)
ἴασπις 110:7, 137:22
ἰάσω με 110:13
Ἰασων 140:13
ἰατρεία 124:16, 556:11
ἰατρός 110:20, 123:21, 124:12, 823:5, 833:8, 845:8
ἰατροσοφιστής 123:22, 197:24
Ἴβηροι 110:21, 24, 147:21
ἶβις 626:9, 834:11
ἰβίσκος 181:3, 409:27, 604:6, 626:24, 654:23
ἰγδίον 23:15, 111:7
ἰδαία 114:20, 527:25
  ῥίζα 113:2
ἴδε 112:20
ἰδιαίτερον 37:14
ἴδιον 37:11, 115:14
ἰδιότητα (ἰδιότης) 200:15
ἰδιώματα 290:23
ἰδού 113:8, 599:4
ἰδύμενοι 114:24
ἵδρωσις 42:6–7
ἱδρῶτος (ἱδρώς) 42:6–7, 199:23
ἱερά 115:19, 147:3
  βοτάνη 115:15
  Ἰούστου 148:10
  πικρά 147:3, 1558:8
ἱερακίτης 148:22
Ἱέραξ 148:23
ἱεράπολις 150:7
ἱερατεῖον 114:16, 149:3, 149:9?
ἱερατικόν 149:6, 2086:12?
ἱερεύς 115:24, 147:5, 150:1, 279:15
ὁ ἱερός 7:9–10
Ἰησοῦς 139:2, 847:21
  νίκη 847:22
ἱκετεύσω 146:5
ἱκέτης 146:7
Ἰκόνιον 146:14, 146:18
ἴκτερος 572:5
ἱλαρία 130:3
ἱλαρῦναι 129:27
Ἰλλυρικὴ ἶρις 130:8
Ἰλλυρικόν 170:12?
ἰλύς 130:1
ἱμάντας 136:3
ἱμάντιον 185:6?, 192:23?
ἱμάς 133:4, 136:3

ἱμάτιον 133:26
ἱματισμός 133:27
ἵνα τί 137:3
ἰνδικόν 137:12, 640:16
ἰνδικτιῶνα 110:1, 199:10
ἰνές 137:4
ἰνώδης 137:5
ἰξευτής 126:3
ἰξός 126:2
ἴον 118:3, 686:27, 842:7
ἴονθος 152:7
Ἰόππη 843:3
ἰός 35:24, 118:10, 118:18, 241:15, 687:24
σιδήρου 118:18
ἰουδαϊκός (λίθος) 210:9, see λίθος (ἰουδαϊκός)
ἰουδαΐσαι 838:1
Ἰουλιάνιον 130:26
Ἰουλιανός 117:24
Ἰούλιος 117:28, 841:6
δικτάτωρ 112:27
Ἰούνιος 118:8
Ἰοῦστος 842:16, 847:21
ἱππάκη 143:13
ἱππίατρος 144:8, 196:10, 301:23, 1229:7, 1543:4, 1579:22
ἱππικὸς
νόσος 260:20?, 260:21?
ἀγών 260:21, 528:1
ἱπποδρόμιον 142:6
ἱππόδρομος 259:18
ἱππόκαμπος 141:18, 144:11
ἱπποκάμπου (ἱππόκαμπος) 213:11
ἱπποκένταυρος 143:3, 619:7, 632:28
Ἱπποκράτης 143:6, 619:16, 843:2
ἱππομανές 828:19
ἱππομάραθον 132:8, 142:2
ἱππομάραθρον 80:13, 142:4, 142:16
ἱπποσέλινον 141:5, 142:11, 213:12
ἵππουρις 141:16, 141:25, 144:23
ἄλλη 143:8
ἱπποφαές 144:4
ἱππόφαιστον 144:14
ἴρινον 114:5, 148:18, 290:26
ἴρινον (μύρον) 70:19–20, 148:5, 851:22
ἶρις 139:16?, 147:8, 149:1, 851:21
ἀγρία 150:5–6
ἴς 137:4
ἰσάτις 138:7, 140:17
ἰσατώδης (χόλη) 140:20
Ἰσαυρία 137:18
ἰσημερία 139:12
ἰσθμὸς (Κορίνθιος) 245:23
ἴς κιθάρας 217:15?
Ἰσπανία 235:22
ἰσογώνιος 138:5–6
ἰσόμετρα (ἰσόμετρος) 229:18
ἰσόμετρον (ἰσόμετρος) 218:27
ἰσόπυρον 139:4–8
ἰσοσκελής 138:5–6, 643:27
(ἰσ)ότονος 106:24?
ἰσόψυχος 140:3
ἱστοκεραία 178:18, 1379:14
ἱστόποδα (ἱστόπους) 222:9
ἱστόποδες (ἱστόπους) 270:17
ἱστορία φιλοθεΐας 222:6
ἱστορικόν? 242:14
Ἰστρικόν ἔλαιον 210:7, 222:3
ἱστῶν 140:4
ἰσχίας 932:16
ἰσχιάς 242:19
ἰσχυρός 7:9–10, 140:8, 240:15, 567:24, 1344:26, 1384:8

ἰσχύς 140:21
ἴσχυσε 140:10
Ἰταλία 123:20
ἡ Ἰταλική 123:17, 123:19
ἰτέα 123:22, 165:20, 171:12, 845:9
Ἰτουρία 124:5
ἴτρια 124:18
ἴτριον 109:18, 124:9, 224:18
ἴτρον 124:13, 1161:2
ἰχθύς 126:7, 1645:13
ἰχνεύμων 1314 n. 16, 1861:11, 1862:3
ἴχνη 125:26
ἴχνος 125:26
Ἰώ 116:2
Ἰωάννης 110:15, 839:13
ἰώμενος 110:9
Ἰώνιος 403:2
ἰωνίτης 203:14
Ἰώπολις 118:16?
ἰῶτα 840:16

K

κάγκαμον 1699:18, 1700:11
καγκελλάριος 1812:12
κάγκελλος 1812:13
καδμεία 238:15, 535:14, 1687:15
καθαίρεσις 1706:2, 1856:13
κάθαρμα 1860:1
καθάρματα 1704:6, 1859:3, 1860:1
καθαροί 1858:17
καθαρός 1856:20
καθαρότης 1706:7
κάθαρσις 1706:2, 1856:13
καθαρτικόν 1706:1, 1859:5
καθέδρα, -ων 1859:7
καθέδριον 1859:7
καθεῖλες 1706:9
καθείλοσαν 1706:11
καθέξουσιν 1706:13
καθὲς κύριε 1858:8?
καθετήρ 1705:18, 1859:4
καθέτης 906:2?
κάθετος 906:2?, 1697:18, 1705:15, 1706:6, 1860:2
καθήλωσον 1705:13
καθολική 1706:4, 1857:1, 1857:12
καθολικός 288:6?, 1857:4
καί 1697:19
καικίας 1703:4, 1718:4
καινός 1700:17
καινοτομία 1701:4
καίριον 865:24?
καιρός 1697:22, 1775:8, 1780:15, 1843:14
Καῖσαρ 1717:10, 1817:3
Καισαρεία 1817:7
κακὴ ἄρσις 1829:17
κακόν 1703:3
κακοπραγμονεῖ 1830:5
καλάϊνον (electrum) 1788:9
καλαμάγρωστις 1698:10
καλαμάριον 1846:3
καλάμη 1699:7
καλαμίνθη 1698:12, 1698:20, 1698:22, 1793:7
κάλαμος 1699:9, 1699:11
  ἀρωματικός 1698:14, 1698:25, 1787:2
  φραγμίτης 1698:23, 1783:4
καλάνδαι 1698:8, 1789:1, 1794:3
καλὴ ἄρσις 1783:10
καλιγάριος 1788:6, 1788:15
καλίγιον, -α 1788:7
καλκῖτις 1797:7, see χαλκητάριν
καλλίας 443:10, 456:26, 498:23

καλλιβλέφαρον 1788:12
Καλλίνικος 898:19?, 1699:17, 1791:3, 1794:11
κάλλιον 1699:16
κάλλιστος 1699:5
καλλίτριχον 1699:3
καλλονή 1699:13
κάλλος 1699:15
καλός 1785:15
ἄνθρωπος 1786:20
ἵππος 1791:21?
καλοῦσιν ἰλιακόν 1744:11
κάλπη 1796:6
κάλπιον 1796:6
κάλπις 1792:1?, 1796:6
καλώνυμος 1793:19
καμηλοπάρδαλις 444:3
κάμηλος 501:1
κάμινος πυρός 1801:3
κάμπη 1699:25
καμπτός 698:14, 1800:14
καμπτύς 698:14, 1430:2
καμψάνεμα 967:14
καμών 1799:12
κἄν 1802:8
κανάλης 1700:20
κανάλιον 1772:4, 1811:19
κανθαρίδες 1700:21, 1813:10
κανίσκιον 1807:14, 1811:21
κάνναβις 1701:1, 1802:14, see ἀγρία κάνναβις
ἥμερος 1701:2
κανοπικόν 1485:9
Κάνωπος 1806:20
καπηλεῖον 1822:13, 1823:9 (-α)
κάπηλος? 83:22, 1821:11, 1821:16, 1822:11
καπνός 1702:6, 1702:12, 1702:20, 1745:3
κάππα 1702:5?
Καππαδοκία 1702:10, 1819:13, 1820:20 (λίθος φρύγιος... γεννᾶται ἐν Καππαδοκίᾳ) 864:3, 864:18, 970:11
κάππαρις 828:16–21, 1702:3, 1702:16, see ὀλόφιτον?
κάπρος 1825:3
καραβώδης? 278:22
καρβωνία 1751:17
καρδαμίνη 1318:14, 1345:13
κάρδαμον 1688:1, 1688:4, 1703:20, 1750:15, 1751:21, 2068:20 (confused with θλασπέως)
καρδάμωμον 603:10, 1688:3, 1703:18, 1750:16
καρδία 1703:21
Καρία 1704:7
καρίδες 1704:22, 1843:12
Καρκηδών 1792:18?
καρκίνοι 1485:21
καρκῖνος 1703:11, 1705:6, 1779:23
κάρος 1704:1, 1704:3, 1704:9
καρούχα 1835:3
καρπήσιον 1704:17
καρποβάλσαμον 1837:9?, 1839:23
καρπός 1702:18
τήλεως 1624:12?
καρποφορία 1703:22
καρποφόρος 1703:22
Κάρραι 1688:14, 1704:10, 1780:6
καρτερία 1840:11
κάρυα 1687:12, 1704:24
βασιλικά 1703:12
ποντικά 1703:15
καρυόφυλλον 302:8, 1837:10, 1849:1
καρυωτὸς φοίνιξ 1818:14?
Καρχηδών 1633:23?
καρωτίδες 1705:2

κασσία 1324:15, 1701:17, 1701:23, 1816:15
κασοῦλα 1741:23
κασσίτερος 677:24, 911:19, 1814:10, 1816:1
κασσύματα 1701:19
καστάλια 1816:7
καστανέα 1701:22
κάστανον 1701:15
καστόριον 1701:13, 1815:7
καστρησιανός 1816:11
καστρήσιος 1816:13
κάστρον, -α 1815:18
κάστωρ 444:16, 515:22, see ὄρχεις κάστορος
κατά τοῦτο 1695:25
καταβαίνει 1692:16
καταβήσεται 1692:20
καταβιβάζων 194:21, 1760:12
καταγένος 1690:1
καταγελασάτωσαν σου 1692:22
καταγραφή 1689:18, 1690:6 (-ήν), 1760:1, 1760:6
κατάγω 1692:24
καταδιεῖλε 1692:18
καταδιείλοντο 1693:2
καταδικασεταί σου 1693:4
καταδίκη 1690:8, 1693:1, 1760:18, 1762:11
κατάδικος 1692:25, 1760:18, 1762:11
καταδιώξει 1693:6
κατάθεσις 1759:18
καταθλασθῆναι 1695:11
καταιγίς 1693:8
κατάκαρπος 1694:11
κατακλυσμός 1694:13, 1766:14
κατακυριεύσει 1694:17
κατακυριεύσωσι 1694:19
καταλάβοι 1693:13
κατάληψις 1693:11, 1697:17
καταλήψομαι 1694:3
κατάλοιπος 1693:16
καταλύπειν 1693:18
κατάλυσις 1765:7
καταμόνας 1693:20
κατανάγκη 1701:6
κατανοεῖ 1693:22
κατανοεῖς 1693:24
κατάντημα 1693:26
κατανύγητε 1694:1
καταπατήσει 1694:5
κατάπλασμα 1766:9
καταπλάσματα 1693:10
καταπίεταί με 1695:3
καταποντισμός 1694:7
καταπόντισον 1694:9
κατάρα 1694:15
καταραχθήσεται 1694:26
καταρράκται 1694:23, 1767:19
καταρράκτης 1694:21
καταρτίζουσα 1695:1
καταρχή 1697:15, 1768:16
κατασκευή 1692:1, 1765:19
κατασκηνώσεις 1695:5
κατάστασις 1691:23, 1760:8, 1761:7, 1765:16
κατάστησον 1695:7
καταστικοί 1692:9
κατάστρωμα 1815:12
κατάσχεσις 1695:9
κατατέρπου 1695:27
κατατοξεῦσαι 1695:23
κατατρεπόμενοι 1767:9
κατάφασις 987:18, 1477:22, 1588:17, 1689:5, 1766:8
καταφονική 1692:14?
καταφορά 169:19

καταφυγή 1696:1
καταχθείησαν 1696:3
κατεκάμφθη 1696:5
κατέκαμψαν 1696:7
κατέλαβόν με 1696:9
κατελάλεις αὐτοῦ 1696:13
κατέναντι 1696:11
κατεπανουργεύσαντο 1695:13
κατεπίομεν 1696:16
κατεπόθη 1696:18
κατέρρηξας 1696:20
κατεστάθην 1696:22
κατέστησας 1696:24
κάτεσχεν 1696:26
κατεύθυνε 1696:27
κατευοδωθήσεται 1695:17
κατεφίλησαν 1695:19
κατηγόρημα 1689:15
κατηγορία 111:9, 1318:11, 1689:16, 1727:1, 1727:20, 1759:20, 1759:21
κατηγορίας 1689:16, 1698:20, 1759:21
κατηγορικός 1760:4
κατήγορος 1760:2
κατηγορούμενος 1759:25
κατήρτισε 1695:15
κατηρῶντο 1695:21
κατήχησις 1692:13
κατοικητήριον, -ια 1696:29
κατοικῶν 1697:1
κατοπτήρ 1229:9?
κατοχή 1691:22
κατοχόμενοι 1692:8
κάτοχος, -ή 1691:20, 1692:6, 1697:9, 1697:12
κάτω 1697:3
καυκαλία 1703:7
καυκαλίδες 1689:3?
καυκαλίς 1479:3, 1689:1
καῦσος 1688:10
καυτήρια 1029:23
καυχᾶσθηε 1687:1
καύχημα 1728:17
καυχήσονται 1687:3
κάχληξ 1796:18?, see κόκλος, κόκλαξ
κάχρυον 1698:2
καχρύς 964:22, 967:14
καψάκη 683:26
Κεγχρεαί 1811:17
κέγχρος 1361:20, 1716:4, 1716:18, 1811:18
κεδρέα 1715:13, 1718:21
κέδριον 1715:10
κεδρίτης οἶνος 1715:15, 1718:22
κέδρος 1715:17, 1718:17, 1832:19
κέδρωστις 1541:8
κειμήλιον 1799:6
κελτική (νάρδος) 1788:18
κεκαθαρισμένη 1718:8
κεκαλλωπισμένη 1718:9
κεκαύμενος 1697:20
κεκόλληται 1718:11
κεκραιπαληκώς 1718:12
κεκρίτης 1719:9?
κεκρυμμένη 1718:14
κεναγγία 1717:5
κενεών 1161:4
κενόν 1700:15, 1716:20, 1717:7
κενότης 1769:10
κενταυρικός? 366:1
κενταύριον 1231:5, 1460:18, 1807:23
λεπτόν 1700:23
τὸ μέγα 1716:25
κένταυρος 1809:11
κέντημα 1808:8, 1808:8

κεντηνάριον 1807:20, 1808:3
κέντρα 1808:15
κέντρον 1715:25, 1716:19, 1716:23, 1808:12
κεντυρίων 1717:9, 1808:19
κεραία 1379:14, 1386:15, 1719:15
κεραμεύς 1110:23, 1719:11
κεραμίς 1845:21, 1846:6
κέρας 1718:20 (-άτων), 1719:6, 1849:10 (-ατος)?
κερασία 1718:24, 1719:7, 1781:16
κερασός 1719:7, 1781:16
κεράστης 1850:19, 1851:18
κεράτια 242:22–3, 1719:1, 1780:22, 1839:10?, 1844:18 (confused with creta)
κεράτιον 1780:10, 1839:12
κερατίσομεν 1719:13
κερατοειδής (χιτών) 1781:1
κερατωνία 1719:3
κεραυνός 1718:16
κερδαλέος 1833:23
κέρκουρος 1850:13
κέστρον 1717:16, 1816:3, 2058:17
ψυχότροφον 1717:14, see ψυχότροφον
κεφάλαια 1717:21
κεφάλαιον 541:7, 1702:24, 1718:1, 1823:15
κεφαλαΐον 797:6?
κεφαλαλγία 1562:9?
κεφαλή 1702:19, 1717:23
κεφαλίδες 384:21
ἐν κεφαλίδι 198:1
κέφαλος 1717:24
κεφαλωτόν 1717:19, 1822:7
κεφαλωτός 1823:6
κηκίδων 85:21
κηκίς 85:21, 1779:14, 1802:11, 1811:9
κῆμος 1774:7 n. 21
κημός 1700:1, 1774:7
κῆνσος 1776:6
κηπαία 1812:5
κηρίον 1781:22
κηρίων 1841:12
κηρός 1780:12, 1833:5
κήρυκες 916:19, 1704:19, 1780:17, 1781:7
κήρυξ 1519:20?, 1780:17, 1781:5
κηρωτή 1834:10
κῆτος 1690:16, 1697:4, 1715:23 (-εα), 1771:5
κίδαρις 1769:1
κιθάρα 1782:15
κιθαρίστης 1782:19
κιθαρῳδίς 1782:19
κίκεως καρπός 812:1–2, 1558:5
κίκι 1779:16, 1793:21
κίκινον (ἔλαιον) 1779:17
Κιλικία 1771:14
κιμωλία 300:19
γῆ 1378:24, 1774:1, see γῆ (κιμωλία)
κινάρα 879:7, 891:3, 905:17, 1775:3, 1803:9
κίνδαξ, -ακος 1737:18?
κίνδυνος 1737:11, 1769:11, 1775:7
κιννάβαρι 502:8?, 502:24?, 1709:6, 1775:13, 1803:14
κινναμώμινον (μύρον) 1775:16
κιννάμωμον 1665:4, 1740:7, 1775:1
κινυριστής 907:25
κιρκαία 1781:12
κιρκήσια 1781:18, 1850:20, 1853:1
Κιρκήσιον 1782:1
κίρκινος 1852:10
κίρκος 1850:20, 1853:1
κίρσιον 1841:23, see κρίσσιον
κιρσός 577:2, 1781:9, 1848:18
κίσθαρος 1779:5

κίσθος 1776:7, 1778:24, 1818:16

κίσσηρις 1778:20

κισσός 1586:12, 1779:1, 1779:5

κίστος 1557:11?, 1779:1

κιστώ 1701:26

κίτρια 1070:26, 1084:27, 1767:18

κίττα 1770:23

κίχλη πετραία 891:16?

κιχρῶν 1771:12

κιχώριον 1811:10

κίων (-ονος) 1802:17

κλαυδίανον 895:16, 1785:19

Κλαυδία 1785:23

Κλαύδιος 1785:23

κλαυθμός 1783:7

κλαυσθήσονται 1783:10

κλεῖδες (κλείς) 276:12

κλειδός 1788:10

κλείς 897:3, 1788:10

κλεισοῦραι 1792:3

Κλέονος (κολλύριον) 1784:24

Κλεόπας 1788:14

Κλεοπάτρα 1716:16

Κλέος 1788:3?

κλέπτης 1784:26

κλεωνία 1793:14

κληδόνες 1785:18?

κλῆμα 1509:9, 1571:4?, 1785:1

κληματίς 1789:15

καθαρτική 1790:1

κληρικοί 1790:17, 1791:8, 1844:20

κληροδοσία 1791:14

κληρονομία 1791:1, 1791:10

κλῆρος 1790:21, 1798:19

κλίβανος 1788:5, 1788:13

κλιμακάριον 1790:9?, 1793:16?

κλιμακτήρ 1790:11

κλίμα 1789:12

κλίματα 1782:22, 1793:22

κλίνη 1791:13

κλῖνον 1791:16

κλινοπόδιον 1792:12

κλιτύς 1788:21

κλύδονες 1786:17?, 1787:9?

κλύμενον 1786:12

κλυστήρ 493:17, 494:13, 507:11?

κλωβίον 1785:6

κλωβός 1785:4

κνέωρον 2046:18

κνήμη, -ην 1811:3

κνηστόν 1812:1?

κνῆστρον 2046:17

κνίδη 1810:7, 1810:11

κνίδινον (ἔλαιον) 1810:8, cf. 1606:19

Κνίδος 1809:21, 1810:11

κνικέλαιον 1810:8

κνίκιον 1582:10

κνίκος 1736:16, 1779:18, 1810:1, 1810:18

κνισμός 1810:20

κόγχη 1728:15, 1811:7

κοδράντης 1723:5?

κοῖλα 1769:13

κοιλάδες 875:27

κοιλάς 1731:19

κοίλη (φλέψ) 1729:12

Κοίλη Συρία 1324:4

κοιλία 1731:17

κοίλωμα 1730:16

κοιμητήριον 1735:1, 1774:9, 1800:20, see κωμητήριον

κοινίον 1774:19

κοινοβάριος 1803:19

κοινόβιον 1807:1
κοινόν 1775:12?
κοινωνία 1738:13, 1740:21, 1775:10
κοινωνός 1775:11
κοίτη 1725:19
κοιτών 1687:6, 1688:8, 1770:16
κοιτωνίτης 1782:14
κόκκαλος 1748:3
κοκκομηλέα 1748:8, 1749:9
κόκκος
βαφική 1519:25, 1748:6, 1749:11
κνίδος 1748:4, 21
κολαφισμός 1729:11
κόλλα 1732:12
κολλίσκιον 493:2?
κολλοκασία 1720:12
κολλύρα 1787:6
κολοβίων 1731:6, 1785:7, 1731:16, 1806:22
κολοβός 1730:14, 1785:14
κολόβωμα 1729:17
κολοκασία 1787:4, 1797:4
κολοκύνθη 1731:3
ἀγρία 1729:21, 1730:12
κολοκυνθίς 1509:2, 1729:19
Κολοσσαί 1730:21
κολοσσός 1729:23
κολούσω 1729:25
κολοφωνία 545:2, 1731:1, 1796:3, 1898:16
κόλπος 1732:1
κολυμβάδες 1729:14
κολχικόν 1732:19
Κολωνία 1731:22
κόμαρος 1733:14
κόμης 1734:6, 1734:12, 1734:18
Σέλευκος 1734:13
κόμητες 1734:22
κομήτης 1517:1, 1734:16 (-αι), 1800:2 (-αι)
κομισάσθωσαν 1735:11
κόμμι 1733:11, 1734:4, 1735:17, 1737:1, 1799:13, 1846:11
κωνείου 1739:22, see κώνειον
κομμίδιον 1737:1
κομμωτικὸν (ἔλαιον) 1736:3
κονδῖτος (οἶνος) 1615:21, 1633:18, 1738:9, 1804:9
κονδρίλλη 878:19
κονδυλώματα 1737:20
κονία 1738:12, 1739:23, 1740:22, 1741:3
κοντάριον 1732:7, 1739:14
κόνυζα 1728:8, 1738:1, 1738:18, 1850:6
κοπάδιον 1745:15, cf. 1743:3
κοπετός 1743:18
κοπίσκος 626:5, 976:21, 1747:20
κόπος 1743:1, 22, 1745:9
κοπρία 1746:11
κόπρος 673:24, 1746:4
κοπτή 1745:14
κόραξ 1162:13 (-ακος)?, 1750:4, 1832:13 (-ακος), 1851:21 (-ακες)
κοράλλιον 918:13, 1522:8, 1750:6, 1754:20, 1834:22
κόρεις οἱ ἀπὸ κλίνης 1753:2
κόρη 1753:8
κόρην 353:18
κορίαννον 1570:8, 1722:17, 1753:5
κορίανον 957:2?
κορίνθινον 1838:7?
Κόρινθος 1753:16, 1754:12
κόριον 1753:10, see κορίαννον
κόρις τὸ φυτόν 1752:23
κορύβαντες 1750:12
κορυδαλός 1752:1, 1752:8

κόρυδοι 1751:19

κόρυδος 1523:13, 1751:18

κόρυζα 1752:2, 1754:7, 1757:18

κορύνη 1755:9

κορυφή 1754:5

κορώνη 1731:11, 1835:14

κορωνοπόδιον 1835:17

κορωνόπους 1523:11, 1753:21, 1755:7, 1755:14

κοσμητός, -ή 1742:7

κοσμικός 1724:7, 1742:6

κοσμοκράτωρ 1724:10, 1733:10, 1742:16

κόσμος 1724:4, 1742:1, 1742:17

κόστος 1690, note 1, 1701:12, 1702:1, 1741:8

κότε 1717:12?

κότινος 1728:1

κοτύλη 1725:6, 1725:13

κοτυληδόνες 1727:17, 1761:5

κοτυληδών 1308:3, 1726:20

ἄλλη 1725:14

κουβικουλάριοι 1687:7

κουβικουλάριος 1707:4

κουεστιονάριος 1815:9

κουράτωρ 1752:10

κούρητες 1750:20, 1752:18

κοῦρμι 1749:19

κοῦσπος 1742:12

κουστωδία 1741:15

κουφόλιθος 1643:21

κοφινάριον 1745:7?

κόφινος 1703:6, 1745:4, 1746:12

κόχλαξ 1796:18?, 1798:15, cf. 378:11, 770:4, see κάχληξ, κόχλος

κοχλίας 1724:14, 1728:19

κόχλος 1796:18, 1798:15, cf. 378:11, 770:4, see κάχληξ, κόχλαξ

κράββατοι? 491:26

κράββατον 1687:6?, 1688:8?

κράζειν 1831:5

κράμβη 1831:19

ἀγρία 358:16, 1845:15, see ἀγρία κράμβη

ἥμερος 1832:5

(θαλασσία) 1832:7, 1845:16

κρανία 1831:15

κράξω 1852:7

κρᾶσις 1848:19

κραταία 1758:15

κραταιόγονον 1781:3, 1832:1

κραταιός 1831:8

κράτιστος 1831:11

κράτος 1831:13

κρατυνέτω 1831:10

κραυγή 1831:14

κρέας 1834:5, 1840:14

κρέεα 1834:5

κρείσσων 1834:7

κρημνός? 146:4

κρήνη, -ας 708:14?

Κρήτη 1839:8

κρητική γῆ 1847:4

κρητικός (οἶνος) 1842:22

κρίθη 1841:13, 1842:12,1848:1

κριθήτωσαν 1844:6

κρίθμον 1841:19, 1842:8

κρῖμα 1843:22

κρίνει 1844:1

κρίνον 148:18, 268:22, 290:26, 1844:1, 1844:3

κρίνων 1844:1

κριός 268:28, 1842:9, 1844:8

κρίσις 1844:9

κρίσσιον 1841:23, see κίρσιον

κρίτης 1843:23

Κρίτων 1843:1
Κροῖσος 1836:13
κρόκινον (ἔλαιον) 1838:4
κροκοδείλιον 1837:21
κροκόδειλος 1750:21, 1755:13, 1756:15, 1757:11, 1838:1, 1851:15
κρόκον 517:22
κρόκος 882:16, 1757:10, 1837:17 (-ου)
κρόγου μάλαγμα 1837:19
κρόμμυον 1835:1, 1845:14
κρόνιον 1836:5?
Κρόνος 1836:7
κροσσωτός 1834:20
κρόταφοι 1834:16
κροτήσατε 1834:18
κρότων 1609:8
κρουνοί 1813:1, 1835:20
κρουνός 1803:11
κρουνούς 1813:1, 1835:20
κρυσταλλοειδές (ὑγρόν) 1836:16
κρύσταλλος 918:7, 1836:18, 1844:13
Κτησιφών 1763:1
κτητική 146:9?
κτητικόν 1763:3
κτίστης 1762:10
κύαθοι 1110:16, 1719:21
κύαθος 1719:21, 1720:9, 1758:13
κύαμος 1720:1
  αἰγύπτιος 1720:12, 1736:1
κυανός, -οῦ 1720:3
κυάνωσις 1741:17
κυβερνήτης 1721:23
κύβος 1721:3
κυδωνίτης οἶνος 1723:11
κυκλάμινος 1720:17, 1748:15
κυκλόθεν 1769:17
κύκλος 1748:10, 1749:3, 1770:14, 1779:21
κυκλώσει 1770:3
κυκνάριον 1748:13
κύκνος 1747:18, 1749:1, 1749:16, 1780:2, 1829:16
κύλινδρος 1731:20, 1732:9
κυμβάλιον 1726:24
κύμβαλον 1769:20
κύμικον 303:6–11
κύμινον
  ἥμερον 1734:7
  ἄγριον 1734:8
  ἄλλο 1734:10
κυνάγχη 1740:18, see συνάγχη
κυνανθρωπία 1736:20
κυνάνθρωπος 956:24, 1163:5, 1809:3
κύνειον 1731:15
κυνηγία 1737:8, 1738:7
κυνήγιον 1715:9, 1802:23
κυνηγός 1737:4
κυνίδιον 1750:21
κυνικοί 1737:14
Κυνικός 1739:7
κυνικός 1163:5
κυνικός (σπασμός) 1741:6
κυνόγλωσσον 1737:11
κυνοκράμβη 85:16
κυνομόριον 375:13–15
κυνόμορον 85:16, 148:8, 1729:15, 1776:4, 1960:23, cf. 148:8?
κυνόμυια 1769:22
κυνός 1740:17, 1768:21
  ὄρχις 1739:5, 1749:8
κυνόσαργες 1738:5, 1739:10, 1740:24?, 1775:18?
κυνόσβατος 828:18, 1739:1

δὶα κυνῶν 572:3, 1731:15
κυπάρισσος 1743:20, 1746:14
κυπειρίς ἰνδική 1743:13
κύπειρος 1517:8, 1718:3, 1742:23, 1743:17, 1745:21
κύπρινον (ἔλαιον) 1746:8, 1746:15
Κύπρος 1746:5
κύπρος 1746:2
Κυρήνη 1754:12, 1754:14?
κυριακή 1754:11
Κυριακός 1754:1
κυριακός 214:7, 274:15
κύριε 1753:12, 1770:6, 1770:9
ἐλέησον 1753:15
Κύριλλος 1754:9, 1754:22
Κυριναϊκός (ὀπός) 1770:10
Κυριναῖος 1753:20, 1770:7
κύριος 1724:13, 1754:2, 1770:5, 1770:12, 1843:14
Κυρρηστικοί 1752:6
Κύρρος 1752:6
κυρτός 604:3?, see ἀμφίκυρτος
κύτινος 351:10, 1725:12, 1727:5, 1727:13
κύτισος 1727:14
κύφι 1744:16, 1744:22 (ἀντίδοτος) (-εως)
τὸ μέγα 1744:11
κῦφος 1742:12
κύφων 1743:24?
κύψει 1770:1
κύων 1740:17, 1768:21
κωβιός 1720:24, 1739:20
δὶα κωδίων 554:4–7, 571:22
κώδυα 1722:5
κώδυον 1720:10
Κωκυτός 1726:17, 1830:3
κῶλα 1729:7
κῶλον 1125:22, 1730:25
κῶμα, -ατα 1733:12
κώμαρις 1735:5
κωμητήριον 1734:3, 1735:1, 1800:20, see κοιμητήριον
κωμικός 1735:21
κωμῳδία 819:6, 1734:5, 1735:19
κωμῳδός 1734:20
κωνάριον, -ια 1736:19
κώνειον 363:3, 387:1, 1738:15, 1739:23
κωνεῖον 363:3, 1737:22?, 1739:23
κῶνοι 1737:15, 1737:8 (κῶνος)
κῶνος 277:10?, 1333:18, 1457:1, 1521:4, 1738:8, 1738:20
Κωνσταντῖνος 1741:12
κωφός 1743:22

Λ

λάβραξ, -ακος 940:22
λαβύρινθος 375:22
λάγανον 932:8, 942:11
λαγών, -όνες 932:5, 1161:8
λαγωὸς
θαλάσσιος 931:14
χερσαῖος 931:15
λαγώπους 931:18
λαγωφθαλμόν 931:24, 932:9
λάδανον 409:15, 932:14, 943:9
λαθυρίς 933:9, 936:5
λάθυρος 936:10
λαϊκός 969:1
λαιμαργία 967:6, 969:3
λάκκος 935:17
λαλήσει 933:26
λαλία 974:3
λαμπάς, -άδα 976:5

κυνανθρώπου 954:21, 2008:8
λαμπήδων 934:3
λαμπρότατος 934:12
λαμπρότης 934:14
λαμπτήρ 422:8?, 976:4
λάμπων 934:1
λαμψάνη 934:19
λαξευτήριον 933:24
Λαοδίκεια 932:24, 943:8, 949:11
λαός 933:1, 954:11
λάπαθον 935:13
λάρυγξ, -υγγος 518:8, 935:21, 965:10
Λαῦσος 954:12?
πραιπόσιτος 954:13
λάχανα 933:21
λέβης 944:3
λέγετε 944:6
λεγεών 941:13
λέγουσι 944:8
(λει)εντερία 205:21
λειμώνιον 967:3
λείξουσιν 966:5
λειοτριβήσει 943:20
λεῖπον 968:24
λειπυρία 968:6
λείρινον μύρον 174:2
λειριόμυρον 174:2
(ἐν) λειτουργίᾳ 398:11
λειχήν 205:16 ([λειχήν ὁ] ἐπὶ [τῶν] πετρῶν), 963:10 (ὁ ἐπὶ τῶν πετρῶν), 965:20?, 965:24, 966:8 (ὁ ἐπὶ τῶν πετρῶν)
λειχῆνες 965:21 (ἵππων), 965:24, 966:6
λειχηνικόν (ἔμπλαστρον) 966:3
λειῶ 943:23
λεκάνη 969:2, 981:11
λεκτίκιον 935:18, 946:5, 980:8
λεξικόν 945:20, 973:6
λέξις 945:17, 973:1, 1610:19
λεοντοπέταλον 783:5 ([λεοντοπέ]ταλον), 944:16, 1463:19
λεοντοπόδιον 944:16–17, 963:1
θορύβηθρον 1463:20
Λεόντιος 932:25
λεπίδιον 946:3, 960:13, 968:12
λεπίδος ἄνθος 943:12?
λεπιδωτή 968:8
λεπίς 945:26, 968:26
χαλκοῦ 946:1
λέπρα 945:27
λεπτά 979:8
λεπτοκάρυα 1703:17, see κάρυα
λεπτότης? 581:3
λευκάκανθα 945:3, 945:6, 957:9, 958:18, 1475:19
λευκάς 944:22
λευκή 944:15, 945:9, 956:18, 956:20, 1374:24
ἄκανθα 615:4, see ἄκανθα λευκή
λευκογραφίς 945:10, 958:25
λευκόϊον 945:4
λεύκωμα 944:20
λέων 932:21, 934:22
λήθαργος 969:18
λημνία
γῆ 966:15, 966:19?
γῆ καὶ λημνία σφραγίς 967:7
σφραγίς 787:14, 934:24, 966:15, 966:20, 975:9, 1092:1, 1108:20
λῆρος 935:23
λήψεται 968:15
λίβα 963:14
λίβανος 963:17, 963:22, 964:18
λιβανωτίς 964:19, 967:12, 1698:6

λιβανωτός 718:23, 963:19, 963:21, 964:18, 968:21, 976:18
Λιβερτίνων 576:8, 947:1
λιβόνοτος 963:25
Λιβύη 938:4, 939:7, 946:21, 963:13
λιγνύς 965:5
λιγυστικόν 947:3, 964:5, 965:3, 973:7
λιθάργυρος 969:21
λιθοκόλλα 972:1
λίθος 946:6, 969:12, see ἀγήρατος (λίθος), ἀδαμαντικὸς (λίθος), ἀδάμαντος (λίθος), ἀλιστὸς (λίθος), ἀφροσέληνος (λίθος), εὐτύχιος (λίθος)
 αἱματίτης 970:8, 970:18, see αἱματίτης (λίθος)
 ἀλαβαστρίτης 971:7
 ἀμίαντος 971:13, see ἀμίαντος (λίθος)
 ἀραβικός 970:27, see ἀραβικός (λίθος)
 γαλακτίτης 971:1, see γαλακτίτης (λίθος)
 γαγάτης 970:22
 γεώδης 972:8, see γεώδης (λίθος)
 θρᾳκίας 970:24
 θυΐτης 971:9
 ἰάσπις 971:23, see ἰάσπεως
 ἰουδαϊκός 971:11, see ἰουδαϊκός (λίθος)
 μαγνῆτις 970:26, see μαγνῆτις
 μελιτίτης 971:3, see μελιτίτης (λίθος)
 μεμφίτης 971:18
 μόροχθος 971:5, see μόροχθος
 ναξίας ἀκόνης ἀπότριμμα 972:13
 ὀστρακίτης 972:4, see ὀστρακίτης (λίθος)
 ὀφίτης 971:25
 ἀπὸ τοῦ ποταμοῦ Πόντου 863:24
 πυρίτης 970:3, 970:4, 970:6, 970:15, see πυρίτης (λίθος)
 σάμιος 972:10
 σάπφειρος 971:16
 σεληνίτης 971:20
 σμύρις 972:6
 σπογγίτης 971:27
 σχιστός 970:20
 φρύγιος 970:11, see φρύγιος (λίθος)
λιθόσπερμον 970:10
λιμήν 966:17, 974:12
λιμητόν 967:16
λίμνη 966:18
λιμνῆστις 438:16, 966:22
λίμος 966:13
λινάριον 967:23
λινόζωστις 964:15, 967:17
λινοποιός 967:24
λινόσπερμον 967:21, 967:25, 1244:20
λιπαροί 968:5
λιπυρίας 968:6
λιτανεία 951:5, 965:12
λιτανεύωσι 965:13
λίτρα 965:17
λίτρον (νίτρον) 180:18
λίψ 940:17, 963:14, 963:15, 968:16, 968:18, 979:10
λόβια 946:24
λογάριον, -ια 948:7
λογάς, -άδος 947:5
Λόγγινα 948:20
Λόγγινος 948:4
τὰ λόγια 947:8, 948:10
λογίατρος 947:6
λογική 564:12, 947:13, 947:15
λογικοί 947:22, 948:3
λογικός 947:20
λόγιος 947:24?
λογιότατος 947:19

λογίσεται 947:23
λογισμός 947:11
λόγος 947:9, 948:10
λόγους 947:21
λόγχη 954:9
λογχῖτις 953:6 (ἑτέρα), 954:2
λοιμός 953:24
λοιμώδης 953:25
λουδάριοι 949:2
λουκανθήσομαι 944:1
Λουκᾶς 957:14
λούσω 946:10
λοχευομένη 951:19
λύγος 948:18
λύκαινα, -αι 956:6?
λυκάνθρωπος 956:24, 1809:5
λύκειον 958:16
λύκειος (νόσος) 956:24
λύκιον 956:11, 957:4, 958:15
λυκοκτόνος 232:18, 956:15
λύκος 958:21
λύκοψις 210:22–3, 956:9, 958:22
λυμαινόμενος 946:8
λύρα 959:1
λυριστής 959:2
Λυσανίας 954:23
Λυσίας 955:1
λυσιμάχιον 954:17, 954:21
λυσσητής 954:25?
λυσσῶντος? 226:6
Λύστρα 954:27
λυτρώμενος 965:8
λυτρωτής 965:9
λυχνίδιον 953:1
λυχνίς 952:23, 953:18
  ἀγρία 952:24
λύχνος 965:7, 966:4
λῶος 946:11
λωρότομος 969:5
λῷστος 954:25?
λώταξ 950:14
λωτάρια 950:15
λωτός 950:22, 954:20
  ἄγριος 950:17
  ἥμερος 950:19
  ὁ ἐν Αἰγύπτῳ 950:9
  τὸ δένδρον 950:15

M

μαγάς, -άδα 985:15
μάγγανον 989:18, 1005:19
μάγειρος 985:12, 1007:18
μαγιστριανοί 1007:5
μαγιστριανός 1002:13
μάγιστρος 985:9, 1002:13
μαγνῆτις 297:3–4, 660:17, 863:6, 1006:15, see λίθος (μαγνῆτις)
μάγος 1000:28
μαδάρωσις 986:9, 993:5, 994:7
μάδελκον 986:11
μαελέθ 1023:9, 1029:17
μᾶζα 986:17
μαθήματα 995:5
μαθηματική, -ῶν 1194:8
μαθηματικοί 995:3
μαθηματικόν 995:4, 7, 1181:5, 1185:21, 1194:9
μαινίς 1023:20
Μακαρία 1148:24
Μακάριος 992:8, 1143:3, 1148:18
μακεδονικόν 992:2
Μακεδωνία 1145:1

μάκελλον 993:4, 1146:14
μάκερ 992:12, 992:18
μακράν 992:10
μακρόθεν 992:6
μακροθυμία 1148:4, 1148:9
μακρόθυμος 992:14, 1148:6
μακροτράχηλος 1148:7
μαλάβαθρον 1087:15
μάλαγμα 1088:1
μαλάχη 1021:13, 1032:1
μάλιστα 1093:7
μᾶλλον 988:1, 1089:15
μανδήλιον 1103:26
μάνδρα 990:10
μανδραγόρας 933:7, 990:12, 1068:11, 1104:5
μανία 989:15
μάραγνα 1150:24
μάραθρον 993:10, 1164:9
μαρασμός 993:7, 993:19
  φθινώδης 993:20
Μάργος 1149:17
Μάρκελλος 994:1
Μαρκίων 1162:1
Μάρκος 1161:26
μαρμαρίτης 1689:3
μάρμαρον 1159:11
μάρον 994:11
μαρσύπιον 1159:24
μάρτυρ, -ος 798:16
μαρτυρία 993:14, 1155:5
Μαρτύριος 1156:7
Μαρτυρόπολις 994:2
μάρτυς, -υρος 993:16, 1156:6
μασθός 991:10
μάστιξ, -ιγος 991:13
μαστίχη 990:26
μαστίχινον 991:3
ματαιότης 987:11
ματαιοτήτων 987:19, 1060:17
ματαίως 987:13
Μαύσωλος 1037:11
μαχαιρώνιον 866:1
μέ 1017:8
μεγαλεῖον 187:12–14, 1017:16
μεγάλη 1017:18
μεγαλοπρέπεια 1017:21, 1068:1
μεγαλοπρεπέστατος 1068:3?
μεγαλορρήμων 1017:23
μεγαλοσύνη 1004:6
μεγαλυνθησόμεθα 1018:1
μεγαλύνομεν 1018:5
δὶα μέθης 565:16
μεθοδικός 1025:6
Μεθόδιος 1186:16
μέθοδοι 995:9, 1181:9
μέθοδος 1025:3, 1180:2, 1186:3, 1186:11
μεθύσκων 1025:9
μεθύων 1025:2
μελαγχολία 990:14, 1021:15, 1021:20, 1085:3
μελαγχολικά 1017:10, 1021:16
μελαμπόδιον 1073:13
μελάμφυλλον 271:11–17
μέλαν 1022:6, 1073:17
  σπόδιον 1071:1, see σπόδιον
μελάνθιον 1023:3, 1071:13
μελαντηρία 1022:4
μελέτη 988:7, 1022:7
μελετήσει 1022:11
μέλι 1023:7, 1070:21 (-ιτος), 1072:12
μελία 1021:22, 1023:4, 1073:15
μελικηρίδες 1022:20
μελικηρίς 1072:15?

μελίκρατον 1022:13, 1091:27, 1093:9
μελίλωτος 1022:2, 1071:3
μελίμηλα 1073:7
μελίνη 1473:3
μέλισσα 1022:1
μελισσόφυλλον 1022:18, 1072:25, 1093:11
μελίτεια 1070:15?
Μελίτη 1070:24
μελιτίτης (λίθος) 865:10, 1072:16, see λίθος (μελιτίτης)
μελιτώματα 1022:3
μέλος, -εα 1091:17
μελωτή, -ήν 1070:25
μενδήσιον 1023:17
μένει 1023:16
μέριμνα 1024:14
μεριμνήσω 1024:23
μερίς 1025:1, 1025:8 (-ίδος)
μεριστική (τέχνη) 1077:11
μερολογία 1040:1
μέρος 993:17
μεσαραϊκαί (φλέβες) 991:1, 1024:1
μεσάραιον 668:24, 990:24
μεσεντέριον 669:3, 1024:3
μεσημβρία 1024:5, 1075:20
μεσημβρινός 1113:1
μέσον 1023:23
μεσοπόρφυρα 990:19
μέσπιλα 1023:24
μέσπιλον 991:8
Μεσσίας 991:5
μετὰ τοῦ 1019:7
μετάθεσις 252:7, 581:4, 987:17, 1066:7, 1689:5
μεταλλικά 1018:13
μεταλλικοί 987:16
μέταλλον 1063:1, 1091:5
μετάνοια 1069:9
μεταστήσης 1018:23?
μετατίθεσθαι 1019:1
μετάφρενα 1019:8
μετεμελήθη 1019:12
μετεώρισις= μετεωρισμός 1019:16?
μετεωρισμοί 1019:13
μετεωρολογία 1019:18
μετεωρολογικών 91:4
μετέωρος, -δοτός 1203:1
μετῆρας 1019:10
μετόχη 1018:16
μέτοχος 1019:14
μέτρα 987:15, 1069:24
μετρητὰς ἐλαίου 1019:6?
μετρητής 1019:3, 1203:12, 1868:24
μέτρον 1053:9?
μετώπιον 858:16, 1543:6
μετώπιον (μύρον) 1168:11
μή 1066:10
μηδικά 1084:27
μηδική 1012:6, 1068:13
μήδιον 1068:15
μήκων 1076:10
    ἀφρώδης 1076:10
    Ἡράκλεια 1076:10
    κερατῖτις 1076:10
    ῥοιάς 992:16
μηκώνιον 1076:21
μῆλα, 1071:12, 1084:25
    ἀρμενικά 1071:20
    κυδώνια 1071:7
    μηδικά 1071:24
    περσικά 1071:16
μήλη 238:24
μήλινον (μύρον) 1072:18, 1168:1, see μέλαν

σπόδιον
μηλόμελι 1073:7
μηλωτή 987:21, 1519:10
μήν, -ας 1068:19, 1074:5, 1108:20 (-ος)
μηναῖον 1076:26
μήνιγγες 1074:15, 17
μηνιγγοφύλαξ 1074:19
μηνίει 1074:20
μῆον 1068:26
μητέρα 185:7
μήτηρ 1065:12, 1069:23, 1106:7
μήτρα 1065:10, 1069:24
μητρόπολις 1065:20, 1070:5
μητροπολίτης 1065:16
μηχανή, -ας 988:5, 1070:8, 1078:22
μηχανική 1021:12
μηχανική (τεχνή) 1081:27
μίαν 178:24
Μιθριδάτειος 1744:23
Μιθριδάτης 1202:27
μικρο- 1148:13
μικτόν
ἔμπλαστρον 188:23, 191:8, 1145:11
φάρμακον 185:6?, 192:23?
μιλήσιον 1073:11
Μίλητος 1070:19
μιλιάριον 818:25, 824:22, 1071:25
μίλιον, -ια 1068:6, 1071:9, 1072:3?
μίλτος 1099:4, 1797:7
σινωπική 1073:9
μίλφωσις 993:5, 994:22, 1072:1
μιμαίκυλα 1733:14
μιμνήσκεις 1073:18
μιμνήσκεται 1073:20
μίνθη 1075:1
μίσεως 1075:2
μίσυ 1035:12, 1035:15, 1075:2, 1075:12
Μιτυλήνη 1070:3
μνήμη 1104:13
μνημονεύει 1108:18
μνημονευτική 1074:12
μογίλαλος 1068:5
μόγις 974:25, 1000:12?, 1026:25
μοῖρα, -ας 1039:10, 1040:10, 1040:12,
1077:2?, 1077:10
μοίρας 1037:23
μοιρολογία 1040:1
μή μοιχεύσεις 1070:6
μοιχός 1068:24, 1448:19
μολόχη 1032:1, 1086:3, 1089:13
μολόχινον (ἔλαιον) 1032:10
μολύβδαινα 1030:27, 1031:6, 1032:11,
1039:24, 1382:11
μολυβδοειδής (λίθος) 1031:20
μόλυβδος 1031:9, 1031:11
πεπλυμένος 1031:18
μονάζων 1034:6
μοναρχία 1103:2
μοναστήριον, -ια 1034:19, 1069:3, 1105:12
μοναστικός 1034:22
μοναχικός 1030:1
μοναχός 1034:3, 1146:3
οἶκος 1029:27
μοναχῶν ναός 1029:27
μοναχῶς 989:17?
μονήτα 1034:9, 24?
μονητάριοι 1034:12, 1035:3
μονητάριος 1034:24?
μόνιος 1034:15, 1035:6
μονογενής 1034:17
μονοήμερα 1035:5
μονοήμερον 1033:24

μονοκέρατοι 1034:24?
μονοκέρως 1035:10
μονότροπος 1034:1
μονοούσιος 1034:23
Μοντανισταί 1035:1
μορέα 1039:21, 1041:13
μόροχθος 958:26, 1041:9, see λίθος (μόροχθος)
μορφή 1042:14, 1160:22
δὶα μόρων 553:15, 565:14
μοσυλίτις 1037:10
μόσυλον 1037:8
μόσχος 1035:16, 1035:17, 1037:14, 1037:20
μοῦσα, -ας 1037:22
μοῦσαι 1977:6
μουσεῖον 1036:12
μουσικάριος 1036:22, 1037:18
μουσική 1036:6, 1037:16
μουσικός 1033:10, 1042:12
μουσουργός 1035:21
μόχλος 423:8, 1030:17
μπόμβυξ= βάμβαξ 1576:11, see βάμβαξ
μύαγρος 1026:5
μυακάνθινος 1026:13
μυάκανθος 122:5?, 239:18–20, 1026:21?
μύακες 1025:22
Μυγδονία 999:12, 1008:9
μυδρίασις 67:12, 184:18, 1028:3
μυέλος 1028:10, 1069:5
μυές 1028:14
μύκητες, -ήτων 1038:25
μύλη 1032:6, 1068:25, 1072:11 (-ας), 1894:18
μυλλός 1031:15?, 1033:4, cf. 1031:13
μύλλω 1031:15?, 1033:4, cf. 1031:13
μύλος 1032:6
μυλών 1031:17
μυογάλη 1027:2
μυοκτόνον 273:4–5
μυός
  ὦτα 1026:3
  ὠτίς 1026:11
μύουροι 1025:18
Μύρα 1039:23
μύρα 1077:7?
μυρίας 1069:1
μυρική 1040:21, 1458:7, 1480:4
μυριόφυλλον 1042:20, 1044:1
μυρμηκία 1041:15, 1042:10 (-αι, -ων)
μυροβάλανος 351:1–3, 411:4, 1041:10
μύρον 1040:3, 1043:19, 1068:20, 1077:7?, 1077:8, see δάφνινον (μύρον), ἐλάτινον (μύρον), ἡδύχρουν (μύρον), ἴρινον (μύρον), κινναμώμινον (μύρον), λείρινον μύρον, μετώπιον (μύρον), μήλινον (μύρον), νάρδινον (μύρον), ναρκίσσινον (μύρον), σούσινον (μύρον), σχοίνινον (μύρον), τήλινον (μύρον), ὠκίμινον (μύρον)
μύρρα 1042:23, 1043:24, 1068:9 (-αν)?
μυρρίς 1042:23, 1043:24
μυρσίνη 1041:8, 1043:9
  ἀγρία 1043:13
μυρσίνινον 833:10
μυρσινίτης
  οἶνος 1041:16
  τιθύμαλος 1044:4
μυρσινοειδές 1789:17
μύρσινον (ἔλαιον) 1043:10
μυσαρία 1037:5
Μυσία 1037:21
μῦσος 1035:20?
μυστήρια 1037:15
μυστικός 1033:10?, 1042:12?

μύστρον 1036:17, 1036:21, 1053:9?

μυωπίασις 1025:11, 1025:25, 1036:13

μύωψ 1025:20

μύωψες 1025:24?

μῶλυ 1031:2, 1032:4, 1032:8

μώλωψ, -ωπος 1031:14

μωροί 1041:7

μώρωσις 1041:18

N

ναός 1208:6, 1228:17

νᾶπυ 1209:6

σίνηπι 1209:7

νάρδινον (μύρον) 1210:3

νάρδος 1040:4, 1068:20

ἀγρία 1277:3, cf. 1277:10

κελτική 1209:18, 1276:16, 1277:1, 1277:11, see κελτική (νάρδος)

ὀρεινή 1209:20, 1276:19

ναρδόσταχυς 1209:16, 1277:13, 1930:21

νάρθηκος 71:9

ὀπός 183:11–12

νάρθηξ 71:9, 1210:5 (-ηκος), 1279:7, 1787:17

νάρκη 1209:26, 1210:7, 1278:23

ναρκίσσινον (μύρον) 1210:11

νάρκισσος 459:22, 1209:24, 1279:4

νάσκαφθον 1208:18

ναυαγῆσαι 1224:15

ναύκληρος 839:4, 843:9, 1230:10

Ναυπλίου Ευβοέως 1372:6

ναῦς 839:4, 1222:14

ναῦται 18:8–9

ναύτης 1207:18, 1222:16

νεᾶνις 1220:16, 1517:14?

νεανισκαί 1541:20

Νεάπολις 1209:12, 1220:23

νεέλασσα 1927:23

Νεῖλος 1213:4?, 1244:4

νεκρός 1222:7

Νέμεα 1250:5

τὸ πρὸς τὴν γῆν νενευκός 1607:9

νεομηνία 1220:14, 1227:1, 1244:6

νέος 1208:7

νεοσσιά 1228:26

νεόσσιον, -ια 1228:26

νεότης 1220:19

νεόφυτος 1220:21

νερόν 1210:17

Νεστόριος 1256:7

νευρά 1221:9 (-ᾶς), 1231:5

νεφέλιον 1222:3

νεφριτικοί 1265:17

νεφρῖτις 1209:14, 1222:5, 1243:20, 1245:12

νεφροί 1222:1

νεφρός 1222:1

νεώτερος 1220:17

νῆμα 1244:7

νήπιον 1244:22

νήριον 352:18, 1245:23, 25, 1277:20?

νῆρις 1276:21, 1609:5?

νῆσσα 1244:18

νηστεία 968:1, 1244:19

Νικάτωρ 1245:22

νίκη 1245:6

Νικήδορος 1245:21

Νικόλαος 1245:4, 1245:7

Νικόμαχος 1245:16

νίτρον 180:18, 965:14, 1244:3, 1245:3?, 1684:23, see βερενίκιον (νίτρον), λίτρον (νίτρον)

νιτρονικόν 1064:10?

νίψομαι 1244:23

νομή 1226:21, 1227:25
νομικός 1251:21
νόμισμα 1123:16, 1227:3
νομοθέτης 1227:26
νόμος 1226:21, 27, 1227:1
νομός 1226:21
νόσημα 1257:4?
νοσοκομεῖον 1243:14
νόσος 1228:22, see λύκειος (νόσος), ἱππικὸς νόσος, ὀφθαλμικὸς (νόσος), στομαχικός (νόσος)
νόστος, -οι 1256:9
νοτάριος 1225:24, 1226:1, 1227:13, 1251:21
νότος 1225:21
νούμερα 1227:10?, 1227:16, 1228:1
νούμερον 1250:8
νυκτάλωψ, -ωπος 1225:11, 1230:1, 1383:11
νυκτίκοραξ 1243:16
νυκτός 1243:18
νυμφαία 841:22, 1228:2
νύμφη 847:6, 1227:4, 1244:11
νύμφιος 847:6, 1243:19, 1244:10
νῦν 1243:13
νύξ 1243:21
νῶτος 1225:26

Ξ

ξάνθιον 908:22, 909:1
Ξάνθος 909:26
ξειρά? 574:22
ξενία 160:9, 162:13
ξενοδοχεῖα 160:5, 162:20
ξενοδοχεῖον 159:18, 165:10, 165:18
ξενοδόχος 162:22, 910:22
ξένος 909:4
Ξέρξης 912:3
ξέστης, -ην 910:12, 1814:20
ξηρανθήσονται 910:14
ξήριον 702:4?, 910:16
ξηροφθαλμία 910:20
ξίφιον 866:1, 1371:12
ξιφίον 910:10
ξύλα 909:6
ξύλον 908:20
ξυράφιον 910:8
ξυρίς 61:1, 909:18
ξυρόν 910:8
ξυστάριον 452:22?
ξυστός 452:22, 909:7

O

ὀβολός 12:13, 49:10–22, 50:4, 953:21, 1985:8
ὀβρύζατον 75:28?
ὄβρυζον 20:25, 75:28?
ὄγκινος 85:22, 85:25, 85:29, 86:19
ὅδε 47:20
ὁδήγησον 53:4
ὁδηγητής 53:9
ὀδόντα 95:27
ὀδόντια 52:18
ὁδοποιησάτε 52:11
ὁδός 52:17
ὀδούς 52:20
ὀδύνας (ὀδύνη) 52:24?
ὀδύνη 52:24
ὄη 47:14, 47:17, 47:19
ὀθόννα 98:4, 670:12
οἴδημα 52:21, 53:1, 1384:4, cf. 53:22
οἰδήματα 53:22, cf. 52:21, 53:1
Οἰδίπους 52:26
οἶδος 112:26

οἰκοδεσπότης 145:25, 572:1
οἰκοδομηθήσονται 48:10
οἰκόδομος 145:8
οἰκονομικοί 276:19
οἰκονομικόν 146:17, 273:8
οἰκονόμος 145:12, 275:10?
οἶκος 48:12, 145:11
ἡ οἰκουμένη 48:19, 274:17
οἰκτιρμός 48:15, 48:17
οἰκῶν 48:14
οἰνάνθη 75:6
ὀστράκων 70:27?
οἰνάνθη (τὸ φυτόν) 59:9
οἰνάνθινον (ἔλαιον) 665:8, see οἶνος οἰνάνθινος
οἰνάριον 69:12, 196:21
οἰνόμελι 71:13
οἶνος 69:12, 666:13, see ἀπίτης οἶνος, ἀψινθίτης οἶνος, θαλάττιον οἶνος, κεδρίτης οἶνος, κονδῖτος (οἶνος), κρητικός (οἶνος), κυδωνίτης οἶνος, μυσινίτης οἶνος, ῥοδίτης οἶνος, ῥοΐτης οἶνος, σκιλλητικὸς οἶνος, Σκυβελλίτης (οἶνος), στροβιλίτης οἶνος, σχίνινος (οἶνος), φοινικίτης οἶνος, χαμαιδρυΐτης οἶνος
ἀγριοναρδίτης 73:19
ἀκορίτης 74:3, 85:19, 85:24, 275:13, 278:9
ἁλοσανθίτης 74:7
ἀρωματίτης 73:8
ἀσαρίτης 73:17
βουνίτης 72:10
γληχωνίτης 73:3
δαυκίτης 73:22
δικταμνίτης 72:12
ἑλελισφακίτης 73:24
ἑλλεβορίτης 74:23
θυμβρίτης 72:22
θυμελαΐτης 74:16
θυμίτης 72:19
καλαμινθίτης 72:27
καταρροϊκός 73:13
κέδρινος 71:23
ἐκ κέστρου ψυχοτρόφου 72:3, 75:1
κονυζίτης 73:5
μανδραγορίτης 74:21
μαραθρίτης καὶ ἀνηθίτης καὶ πετροσελινίτης 74:11
μελιτίτης 71:11
ναρδίτης 73:10
νεκταρίτης 73:15
οἰνάνθινος 71:19, see οἰνάνθινον (ἔλαιον)
ὀριγανίτης 72:24
πανακίτης 73:27, see πάνακες
πισσίτης 71:21
πρασίτης 72:15
ῥητινίτης 72:17
σελινίτης 74:5
σκαμμωνίτης 74:26
στροβίλινος 136:17, 222:11
στυράκινος 136:17??, 222:11??
τραγοριγανίτης 72:7
ὑσσωπίτης 72:1
χαμαιλαΐτης 74:19
χαμαιπιτυΐνος 74:19
φθόριος 74:9
οἴσυπος 77:21, 234:18?, 616:30, 665:14
οἴσω 48:6
ὄκλαξ 1386:6
ὀκτώ 61:3
ὅλη 64:11
ὀλιγώθησαν 64:19
ὀλίσθημα 64:21
ὀλισθήσετε 64:25?

ὁλκάδιον 173:12, 180:6
ὁλκάριον 173:12
ὁλκή 65:13
ὁλοθεῖος 64:3?
ὁλοκαύτωμα 63:12
ὀλολυγών 170:8
ὁλόστεον 63:14
ὁλόφιτον 62:22
ὁλόφυτον 203:17, 828:18
ὀλυγκεὺς ὀξυδερκικός 88:2
Ὀλύμπια 168:21, see Ὄλυμπος
ὀλυμπιάς 168:21
Ὀλυμπιόδωρος 63:23, 65:5, 169:8
Ὀλύμπιον 65:1
ὀλύμπιος 169:5?, 170:20, 177:11
Ὄλυμπος 63:18, 158:5, 170:26, see Ὀλύμπια
ὄλυνθοι 63:21, 64:1
ὄλυρα 63:25
ὀμβρίζειν? 64:13
ὄμβρος 66:9
ὅμηρα 638:5
Ὁμηρίσματα 193:5
Ὅμηρος 66:3
ὁμιώματα 261:22?
ὄμμα 66:1
ὀμμάτια 66:1
ὀμνύων 66:11
ὁμοιοπαθής 66:26
ὅμοιος πατρί 1351:14?
ὁμοιούσιον 67:1, 185:2, 185:3, 616:1, 616:2
ὁμοιούσις 543:21
ὁμολογία 66:12, 183:23, 187:6
ὁμοούσιον 615:30
ὁμόπατροι 183:19?, 191:24?
ὀμφάκινον (ἔλαιον) 79:9
ὀμφάκιον 67:6, 189:6, 189:11, 1264:24
ὀμφακῖτις 1504:11, 1811:9
ὀμφακόκαρπος 272:6
ὀμφακόμελι 67:2, 191:1, 1264:22
ὄμφαξ, -ακος 1264:21
ὁμωνυμία 66:25, 616:28?
ὁμωνυμίας 68:11
ὁμώνυμος 66:24, 184:15, 616:29
ὄν 55:13, 68:1, 121:18
ὄναγρα 68:13
ὄναγρος 68:9
ὀνειδισμός 70:22, 306:29?
ὀνειδιστής 202:6
ὄνειδος 70:21, 1243:12
Ὀνήσιμον 211:22
ὀνίσκος 75:17
ὀνοβρυχίς 68:8?, 69:8
ὄνοι 69:22
  ὑπὸ ὑδρίας 666:4
ὀνόκλεια 69:26, 210:22–3
ὄνομα 68:27
ἐξ ὄνομα 352:20?
ὄνοσμα 70:6
ὀνοχειλές 210:22–3
ὄντως 208:13
ὄνυξ 69:17, 69:18, 666:14
ὄνυχες 69:17
  αἰγῶν 666:8
  ὄνων 666:8
ὀνύχιον 69:17, 20, 71:4, 817:17
ὄνυχος 202:4
ὀνωνίς 69:14, 202:19
ὀξάλμη 60:15
ὀξεῖα 60:23
ὄξος 61:7, 155:4, 665:16
ὀξυάκανθα 60:25, 187:10, 187:11, 870:21, cf. 182:12

ὀξύβαφον 60:13, 76:22, 159:22
ὀξύγαλα 159:16
ὀξύγγιον 60:7, 140:16, 159:21, 159:26
ὀξυγράφος 61:9
ὀξύκρατον 60:21
ὀξύμελι 61:5, 159:2
ὀξυρρόδινον 909:16
ὀξύφυλλον 909:21
ὀξύχολος 163:11
ὄπιον 260:3–5
ὀπισθότονος 84:8
ὀπίσω 82:2
ὁπλαί 83:26
ὅπλον 1568:18
ὅπλον 83:27
ὀποβάλσαμον 129:5–6, 233:19, 250:8, 263:21, 1486:11, 1573:4
ὀποπάναξ 667:4, see πάνακες
ὀποπάνακες 265:24
ὀπός 81:7, 208:26, 666:28, 667:3
  κυρηναϊκός 667:1, cf. 447:23, 545:9
ὀπῶρος 61:23
ὀπωροφυλάκιον 81:5
ὅπως 81:9
ὅρασις 51:24
ὄργανα 88:4–5, 88:25
ὄργανον 88:4–5
ὀργή 87:26
ὀργίλος 88:1, 214:17
ὀρείχαλκος 295:11
ὀρεοσέλινον 94:11, 94:16, 94:27, 285:21, 579:28?, 1353:26
ὀρέστειον 94:23
Ὀρέστης 96:3, 622:13?
ὄρη 91:5–6, see ὀρός, οὖρος, οὐρός
ὄρθιον 670:4
ὀρθογραφία 95:11
ὀρθοδοξία 304:11
ὀρθόδοξος 304:3, 304:10
ὀρθόπνοια 95:5, 95:9
ὀρθρίζω 95:7
ὅρια 92:7
Ὀριβάσιος 1433:5?
ὀρίγανον 89:19, 89:25, 289:5
  Ἡρακλεωτικόν 92:18
ὀρίγανος 669:12
  ὀνῆτις 92:13
ὁρίζων 91:27–9, 92:8, 148:14
ὅριον 92:7
ὁρίσαντα 92:16?
ὁρίσας 92:16?
ὅρισμα 93:18?
ὁρισμός 52:1, 90:18, 91:27–9
ὅρκος 52:13, 95:4
ὅρμινον 93:21, 791:11
ὅρμος 1523:26
ὄρνιθες 93:28
ὀρνιθόγαλα 94:1
ὀρνιθόγαλον 94:1
ὄρνις 291:18
ὀροβάγχη 90:25, 93:1, 95:1, 292:8, 668:18
ὀροβάκχη 1449:9
ὄροβοι 91:12
ὄροβος 91:11, 668:17
Ὀρόντης 94:3, 96:1, 538:28, 549:11
ὀρός 91:5, see ὄρη, οὖρος, οὐρός
ὅρος 91:7, 95:22
ὀρρῶδες 54:4, 279:18
ὀρτάρια 91:17, 666:16
ὀρτυγομήτρα 90:8
ὀρύγγιον 89:21, 148:7
ὀρυγῇ 90:7

ὄρυζα 91:1

ὀρφανός 94:29

ὄρχεις 94:10, see ὀρχίδια

κάστορος 164:7–10, see κάστωρ

ὀρχησταί 294:15

ὀρχηστής 294:21

ὀρχήστρια 93:3

ὀρχηστύς 294:19, 295:15

ὀρχίδια 93:5 see ὄρχεις

ὀρχίδιον 93:5, see ὄρχεις

ὄρχις 93:7, 309:3

κυνός? 208:21

σεραπιάς 93:13

ὀρῶν 91:5–6, see οὐρός

ὅς 75:26

ὁσία 76:21

ὅσιος 77:17

ὁσιώτατος 77:19

Ὄσσα 1228:24?

ὀστέα 76:1, 223:2

ὀστέων? 70:27, see ὄστρακον

ὀστρακίτης (λίθος) 864:11, see λίθος (ὀστρακίτης)

ὄστρακα 76:6

ὄστρακον 76:5, 76:17, 77:14, 81:10, 228:21, 239:8

ὄστρεα 76:25

ὄστρεον 666:17

ὄσυρις 77:26

ὄσφρανσις 121:19, 143:10

οὐ 48:2

μά? 610:14

μή 48:2

οὖα 47:14, 47:17, 47:19, 664:14

οὖας 48:3

οὐγγία, -ας 1207:14

οὐγκία 70:1, 70:4, 75:12, 75:15

οὐγκίας 965:19

οὐδέ 47:30

οὐδέν μᾶλλον? 53:2

οὐδέτερα 52:3, 535:12, 827:18

οὐδέτερον 52:2–10

οὐδέτερος 610:14, 827:18

οὐδός 53:24

Οὐεσπασιανός 238:20

Ὀυκάνιος 86:6

οὐράνιοι 93:26, see 89:8

οὐρανοί 150:9

τὸν οὐρανὸν τοῦ οὐρανοῦ 2025:3, 2036:15

οὐρανός 87:7, 90:19, 93:27

οὔρη 91:5–6, cf. 89:23, 90:12

οὐρητικός 1433:5?

οὖρον 91:9, 668:15

οὖρος= ὀρός 90:12, 92:5, 95:22 see ὄρη, ὀρός

οὐρός 89:23 (= ὀρός), 92:3, 92:5(= ὀρός), see ὄρη, ὀρός

οὐρῶν 91:5–6 see ὄρη, ὀρός

οὐσία 76:27, 77:1, 77:3

οὐσίας 77:1

οὐχί 48:1

ὀφεί(λου)σα? 82:4

ὄφεως τὸ σῦφαρ 121:11–12

ὀφθαλμία 84:2

ὀφθαλμικὸς (νόσος) 1648:10

ὀφθαλμός 83:14, 269:13

ὀφθήσομαι 83:12

ὀφιόσκορδον 80:7, 828:18

ὀφιοστάφυλον 86:5–7

ὄφις 82:1

ὀφφικιάλιος 266:20

ὄχλος 157:10–15

ὀχυρός 59:21

ὄψ 666:28
ὀψάριον 83:20
ὀψέ 280:9, 1905:13
ὄψσομαι 83:10
ὀψώνια (ὀψώνιον) 264:22–5
ὀψωνίας (ὀψωνία) 264:22–5

Π

πάγις 1472:6
παγίς 1540:21
πάγουρος 1487:10
παγκρατίασμος 1476:10, 1479:17
παγκράτιον 1476:25
πάγχρηστος 1476:6, 1581:14
πάθος 1486:9
παιδεία 1474:16, 1476:19
παιδέρως 271:11–17, 1541:7
παιδεύθητε 1491:24?
παιδεύσας 1491:24
παιδευτήριον 358:18, 1491:20
παιδικά 724:3
παίδιον 1491:21
παιδίσκη 1474:17, 1476:21
παιδίων (πάθος) 882:11, 1492:1
Παιονία 493:22
παιονία 29:11, 1456:18, 1472:19, 1491:8, 1514:23, 1578:4, 1580:10, 1776:10
παῖς 1474:19
παλαιστή 1475:27
Παλαιστίνη 1548:9, 1573:14
παλαίστρα 368:15?, 400:3
παλαιστρικοί 1475:25
παλατῖνος 1569:21
παλάτιον 1475:8, 1569:17
παλιγγενεσίς 1475:3
παλίουρος 1476:2
Παλλάς, -άδος 1475:12
Παλμανώθης 1572:15
Παλμυρά 1475:5
Παμφυλία 1576:7
πᾶν 1576:13
πανάκεια 1476:17
πάνακες 265:24, 1582:9 see οἶνος πανακίτης
Ἀσκληπιόν 1474:10, 1477:5
Ἡράκλειον 1474:13, 1477:11
Χειρώνιον 1474:11, 1477:9
πανδέκτης (πανδέκται) 1576:18
πανδόκιον 1576:17
πανδοῦρα 1489:9–10
πανδοχεῖον 1541:4
Πανεάς 1476:12
Πάνθεων 1476:14
πανθήρ 354:27, 1578:11, 1578:15?, 1583:13
πανουργία 1476:23
πανσέληνος 1476:7
παντά 1476:1
παντοκράτωρ 1578:3, 1620:19
παντοπώλης 1477:17
δὶα παντός 555:24
πάντως 1543:3, 1543:15, 1579:1
πάππας 1478:21
πάππια 1594:17
πάππιας 1594:17
πάππος 1478:23, 1594:9
πάπυρος 1467:4, 1478:24, 1594:12
παρ᾽ἐμοῦ 1483:9
παρά
μικρόν 1482:7
μίν 1628:1
τό 1482:25
παραβαίνων 21:4
παράβασις 1481:11

παραβάτης 1485:15, 1485:22?, 1603:9, 1603:14

παραβατοί 1485:13?

παραβατώδης 1485:22

παραβολή 1481:13

παράγουσιν 1481:14

παραγραφή 546:10, 1601:24

παράγωγος 1484:13

παράγων 1481:20

παράδειγμα 1559:16, 1604:20, 1606:20, 1622:1

παραδείγματα 1559:16, 1622:2?

παράδεισος 1604:22

παραδοῦναι 1481:22

παραζήλου 1481:24

παραθήκη 1485:27, 1640:5, 1640:18

παραθήσομαι 1482:3

παρακαλῶν 1481:26

παρακατηγόρημα 1480:15

παρακληθῆναι 1481:28

Παράκλητος 1636:18

παράκλητος 1606:20

παραλαλῶν 1482:1

παράλιος 1473:20?, 1481:2, 1485:9

τιθύμαλος 1475:9?, 1476:4?

παράλληλος 1480:27

παράλυσις 279:25, 1485:7

παραλυτικός 1602:15

παραμονάριος 1572:20, 1627:19

παράνομος 1482:9

παράπεισις 1634:5?

παραπληγία 1480:3

παράπτωμα 1482:11

παραριπτεῖσθαι 1482:13

παράσιτος 1602:6, 1633:10, 1633:23

παρασιωπήσεις 1482:15

παραστάς 1629:14

παρασύμβαμα 1480:2

παρασυνάγχη 1480:8, 1481:6

παρασυνεβλήθη 1483:19

παράταξις 1482:19

παράτεινον 1482:21

παρατηρήσεται 1482:23

παρατήσομαι 1482:17

παραφροσύνη 1480:1, 1489:1, 1602:10, 1602:13

παραφυάς 1482:29

παρδαλιαγχές 272:23, 1485:5, 1606:14?

πάρδος 1604:10

παρεγκεφαλίς 1484:24

παρεκάλεσα 1483:1

παρελεύσεται 1483:3

παρεμβολεῖ 1483:5

παρεμβολή 1483:7

παρεμπίπτων 1480:14, 1481:4, 1486:1

παρενοχλεῖν μοι 1483:10

παρέξ 1483:12

παρέπεται 1484:7

παρεπίδημος 1483:13

πάρεσις 1480:16

παρέστησαν 1483:15

παρέστησεν 1483:17

παρῆλθον 1483:21

παρθενικός 1639:14

παρθένιον 964:16, 1484:29, 1486:3, 1499:8, 1559:13

ἀμάρακον 1481:9, 1486:3, see ἀμάρακον

παρθένος 1483:23, 1639:14, 1639:18, 1640:4

παρίδῃς 1483:24

παροικήσει 1483:25

σοι 1484:1

πάροικος 1483:27

παρονομασία 352:20

παροξύνει 1484:5

παρόρασις 1480:19?, 1606:25

παροχέτευσις 1480:23, 1484:26
παρρησία 1480:21, 1496:8, 1606:25
παρρησιαζομένη 1481:1
παρρησίαν 1481:1
παρρησιάσομαι 1483:29
παρώνυμα 1485:19, see παρώνυμος
παρώνυμησις 1602:21
παρώνυμος 1480:25, 1484:15, 1485:11,
1485:17, 1603:1, 1610:21, see παρώνυμα
παρωνυχία 1481:16, 1485:24
παρώργισεν 1484:3
παρωτίδες 1480:11
παρωτίς 1480:12
παστάδας, -δων 227:4
παστός 1478:19
πάσχα 1477:19?, 1477:25, 1589:16
πάσχων 1474:21
πάτερ ἡμῶν 1473:12
πατέρα 1473:5, 1537:1
πατήρ 7:2 note 5, 1473:5, 1537:1, 1538:5
πατρία 1473:7
πατριάρχης 1473:19, 1539:2
πατρίκιος 1537:4, 1539:13, 1539:16
πατρίς 1180:4
πάτρων 1473:8, 1539:12
πατρωνεία 1361:11, 1539:15, 1539:17
πατρωνική 1473:8, 1592:23?
πατρωνομικός 1473:10
Παῦλος 1507:11
παῦσον 1471:7
παύσω 1471:9
Παφνούτιος 1478:27
πάχνη 1474:22
παχύς 1474:24
πέδαι 1492:3
πέδιον, -ια 1541:5, 1621:3
πεδίον 1491:24?, 1491:26
πεζός 1473:1
πεῖνα 1555:9
πεινάσω 1491:13
πείρασον 1491:14
πειρατήριον 1491:16
πεκούλιον 1558:10
Πελαγία 1565:19
πέλαγος 1562:5
πελεκάν 1493:22
πελεκπίνος 113:18–22, 113:26, 114:7–8
πέλεκυς 1493:20, 1574:22
πελωρίς 1493:26
πένης 1494:6
πένθος 1558:9
πενθῶν 1494:3
πεντάβιβλον 1494:7
πεντάγωνος 1578:9
πενταμερής, -ῶν 1578:16
πεντάς 125:7
πεντάφυλλον 1494:4, 1578:4
πεντάχορδος 1580:13
πεντεκοστή 1579:12, 1741:11, 1741:14
πεντόροβον 472:20, 1472:19, 1543:5, 1580:10
πεπεδημένοι 1494:13
δὶα τριῶν πεπερέων 562:9
πέπερι 1474:15, 1494:22, 1540:6, 1557:21
πέπλιον 1495:2
πέπλος 859:19, 1494:25
πεποιθώς σοι 1494:17
πεποικιλμένη 1494:15
πεπόνατον (σμῆγμα) 1494:21
πεπραγμένα 1595:1
πεπρωμένα 1479:1
πεπρωμένη 1479:1
πεπυρωμένος 1494:19

πέπων 1495:1

πέρας 1495:25

περδίκιον 634:17, 1485:1, 1496:19, 1499:8, 1559:13

περιαργυρουμέναι 1498:19

περιβεβλημένη 1496:1

περιβόλαιον 1498:1

περιβολή, -ῆς 1554:10

περιεβάλοντο 1498:5

περιεκύκλωσαν 1498:9

περιελάβετε 1498:23

περίελε 1498:7

περιεπάτουν 1498:27

περιέπλεκε 1498:11

περιεποίησε 1499:3

περιέσχον 1498:15

περίζωμα 80:24, 1618:13

περιζωννῦσι 1498:17?

περικεκοσμέναι 1498:21

περικεφαλαία 139:14

περικλύμενον 1495:21, 1559:6

περικόμματα 1497:7?

περίλοιπον 1497:1

περίλυπος 1497:3

περίναιον 124:14

περινενευκώς (-ότος) 1496:14

περίνεον 1496:22

περίνευσις 1497:6

περιοδεύτης 1496:3, 1606:22, 1621:5

περιοδευτής 1480:10

περιοδία 1608:1, 1621:1

περιουσιασμός 1498:25

περιοχή 1499:1

περιπατητικοί 1472:9, 1496:9, 1624:24

περίπατος 1559:1

περιπλέκειν 1499:5

περιπλευμονία 1497:9, 1624:22, 1634:7

περισκυθισμός 1497:7?

περισσῶς 1498:13

περιστερά 1499:7

περιστερεών 1495:15, 1559:11, 1630:8, 1909:1

περίστυλος 1586:20

Περίτιος 993:21–2

περιτομή 1559:4, 1622:17

περιτόναιον 1496:5, 1620:17?, 2045:13, 2066:18

περιττός 998:6?

περίφασις 1624:21

περιφρυγής 1495:25

μαρασμός 1495:13, 1497:4, 1497:18, 1497:22

περόνη 1496:17

περσέα 1497:27

περσικόν 549:25

μῆλον 1497:20, 1498:3

πεσσός 468:20, 1494:9, 1518:13, 1584:12

πέταλα 813:11, 1537:8, 1537:9, 1543:18, 1569:15?

πέταλον 1537:17?

πεταννύων 1493:9?

πετασίτης 1492:18, 1578:17

πετεινά 1492:23, see πτεινά

πετηνά, -ῶν 1473:23, 1578:15?, 1580:8?, see πτεινά

πετόμενοι 1492:25

Πέτρα 1473:13

πέτρα 1493:1?

πετραία 828:18, 1808:17

Πέτρε 1493:1?

Πέτρος 1493:2?

πέτρος 1493:2? 1538:19

πετροσέλινον 285:21, 580:2, 1357:3, 1493:3, 1538:13

πετρόφακος 1539:21
πεύκη 1492:4, 1492:13, 1521:4
πευκέδανον 1492:4, 1492:10, 1492:16, 1519:16, 1521:19
πεφυτευμένος 1495:11
πέψις 1494:11, 1594:16
πήγανον 801:25, 827:20, 1540:19, 1558:12?
Πήγασος 1472:3
πηγή 1540:21, 1541:1?
πήγιον 1541:1?
πηδάλιον 1509:9
πηλάριον 1546:5, 1570:18?
Πήλιον 1228:24?
πηλός 1544:11, 1558:1, 1567:10
πήρα 1559:15
πιανάτω 1540:5
πίθηκος 1648:20
πικρία 1558:7
πιλωτάριον 369:21
πιλωτός 1544:9, 1547:5
πιμελή1554:7
πίναξ 1554:25, 1555:5, 1555:6, 1581:13
ποῦ πίνομεν 1541:11
πίομαι 1542:4
πίουρος 1542:19
πισάριον 1592:11
Πισιδία 1555:21
πισκίνη 1591:18
πίσος 1555:12, 1592:11
πίσσα 1557:5, 1587:12
πισσάσφαλτος 1582:1
πισσέλαιον 1429:17, 1556:14, 1584:3
πιστάκια 1556:12
πιστεύω 1587:6
δὶα πίστεως 568:8, 569:15
πιστή 1581:18
πίστις 1504:24, 1543:13, 1555:18, 1580:1, 1581:18, 1587:3
πιστός 1543:7
πίστωμα 1586:17?
πιττάκιον 1649:6
πιτυΐδες 1543:11, see πίτυς
πίτυος φλοιός 1539:7, 1543:16, 1767:1
πιτύουσα 1579:17, see 1771:20
πίτυς 977:2, 1543:8, 1580:14, 1771:6, see πιτυΐδες
πίων 1542:6
πλακὲς λίθιναι 1575:2
πλακούς, -οῦντος 1475:1, 1563:18?, 1563:20
πλανῆται 1572:7
πλανήτης, -αι 1572:1
πλάνος 1570:21
πλανῶνται 1563:2
πλάξ, -ακός 1573:18, 1575:1
πλάσας 1563:14
πλάσις 1567:9, 1573:22
πλασθήνη 1563:16
πλασματίας 1573:12?, see 1573:7
πλασσάριος 1573:12?
πλάτανος 1562:15, 1563:12, 1569:20
πλατεῖα 1563:6
πλατυσμός 1563:10
Πλάτων 1563:4, 22, 1569:16, 1570:7
Πλατωνική 1570:2
πλέθρον 1576:3
πλεύμων 1572:19, see πνεύμων
πλευρῖτις 1519:18, 1545:18, 1566:18, 1567:13, 1571:21
πλευρόν 1566:23
πληγή 1570:16
πλῆθος 1571:5
πληθώρη 351:14

πλημμελής 1571:7
πλήν 1571:9
πλήξων 1562:4
πληρές 1566:25?
πληροφορῆσαι 1571:17, 1575:10
πληροφορία 1571:14, 1575:6
πλήρωμα 1575:9
πληρώσεις 1571:10
πλησίον 1571:12, 20
πλησμονή 1571:13
πλινθίον 1566:17
πλιχάς 1563:8
πλοῖον 1567:18
πλόκος? 263:14
πλούσιος 1567:8, 1567:19
πλοῦτος 1567:21
Πλούτων 1563:5, 1567:23, 1569:16
πλύνε 1568:4?
πλύνῃ 1568:4?
πλυνός 1568:20?
πλυσμός 1568:20?
πνεῦμα 1581:10
ἐν πνεῦμα 235:17
πνευματικός 1577:17
πνευμονικοί? 257:12
πνεύμων 1577:5, 1577:19, 1584:23, cf. πλεύμων
  ἀλώπεκος 1577:10
  χοίριος 1577:8
πνιγαλίων 1513:26
πνιγῖτις γῆ 1581:11
πνοή 1577:12
ποδάγρα 1489:3, 1500:18, 1534:5, 1648:13
ποδαλγία 1648:13
ποδήρης 1491:5, 1500:17, 1622:18?
πόδια (πόδιον) 1523:7
πόδιον 1500:24
πόδρικον (φάρμακον) 1489:4?
πόθεν 1531:5?
ποιεῖ 1515:23
ποιηταί 1472:15
ποιητής 1472:14, 1505:2, 1541:12, 1542:12
ποιητικοί 1505:1
ποιητικός 1472:15, 1577:20
ποιητός 1499:19, 1509:26
ποιμανεῖ 1513:20
ποίμνιον 1513:22
ποῖον 1541:15
ποιότητα 136:13
ποιότης 136:13, 1542:10 (-ητα)
ποιῶν 1472:11
πολειδὴς ἀντίδοτος 1506:1
πόλεμος 1507:15, 1568:21
πολεμώνιον 1511:24, 1547:13
πόλιον 238:3, 472:20, 602:18, 1508:3?, 1510:6, 1543:5
πόλις 1509:27
πολιτεία 1507:22, 1509:4, 1509:24, 1510:11
πολιτευθῆναι 1510:2
πολιτευόμενος 1509:22, 1510:1
πολιτικόν 1508:15, 1510:17
δὶα πολλῆς 569:3
πολλοί 1510:13, 1510:27
πόλος, -οι 1507:17, 1508:17
πολύ 1510:13
πολυάρχιον (μάλαγμα) 1511:22
πολύγαλον 1511:9, 1512:1
πολυγόνατον 932:15, 1511:4
πολύγονον 1456:6, 1511:1, 1547:1
  ἄρρεν 1509:9
  θῆλυ 1509:13
πολύκαρπος 1508:24, 1510:19

πολύκνημον 1512:5, 1521:6
πολύμορφος 79:19, 1568:12
πολυνοειδές 1789:18
πολυπόδιον 1508:3, 1510:6, 1730:23
πολύπους 1508:4, 1512:10 (-οδος)
πολύρριζον 1508:22
πολύτοκος 1510:4
πολυχαρίεις 1509:1
πολυχρονία 1512:8
πολυωνύμως 1507:19
πολυωπός 1519:22?
πομφόλυξ 80:25, 569:4?, 1513:16, 1513:24
πονηρευόμενος 1516:1
πονηρία 1515:26
πονηροί 1517:7
πονηρός 75:5, 1515:27
πόνος 1515:24
Ποντικὸν (φάρμακον) 1579:11
Πόντιος Πιλᾶτος 1516:11, 1579:19
Πόντος 1516:24, 1578:19
ὁ πόντος? 84:1
πορεία 1523:1
Πόρκιος Φῆστος 1637:4
πορνεῖον 1491:23
πορνεύων 1524:4
πόρνη 1524:3
πόροι 772:24, 1522:15
πόρος 1522:21, 1614:18
πόρφυρα 1525:12, 1632:4
πορφύρα 1519:20
Πορφύριος 1525:16, 1632:16, 1632:21
πορφύριος 1525:11, 1632:16
πορφυρίων 212:25–6
πορφυροχίτων 1525:18
ποσάκις 1518:15
ποσαπλῶς 1518:18
Ποσειδῶν 1557:7
ποσόν 1518:22
πόστον ἐστί 1518:17?
ποταμογείτων 1503:24, 1537:6, 1565:25, 1926:14
ποταμός 1503:21, 1534:26
πότε 1503:18, 1717:12?
ποτήριον 1504:18
Ποτιόλους 1503:19
ποῦ 1499:11
ποῦς 1500:27, 1518:20
πραγματεία 1601:22, 1604:4, 1608:19
πραγματευτής, -τευταί 1602:1, 1604:7
πραγματικὸς τύπος 1603:12
πραεῖς 1603:5
πραιπόσιτος, -τε 1602:6, 1633:10, 1633:25, see Λαῦσος πραιπόσιτος
πραιτώριον 1620:6
πρακτικὴ (τέχνη) 1622:15
πρακτικόν 1630:20, 1637:1
πρακτικός 1609:3
πρακτός 1637:12
πράξεως τύποι 1627:2?, see πραγματικὸς τύπος
πράξις 1626:19
πραότης 1602:16
πράσα 1479:21, see πράσον
πράσινος 1630:22, see Βένετοι καὶ Πρασινοί
πράσιον 93:21–2, 791:11, 1093:11, 1302:19–20, 1327:22, 1602:4, 1602:17, 1858:18
πράσον 1603:7 (-α), 1839:15, see πράσα
πρέπει 1607:13
πρέσβυς, -εις 1607:11
πρεσβύτερος 1624:14
πρεσσόριον 1573:6, cf. 1573:8, 1573:10, 1574:15
πρηνές 1607:9

πρηστήρ 227:10–11, 1623:13, 1630:16
πριαπισμός 1621:20, 1780:8
πρῖνος 1624:18
πρίων 1622:9
προανατάξομαι 1607:22
πρόβατα 1607:16, 1608:11
προβατική 1128:20, 1129:8
πρόβλημα 1608:2
προβληματικόν 1618:10
Πρόβος 1607:17, see probos
πρόγνωσις 1608:17, 1615:1
προγνωστικόν 1602:19, 1604:3
πρόθεσις 1489:11?, 1618:5, 1620:11, 1620:14
προθεσμία 1618:1, 1639:9
προθεωρία 1602:11, 1617:21, 1640:21
πρόθυρον 1639:21
πρόλοβος 1500:20?
προλογία 1610:9
προλογισμός 1610:12, 1627:12
πρόλογος 1610:12
πρόμνος 1610:17
προξενηταί 1627:7
προξενία 1627:8?
προοίμιον 866:15, 1607:18, 1610:3, see proemium
προπεσοῦνται 1618:8
πρόπολις 1614:22, 1615:19, 1633:1
πρόπομα 1633:16
προπόματα 1615:21
προπτωσίς 1480:19, 1610:1?
προρρητικόν 1616:15
πρός
  αὐτούς 1611:3
  τι 1609:4, 1613:16
προσδέχομαι 1612:3
προσδιορισμός 1611:10, 1611:15
προσδοκία 1611:6
προσεδέξατο 1612:1
προσελάβετο 1612:5
προσέλαβον 1612:7
προσελεύσεται 1612:11
προσέλθετε (πρόσελθε) 1612:13
προσεύξομαι 1612:17
προσευχή 1611:5, 1612:9
προσήλυτος 1613:6
προσθῇ 1613:14
προσκεφάλαιον 1615:20
προσκεφαλίδιον 1615:20
προσκομίδη 1614:11
προσκόπησις 419:1
προσκόψεις 1613:12
προσκυνήσω 1613:10
πρόσταγμα 1502:9?, 1610:23, 1611:1, 1613:2, 1615:3, 1629:5, 1629:19, 1742:17
προστάς, -άδος 1610:24, 1613:18
προστασία 1611:14, 1612:24, 1615:18?, 1629:14, 1629:18
προστίθεσθε 1613:4
πρόστιμον 1611:13, 1615:6
πρόσφατος 1612:15
προσφορά 1613:15
πρόσφυσις 1615:16
προσφώνησις 1614:16?, 1615:8
πρόσχες 1613:8
πρόσχημα 1627:9?
προσώζησα 1612:19
πρόσωπον 1611:8, 1613:1, 1614:7, 1625:3
προσώχθισε 1612:21
πρότασις 1312:18, 1492:21, 1609:15, 1614:16?, 1614:19
πρόφασις 1489:11?
προφῆται 1615:10

πρόφθασον 1618:12

προφυλακτικόν 1615:22

πρόχοος, -ον 1627:5?, 1627:11?

προωνύμιον 1610:19

προωρώμην 1609:13

Πρωτεύς 1609:6, 1615:14

πρωτόστακτις (κονία) 1614:9

πρωτότοκος 1612:23

πταρμικόν 1533:24, 1538:11, 1538:16, see στρούθιον (πταρμικόν)

πτεινά 1536:22, see πετεινά, πετηνά

πτελέα 1534:13, 1537:10

πτέρις 1493:8, 1534:6, 1539:5

πτέρνα 1534:15

πτερνισμός 1534:16

πτερύγιον 1534:8, 1534:22?

πτέρυξ 1534:18

πτερωτά 1534:20

πτήσεις 1535:6?

πτίλλωσις 1536:12, 1536:16

Πτολεμαΐς 1535:19

Πτολεμαῖος ὁ Λάγου 1537:16

πτώματα 1535:3, 1535:21

πτῶσις 1535:8, 1535:16, 1537:19

πτωτικός 1535:13

πτωχός 1534:25, 1535:5

πυγών 1500:3?

πυθικοί 1531:21

πύθων 1531:21

πυκάζοντες 1520:12

πυκνόκομον 1512:6, 1521:6

πύκται 1521:25

πυκτικοί 1521:17

Πυλάδης 96:3

πύλη 1541:24

πυξάκανθα 956:11

πύξινος 1505:12

πυξίς, -ίδος 1505:17

πῦρ 1542:20, 1558:14

πυργίσκος 1606:9

πυργόβαρις 1542:2

πύργος 1542:21

πύρεθρον 1522:17?, 1529:1

πυρεῖον 1518:25?, 1520:6 (-εῖα)?

πυρετός, see ἑκτικός (πυρετός), ἐφήμερος (πυρετός)

τριταῖος 825:25

πυρίκαυστα 1524:7

πυρίτης 883:3, 1500:21, 1523:5, 1524:16, 1609:22

ἀργυρίτης 1609:11

λίθος 864:16, see λίθος (πυρίτης)

πυριφλεγέθων 1523:24

πύρνος 883:4, 889:1?

πυρόεις 1526:4

πυρός 252:23, 1522:19, 1542:5

ἄχνη 2046:16

πυρράκης 1526:5

πυρσός 1524:22

πύρωθρον 1522:17?

πύρωσις 1615:11?

πύρωσον 1542:7

πυτία 1504:21, 1543:1, 1725:3

πύωσις 1494:23

πώγων 1500:1

Ρ

ῥᾶ 1861:6
ῥάβδος 1861:4, 1863:21
ῥαγοειδής 1869:15
ῥακὰ 1862:14
ῥάμνος 1861:12, 1887:23
ῥαντίσεις 1862:4
ῥαπόντικουμ 1861:6, 1888:20, 1898:1
ῥάπτης 1912:3
ῥαφάνινον 1862:10
ῥάφανος 586:8, 1862:8
ῥαψῳδῆσαι 1912:19
ῥαψῳδία 1912:19
Ῥέα 1861:1
ῥέει 1876:10
ῥεῦμα 533:25, 773:1–2, 1752:3, 1876:12, 1887:6
ῥεύματα 1876:12, 1887:6
ῥήγματα 1880:6
ῥῆμα 666:28, 1899:15
ῥηματικόν 1898:21
ῥῆον 757:24, 1861:6, 1898:1
ῥητίνη 790:13, 1877:4, 1898:15, see Γαλατίας (ῥητίνη), στροβιλίνη (ῥητίνη), τερμινθίνη (ῥητίνη), φρυκτὴ (ῥητίνη)
ῥητορική 562:11, 1878:3, 1885:21, 1898:11
ῥητορικοί 1885:19, 1898:13
ῥήτωρ 552:8, 1878:5, 1898:12
ῥιζαχόσκη 1902:20
ῥίζωμα 1898:6
ῥινάριον 1900:1
Ῥινοκόρουρα 1900:4
ῥίψον 1900:6
ῥόα 1879:10
Ῥόδη 1880:19
ῥοδία ῥίζα 1880:23
ῥόδινον (ἔλαιον) 622:9, 1881:5
ῥοδίτης οἶνος 1881:9
ῥοδοδάφνη 1245:25, 1277:20, 1874:19, 1874:20, 1880:17
ῥοδόμελι 1880:21, 1881:3
Ῥόδος 1881:4
ῥοιάς 720:13, 1879:12 (-άδες)
ῥόϊνος 285:19, 1886:8
ῥοΐτης οἶνος 1879:7
ῥομφαία 1889:2
ῥοπή 1105:16, 1890:14, 1890:21
ῥοσμαρίνουμ 964:24
ῥουβία 1456:25, 26
ῥοῦς 1879:9, 1888:22
ῥουσμαρίνουμ 1816:5
Ῥοῦφος 1890:19
ῥοφέω 1890:19
ῥυθμός 1892:15
ῥυκάνη 1916:19
ῥύπος 1890:18
ῥύσε 1898:4
ῥύστης 1898:5
ῥώθων 1892:12?
ῥώθωνες 1892:14
ἣν οἱ ρωμαῖοι ἐρβαρωβίαν καλοῦσι 656:7
Ῥώμη 1876:11

Σ

σάββατα 1291:6
Σαββατιανοί 1356:14
σάββατον 1933:3
σαβῖνον (ἔλαιον) 1291:7
σαγαπηνόν 258:27, 1291:12, 1299:5, 1301:1
σάκκος 1294:24

σάκρα 1386:9

σάκχαρ 1292:18, 1351:15

σαλαμάνδρα 1292:19, 1354:13, 1357:4?

σάλπιγξ, -ιγγος 1293:3

σαμία (γῆ) 1293:10, see γῆ (σαμία)

Σαμοθράκη 1357:13

Σάμος 1357:12

σάμψυκος? 466:12

σαμψύχινον (ἔλαιον) 1293:9

σάμψυχον 1293:6, 1359:25, 1360:7

σανδαράχη 943:18, 1293:25, 1294:5, 1361:25

σάνδυξ 1294:1, 1361:22, 1588:13

σαπρότης 1294:14

τῶν ξύλων 1609:24

σάπφειρος 1294:15

σάπων 1372:17

σαρακοστή 1295:7

σάρδιον 1387:17, 1387:20, see ἐλατήριον

σαρδόνιος (γέλως) 1295:1

σαρκική 140:11

σαρκοκόλλα 1294:25, 1394:1, 1853:5

σαρκόκολλον 1393:22?

σάρξ 1295:5 (-κός, -κές, -κῶν), 1394:4 (-κός)

σατράπαι 1333:20

σατυρίασις 1292:16, 1329:26

σατυριασμοί 1292:6

σατύριον 309:3, 1292:10, 1329:27

σαύρα 1291:17, 1322:15

σβέννυσθαι 568:17?

σέ 1303:4

Σεβαστή 1298:3, 1303:9

σεβαστός 229:20?, 1303:7, 1351:16

Σεβηριανόν (φαρμακόν) 1303:11

σειρά 574:22?, 773:8, 1180:12 (-ας), 1347:14 (-άς), 1348:23

Σειρῆνες 150:10, 289:9

σειρῆνες 1347:17, 1387:18?

σειρίασις 1347:8

σείριος 1386:22

σεῖστρα 1366:4

Σεκοῦνδος 1381:12

Σελευκίς, -ίδος 1353:12

Σέλευκος 1353:7

σεληναῖος 1207:13

σεληνιακός 1350:19?

σελήνη 1303:4, 1304:1, 1342:1, 1343:16, 1476:8

σεληνικόν καλούμενον 1744:11–14

σελίδες 1342:2

σέλινον 916:14, 967:27, 1304:2, 1353:26, 1357:2

μακεδόνιον 1356:26

σελίς 1342:2

σέλλα, -ην 1385:24

σεμείωμα 1358:4?

σεμίδαλις 1357:26

Σεούηρος 1291:20

Σεραπίων 1393:8, 1393:10

σέρις 1304:27

σέριφον 242:6, 1295:4, 1304:28, 1349:1, 1377:6?, 1566:5?

σέσελι 1304:4 (-εως), 1345:21, 1365:18, 1365:20?, 1661:2 (-εως), 1980:1 (-εως)

σεῦτον 1303:28

σήκωμα 1346:20

σημεῖα 1342:17

σημεῖον 1342:17

σημείωσις 1342:15

σήμερον 1342:14

σηπεδόνες 1346:1

σηπία 1294:17, 1346:3, 1346:15?, 1370:11, 1370:15, 1370:19?, 1370:22, 1371:18, 1393:9

σηπίας, -άδος 1370:22

σηπός 1346:16

σηραγγώδης 1348:21?

σηρικόν 1373:19?

σής 1345:20

σησαμοειδές 1344:19, 1345:15

τὸ μέγα 1345:5

τὸ μικρόν 1345:15

σήσαμον 1344:17

σήψ 1346:16

σιαγών 1335:8

σίαλον 1361:17

σιγή 1336:6

σιγήσεις 1336:11

σιδηρῖτις 32:9?, 33:9?, 148:15–16, 156:18–19, 176:10, 214:15, 1336:27, 1337:6, 1347:12, 1362:4

ἄλλη 1337:8

τρίτη 1337:9

ἀχίλλειος 1337:11

σίδια 1336:24, 1360:6

σίδιον 1337:1

σίκλοι 1341:16

σίκλος 1082:1

σίκυς 1346:22

ἄγριος 1346:25, 1347:6, see ἄγριος σίκυς

ἥμερος 1347:4

σικυώδης 1380:9?

σιλιγνίτης (ἄρτος) 1341:25

σίλουρος 1341:14, 1353:21

σίλυβον 1341:7

σίλφη 1341:18

σίλφιον 545:16, 1293:5, 1341:20, 1354:4, 1355:9

σιμίσιον 1342:21

Σιμωνιακοί 1342:25

σίναπι, -εως 1343:24, 1364:25

σινάπινον 1317:11, 1343:23, 1344:4

σιναπισμός 1343:17

σίνωπις 1362:14

σίον 1335:9, 1337:18, 1343:21, 1345:14, 1660:22

σίραιον 1347:10

σιρικόν 1294:2, 1391:15

σίσαρον 1344:22, 1346:18?

σισύμβριον 302:23, 660:6, 1316:13, 1318:14, 1344:14, 1345:10

σίσων 1343:19?

σιτάριον 109:24, 1340:25, 1360:4?

σῖτος 1341:1

σιττακός 228:8, see ψιττακός

σιτώδη 1362:25

σιτώδης 1362:25

περὶ σιτωδῶν 1362:25

σίφων 1346:9

σκάλα 1385:8

σκαμβός 1379:3

σκαμμωνία 1379:10, 1385:16

σκαμνίον 1385:24

σκάμνον 242:10

σκάνδαλον 927:16, 1294:7, 1378:13, 1379:8

σκάνδιξ 1294:3, 1379:5

σκάρος 1322:12, 1386:18

σκάφη 241:13

σκαφίς 229:13, 232:5, 241:16

σκελετόν 1379:17

σκελετός 2033:18

σκελλός 1378:20

σκέπαρνον 1384:19

σκεπάστης 1379:20

σκέπη 1379:22

σκευάρια (σκευάριον) 241:5?

σκευή 1379:24
σκεῦος 1379:23
σκευσασία ἀβροτονίτης 1379:15?
σκηνή 1383:21
σκήνωμα 1383:24
σκῆπτρον 242:15, 1384:20
σκία 1383:23
σκίγκου οὐρά 1385:22
σκίγκος 240:20?, 242:17?, 1383:26, cf. 771:16, 876:12
σκίλλα 232:18, 241:21, 1384:12, cf. 71:18, 71:20
σκιλλητικὸν ὄξος 1384:14
σκιλλητικὸς οἶνος 1384:10
σκίρρος 1384:4, 1384:23
ἐν μήτρα 1384:24
σκίρρωμα 1385:4
σκιρρώματα 1384:23
σκίρτηρος 1384:25?
σκληρά 1385:10
σκληροφθαλμία 1379:1?, 1385:6
σκολιά 1381:15
σκολιόν 1385:12
σκολιοφθαλμία 1379:1?, 1645:11
σκολόπενδρα 1380:21
σκολοπένδριον 132:17–22, 237:1, 237:2, 583:15, 953:6, 1380:24
σκολοπένδρον 236:26–237:1
σκόλυμος 1380:26
σκόρδιον 1382:15, 2045:18
σκόροδον 1382:20
σκοροδόπρασον 1382:21
σκορπιοειδές 1381:27
σκορπίος 1381:23, 1386:21
θαλάσσιος 1381:24
σκορπίουρον 1382:26?
σκοτεινόν 1380:12
σκοτόμαινα 98:12
σκοτομήνη 1380:14
σκότος 1380:16
εἰς τὸ σκότος τὸ εξώτερον 226:14
σκότωμα? 277:6
σκρίνιον 241:5, 1378:22
Σκυβελλίτης (οἶνος) 1380:8
Σκύθαι 1383:2
Σκυθόπολις 1383:7
σκυθρωπός 1383:19
σκῦλον, -α 1383:16
σκύμνος 1383:18
σκυτάλη 240:10, 1380:17
σκυτάλιον 1726:24
σκύτη (σκῦτος) 240:8, 241:17
σκύφος 240:22, 241:9, 241:25, 870:15
σκώληξ 1381:4, 1383:17, 1385:14
σκωρία 222:5, 240:15, 241:14, 1380:10, 1382:10
ἀργύρου 1382:12
σμαράγδινος 101:12
σμαρίς 1356:7, 1356:12
σμῆγμα 1359:19, see πεπόνατον (σμῆγμα)
δὶα σφέκλης 190:22, see (σμῆγμα διὰ) σφέκλης
σμήλιον 1358:3?
σμῆμα 1359:19
σμίλαξ 1358:11, 1790:4, 2046:4
λεία 1073:3
τραχεῖα 1072:20
σμιλευτός 626:3, 976:20, 1747:21
σμίλιον 1358:3?
σμύρις (λίθος) 1358:1
σμύρνα
βοιωτική 1356:20

τρωγλοδυτική 1039:9, see τρωγλοδυτική (σμύρνα)
σμύρνιον 579:28?, 1356:25, 1357:6
Σογδίανοι 1299:16
σόγχος 660:16, 1314:16, 1315:11
σοί 1308:8
Σόλων 1310:14
σούσινον 1318:1, 1318:4, 1741:21
σούσινον (ἔλαιον) 1294:12
σούσινον (μύρον) 409:5
σοφία 1319:10
σοφίζουσα 1319:8
σόφισμα 1321:4
σοφίσματα 1320:16
σοφιστής 1319:27, 1373:20
σοφιστικοί 1386:1?
σοφιστικός 1320:11–14, 1320:20
σπαθάριος 234:26, 1378:1
σπάθη 238:5
σπαθίς? 260:27
σπαθομήλη 238:24, 239:4, 260:27?
σπάλαξ, -ακος 1475:11
σπανυδρία 1375:3
σπάρτιον 1371:14
σπάσματα 1371:4
σπασμοί 1371:1
σπασμός 78:7, 78:11, 247:19, 258:18
κυνικός 247:19, 258:18
σπασμώδης 1370:25
σπεῖρα 157:10–15, 235:24–236:13, 1250:8, 1374:16
Σεβαστῆς 235:13, 236:16
σπεκουλάτωρ 234:25, 1372:25
σπέρμα 1371:21, 1373:6, 1377:1 (-άτων)
δὶα σπερμάτων 568:3 (φάρμακον), 568:9
σπεῦσον 1371:20
σπήλαιον 235:6, 238:25
σπλάγχνον 1341:5
σπλῆνες 238:22, 265:9
σπλήνια 1088:1
σπληνικοί 238:22, 265:9
σπλήνιον 132:17–22, 237:3
σπληνῖτις 1373:7
σπόγγος 234:6, 8, 1371:22, 1372:9
σποδιακόν 1314:21
σπόδιον 238:15, 1371:25, 1954:2, see μέλαν σπόδιον
σποδός 827:17?, 1372:1
σπουδαῖα 1372:4
σπουδαῖοι 1319:17, 1372:13, 1939:1
σπουδαῖος 234:23
σπουδή 1372:2
σπυρίς 238:1
σπυρίχνιον 881:4
στάβλιον 219:13
σταγών 1327:17
σταδίαι (σταδίης) 227:6
στάδιον 108:5, 219:23, 226:25, 400:3, 1072:3?
στακτή 221:15, 223:11–12, 1168:7, 1328:21, 1333:3, 1680:21, 1738:16, 1740:22
στάσις 219:4–9, 225:25, 1328:11
στασιώτης 226:17
στατήρ 245:10
στατικά 1327:19, 1328:19
στατικόν προσέχιον 1327:19
σταυρός 222:22, 226:16, 228:18, 1330:20
σταύρωσις 225:19
σταφίς 220:8, 275:5
ἀγρία 227:27
σταφυλαί 227:15, 275:5–6, 1333:1
σταφυλή 1328:16
σταφυλὴν ἀπαρτών 1328:14

σταφυλῖνος 220:5, 223:1, 546:27, 547:23, 1328:3
σταφύλωμα 1328:5
στάχυς 1327:22
στέαρ 1329:3
στέατα 1330:26
στεατώματα 1328:7, 1329:5
στεγανός 1329:7?
στέγασις? 223:4
στεγήρης 1329:7?
στῆθος ποδός 1491:26
στελγίς, -ιδος 807:23
στέμμα 1330:28
στεναγμός 1329:9
στενὴ θύρα 1331:5
στερεός 1329:11, 1333:7
στερέωμα 1329:12, 1331:7, 1333:9
στέρνον 1334:1
Στέφανος 222:26, 1328:17
στέφανος 222:27
στῆθος 1331:4, 1394:21
στήλη 1773:24
στήμων 1345:1?
στίβι 1331:1
στίγμα? 76:11
στίγματα 704:1, 1331:8, 1335:27
στίγματος? 76:11
στιλβόν 226:7?, 1331:6
στιλβώσει 1330:22
στίμμεως 222:20
στίμμι 1331:1, 1357:17
στοά 220:11
στοιβή 1329:22, 1329:28
στοιχαδίτης οἶνος 1330:3
στοιχάς, -άδος 1330:1
στοιχεῖα (στοιχεῖον) 220:9, 935:7, 1330:21
στολή 222:17, 227:3
στολίς 227:3
στόλος 1330:14
στόμα 1329:18
στομαχικός (νόσος) 1330:12
στομαχικῶν (στομαχικοί) 221:13
στόμαχος 221:17, 1330:9
στόμωμα 222:24, 1328:9, 1394:22
στραγγαλία 1334:12
στραγγουρία 226:8
στράτα 224:16
στρατεία 224:17
στρατηγός 109:5, 224:22, 1333:28
στρατηλάτης 225:23, 226:22, 1333:15
στρατία 225:13
στρατιώτις 225:9
ὁ ἐπί τῶν ὑδάτων 1334:26
ὁ χιλιόφυλλος 1335:3
στράτωρ 224:18
στρεβλός 1334:14
στρέμματα 1333:17
στρῆνος (στρηνία) 225:20, 226:18
ξηρὰ στροβιλίνη (ῥητίνη) 912:6
στροβιλίτης οἶνος 1333:24
στρόβιλοι 223:23, 1680:17, 1737:15
στρόβιλος 227:10–11, 228:19, 1333:11, 1333:18, 1623:13, 1630:16
στρούθια (μῆλα) 237:23
στρούθιον 139:20, 226:11, 237:23, 1333:13, 1334:3
πταρμικόν 1330:6
στρύχνον 224:21, 568:9, 1334:16
μανικόν 1334:23
ὑπνωτικόν 1334:20
στρύχνος 821:26
στρῶμα 228:5

στύλος 1330:24
στυπίδιον 1330:18
στύπιον 1330:17
στυπτηρία 1330:16,
σχιστή 1332:28
στύραξ 136:17, 222:11, 223:11–12, 1330:10, 1333:4, 1680:20
στω- 1331:15
Στωϊκοί 220:17, 1329:14
στῶμεν καλῶς 1331:13, 1331:19
σύ 1337:16
σύαγρος 976:19, 1305:8
σύγκαμψον 1337:25
συγκοπή 1316:5, 1316:19
σύγκλασον 1337:27
συγκλητικοί 1321:22
συγκλητικός 1316:29
σύγκλητος 1316:23
συγκριτικόν 1340:12
συγχείρισμα 1316:1?
σύγχυσις 67:12, 184:18, 1313:11, 1316:2
συζυγία 1306:23
Συήνη 1305:4
συκαλίς 1321:26
συκαμινέα 1321:16
συκάμινος 1041:13, 1321:18, 1340:14, 1379:10
συκῆ 1321:17, 1340:15
συκίτης οἶνος 1322:3
συκομοραία 1322:1
συκομορίτης οἶνος 1322:5
συκοφάντης 1340:16
συκοφαντησάτωσάν με 1340:18
συκωδής (ὄγκος) 1321:14
σύκωσις 1322:8, 1381:20
συλλαβή, -άς 1309:28, 1315:5
σύλλαβος 977:3
συλλαμβάνωνται 1338:3
συλλογή, -ῆς 1314:9
συλλογίσασθαι 1311:10
συλλογισμός 141:1, 1310:20, 1311:8, 1311:9, 1314:3, 1315:3, 1352:20
σύλλογος 1314:7
σύμβαμα 1311:17
συμβιβῶ σε 1338:5
συμβουλία 1338:7
συμβούλιον 1312:24
συμπέρασμα 1312:18, 1313:8, 1316:8
συμπερασματική 1316:17
συμπλοκαί 1544:18
συμπόσεσταί σοι 1338:9
σύμπτωμα 1338:11
σύμφυσις 1313:1
σύμφυτον 1311:14, 1312:22, 1312:26, 1360:9
μέγα 1312:11
μικρόν 1312:15
πετραῖον 1312:11–17, 1312:26
σύμφυτος 1313:1
συμφωνία 1372:18?, 1675:4
συμψελλικοί 1375:9
συμψέλλιον 1375:5
σύν 1313:9, 1440:24
συνάγχη 1309:12, 1313:12, 1314:19, 1315:20
συναγωγή 1337:3, 1338:13
συναμφότερον 1316:15
συνάντησις 1338:15
σύναξις 1364:18
σύνδεσμος 1340:11
συνδοκτικοῦ πεπραγμένα 1315:17
συνδύασω 1338:19
συνέδριον 254:16?, 257:2?, 1338:17
συνέκλεισαν 1338:21
συνέκλεισας 1338:23

συνέλαβεν 1338:25
συνελήφθη 1338:27
συνελήφθην 1339:1
συνέξει 1339:3
συνεπιτιθέμενοί με 1339:7
συνεπόδισας 1339:5
συνεπόδισεν 120:5
συνεργία 1315:19
συνεργός 1317:8
σύνες 1339:9
συνεσθίω 1339:21
σύνεσις (συνετός) 1318:3
σύνετε 1339:10
συνετιῶ σε 1339:11
συνέτος? 121:21, 1318:3
συνέτρεχες αὐτῷ 1339:13
συνέτριψας 1339:15
συνεφρύγησαν 1339:17
συνηγορία 1362:13
συνήντησαν 1339:20
συνήφθησαν 1339:23
συνθλάσει 1339:25
συνοδία φαληροτόμων 1363:10?
συνοδικόν 1190:16, 1314:23
συνόδιον, -ια 1343:20
σύνοδος 1313:15, 1337:4
συνοδυνώμενός σοι 1338:1?
συνοπτικός 1316:21
συνορισμός 1317:10
Συνουσιασταί 1315:7
σύνοχος 1314:13
σύνοψις 1314:11, 1315:27, 1316:11, 1384:17?
συνταγή 1315:13
συντακτήριον 1315:14
συντακτικός 1315:15
σύνταξις 1315:24
συνταράξει 1339:27
συντέλεια 617:26, 1340:3
συντελέσθητο 1340:1
Συντύκη 55:9
συνώνυμα 1362:22
συνώνυμοι 1316:4
συνώνυμος 1293:26, 1314:14, 1315:9
συὸς ὦτα 1344:6?
Συράκουσαι 1393:20
Συρία 1323:23,1324:19
σύριγγες 1675:3
συριγγίς 1324:15
σύριγξ 29:24, 1324:9 (-γος)
συσσείων 1340:5
σύστασις 1318:17
συστατικόν 1318:18
συστοιχία 1318:11, 1318:18
συστροφή 1340:7
συσχέτω 1340:9
σῦφαρ τοῦ ὄφεως 121:11–12
σφαγή 1370:21
σφαῖρα 235:24–236:13, 235:18, 235:19
σφαιρικά 236:14
σφακελισμοί 1371:6
σφακελισμός 239:1, 242:8
σφάκελος 444:8–12
σφάξαι 1370:23
σφαργάνιον 1371:11
(σμῆγμα διὰ) σφέκλης 1371:6, see σμῆγμα διὰ σφέκλης
σφήν 235:18, 239:14
σφόδρα 1372:5
σφονδύλιον, 237:8, 238:9, 964:23, 1372:14, see φυσαλίδος
σφραγίς 78:14
σφῦρα 1374:8

σχεδία 160:23, 163:10, 232:16, 1351:3, 1379:14?, 1386:15?
σχέδιον 160:19, 232:16 (= σχεδία), 241:22
δία σχεδίου 571:6
σχῆμα 230:9
σχήματα 1350:25
σχίνινον (ἔλαιον) 1350:28
σχίνινος (οἶνος) 1350:26
σχῖνος 818:16, 1350:21, 1384:16?
σχιστὸς (λίθος) 865:14, 970:20
σχοίνανθος 1350:23
σχοίνινον (μύρον) 1167:5
σχοινίον, -ία 1349:27, 1350:7
σχοῖνος 473:4, 603:11, 755:1, 1309:11, 1350:20
  ἀρωματική 1350:11
  ἐλεία 1350:13
σχολάσατε 1349:24
σχολαστικός 231:24, 232:14, 1349:28
σχολή 231:21, 232:12
σχόλια 232:10
σχόλιον 231:19, 232:8, 1350:9 (-ια)
σώζων 1307:3
Σωκράτης 1321:24
σωλήν 1310:10
σῶμα 1311:16
σώματα 218:4, 1311:26, 1488:10
σωμάτιον 1357:19
σῶρι 1323:19, 1324:12, 1386:19 (-εως)
  ἀνθικόν 1324:17?
σωριτικόν 1324:25
Σωσθένης 1318:23
σῶσον 1317:24
σωτήρ 1307:11
  ἡμῶν 1307:21, 1307:24
σωτηρία 1308:1

T

Ταβεννεσιώτης, -τα 787:8
τακτὴν (τιμήν) 784:10
τάλαντον 809:6
ταμεῖον 566:3, 803:12, 811:13
τάξεων 552:9
τάξεως 552:9
τάξις 806:26, 807:15
τάξος 783:15, 1358:16
ταπεινός 594:13, 806:24, 816:26
τάπητα 187:1, 816:17
τάραξις 784:13, 830:5
ταραχή 829:8
ταρίχευσις 830:6?
τάριχος 784:15
ταρσός 452:23, 784:16, 784:21
Τάρταρος 785:3, 790:8, 824:25
ταῦρος 783:11, 1156:9
τάχα 806:23
τεῖχος 802:24
τέλειος 803:3
τελλίναι 789:16
τελλίνη 783:18, 789:18?
τελλινῶν 783:17
τέκτων 805:22, 813:8
τενεισμός 804:1
τέρας 315:22, 790:7
τέρατα 806:13, 827:24
τερεβινθίνη 789:26, 790:5, 790:12, 801:10, 801:13
τερμινθίνη (ῥητίνη) 1898:17
τέρμινθος 274:23, 790:3, 11, 829:17, 1719:16
Τέρτυλλος ῥήτωρ 824:14
τεσσαρακόσια 805:4
τεσσαρακοστός 805:6

τέτανος 788:23, 789:8, 802:13
τεταρταῖος 788:22
τέταρτον 720:2
τετραγωνισμός 801:3
τετράγωνον 789:6, 800:23, 1776:21
τετραετηρικός 800:14
τετραευαγγέλιον 801:1
τετραπλάσιος 801:5?
τετράπους, -οδος 800:25, 817:8
τετράπυλον 800:21
τετράρχης 801:6, 832:15
τετραφάρμακον 789:4, 800:19
τετραχία 789:13
τέτταρα 567:3, 800:27
μαθίσματα 800:28
τέττιγες 788:24
τέττιξ, -ιγος 789:1, 792:16, 802:16, 985:17
τεύθριον 799:23
τεύκριον 788:18, 796:11
τεῦτλον 788:20, 792:10
τέφρα 784:9, 789:25, 827:17?
τέχνη 789:21
τεχνίτης 789:15
τεχνολογία 787:11, 806:25
τέως 783:8, 788:15, 798:9?, 1802:8
τήγανον 788:7, 801:21, 827:20
Τηθύς 299:24
τηθύς 806:22
τηκόλιθοι 801:22
τηκόλιθος 796:2, 797:3
τηλέφια 803:8
τηλέφιον 802:25
τήλινον (μύρον) 803:4
τῆλις 789:18?, 803:5, 1571:1, 1800:6
τήρησις 824:9?
τηρητική 1242:20
Τίγρις 801:26
τιθύμαλλος 805:18, 806:19, 810:20
τιθυμάλων 2051:14
τίμα τὸν πατέρα καὶ τὴν μητέρα σήν 803:21
Τιμαίου Βαρτίμαιος 803:26
τίμη 803:17
τίμησις 811:16
τίμιον? 248:25
Τιμόθεος 803:13
τιμωρία 480:28, 803:19
τιμώτατος 803:16
Τιτάν 802:19
τίτανος 800:11, 802:6, 812:16
τιτίς 789:3, 802:15
τίτλος 800:17, 802:17
Τίτος 800:9
τόκος 797:5
τόμος 794:24
τόνος 795:4
τοξάριον 793:22
τοξευτής 793:20
τοομαῖον 799:10, cf. τροπαῖον
τοπικά 796:14
τοπική 796:13, 1806:17
τοπικός 796:16
τόπος 795:26
τοποτηρητής 57:4, 830:11
τορδύλιον 791:16
τόρνος 464:9, 798:23, 822:23
δὶα τοῦτο 556:9
τραγάκανθα 592:7, 676:1, 783:7, 818:5, 819:21, 820:15
(κόμμι) 821:1?
τράγιον 818:15, 820:18, 821:2
ἄλλο 818:16
τραγισκός 818:10

τραγοπώγων 819:17
τραγορίγανος 819:15, 819:23
τράγος 817:24, 820:29, 821:2
τραγόχειλος 818:13?
τραγῳδία 259:10, 819:2
τραγῳδός 798:8, 819:10, 820:20
Τραιανός 827:7
τράκτατον 831:22
τράπεζα 825:27, 831:11
τραπεζίτης 830:12
τράχηλος 829:7
τραχύτης 819:1
τραχώματα 818:18, 819:13
τραχωματικὸν (κολλούριον) 828:27
Τραχῶνα 829:1
Τραχωνῖτις 818:8
τρεῖς 828:5
τρία 825:3
τριακόσια 826:24
τριᾶς 784:7?, 830:7?
τρίβολος 824:8?, 825:14, 825:21, 826:22
τρίγλα 825:16
τρίγωνον 825:18
ἴτριον 826:21
τρίενος 826:13?
τριέσπερος 825:23
τρίκλινον 832:11
τριμίσιον 824:29, 829:14
τριόβολον 823:1, 824:27
τριόφθαλμος 827:25
τριπλοῦν (φάρμακον) 827:9
Τρίπολις 827:8
τρίπους 816:21 (-οδος), 826:20 (-όδων), 827:17?, 827:26 (-οδος)
τρισκέλης 827:16 (τρισκάλιον)?
τρισμέγιστος 827:28, see Ἑρμῆς Τρισμέγιστος
τρισούσιος 827:11
τριστάτης 502:21, 827:14, 828:23
τριταῖος 133:15–16, 825:25, see πυρετὸς τριταῖος
τριτούσιος? 827:22, see τρισούσιος
τρίφυλλον 826:7, 826:16, 828:9
τρίχα διαστατός 824:11, 826:26
τρίχες 303:26
τριχίασις 821:24, 822:1, 827:4
τριχομανές 826:1, 828:16, 828:19
τριχός (θρίξ) 795:3
τροπαῖον 823:6, cf. τοομαῖον
τροπή 823:29
τροπικός 822:24
τροῦλλα 794:19, 799:17, 808:6, 821:18
τρόφη 802:2, 822:19, 824:6
Τρόφιμος 822:27
τροχίσκοι 829:2
τροχίσκος Ἀνδρώνιος 828:25, see Ἀνδρώνιος (τροχίσκος)
τρυγών 824:3
τρύξ 823:3, 7
Τρωάς 824:5?
τρωγλοδύτης 788:6, 788:16, 821:6, 823:9, 823:18
τρωγλοδυτική (σμύρνα) 821:8, 823:17, see σμύρνα τρωγλοδυτική
τρώξιμα 204:25, 829:10, 1453:3
τρῶμα 822:4
τρώματα 822:5
τύλοι 793:26
τύλωσις 793:24
τυμπανίας 795:6, 795:23
τύπος 795:16, 795:21, 805:20, 813:6
τύπωσις? 546:15
τύραννος 798:10, 822:9

τυρός 797:7
τύφη 796:7
τυφλός 805:14
τυφώδης 805:16
Τυφών 816:11
τυφωνικὸς εὐροκλύδων 795:18
Τυχικός 793:19

Y

ὑάκινθος 48:22
ὑαλέα 58:25
ὑαλοειδής 170:22, 615:6, 2074:9
ὑβρίζειν? 64:13
ὑγιαστικά? 617:3
ὑγίεια 51:10
ὑγιεινός 51:8
ὑγρά 612:12
  πίσσα 612:14
ὑγροκολλούρια 51:11–12
ὑγροκολλούριον 51:14
ὑδατίς 113:1
ὕδατος 112:9–10
ὕδερος 612:20
ὕδνα 33:23, 621:22
ὕδνον 54:6, 664:4
ὑδράργυρος 41:24, 55:3, 610:1
ὑδραύλησις? 609:27
ὕδραυλις 607:25, 609:25, 657:6
ὑδρηλὸν οἴδημα 52:21
ὑδρίον 965:6
ὑδρόγαρον 54:10
ὑδροκήλη 610:9?
ὑδροκέφαλον 80:18–19, 85:8, 610:12
ὑδρόμελι 42:9, 54:13, 285:5, 610:4, 1022:13
ὑδρόμηλον 42:14, 54:17
ὑδρόμυρον 610:3?, 610:6?
ὑδροπέπερι 54:24, 55:1
ὑδρορόσατον 42:8, 360:12, 1889:1
ὑδρόσατον 609:22
ὑδροχόος 117:7, 572:22
ὑδρωπικός 610:10
ὕδωρ 52:15, 112:9–10, see ἀνυπόστατον (ὕδωρ), θαλάττιον ὕδωρ
υἱός 48:8, 118:13, 145:10–11, 202:16
  τῆς ἀπωλείας 140:26, 1331:10
ὕλη 615:1, 615:5 (-ας), 615:10, 624:22, 625:5, 625:6
ὑμῶν 118:1
ὑοσκυάμινον (ἔλαιον) 47:24
ὑοσκύαμος 47:22, 47:26, 78:9, 617:5
ποῦ ὑπάγεις 1499:12
ὕπαρξις 84:20, 617:6
ὑπαρχία 620:1, 620:5
ὕπαρχος 620:2
ὑπατεία 259:1?, 619:13, 646:13
ὕπατοι 619:19
ὕπατος 79:19, 619:13
ὑπέθεντο 118:25
ὑπέλαβές με 118:23
ὑπέλαβον 118:26, 119:13
ὑπερασπιστής 118:27
ὑπερβήσομαι 119:1
ὑπερβολή 620:4
ὑπερεδυνάμουν 119:3
ὑπερηφάνεια 119:7, 143:23
ὑπερηφανεῖν 119:5
ὑπερηφανία 143:23
ὑπερθετικόν 121:7
ὑπερικόν 79:1, 84:5, 617:8, 1631:12
ὑπερορᾷς 119:9
ὑπερῷον 119:11

ὑπήκοον 83:6, 1558:12?
ὑπήνεγμα 119:17
ὑπηνέμια (ᾠά) 119:19, 202:17
ὕπνωσα 119:20
ὑπ' αὐτοῦ 118:20, 118:22
ὑπὸ ὑπάτων 79:29?
ὑπογάστριον 79:15, 569:11, 620:22, 1161:2, cf. ἐπίγαστρον
ὑπογλώσσιον 527:25
ὑπόγλωσσον 80:27, 83:28
ὑπογλωττίδες 81:25
ὑπογραφή 79:12, 142:24, 617:26
ὑπογράφιον 142:24
ὑπογραφῶν 142:24
ὑπόδημα 119:22
ὑποδιάκονοι 1033:9
ὑποδιάκονος 143:18, 617:19, 621:5
ὑποδύτες 80:24
ὑπόθεσις 80:20?, 82:8, 85:3, 85:8?, 618:7, 621:2
ὑποθετικός 618:5, 619:3
ὑποθῆκαι 80:10
ὑποκείμενον 80:9, 618:20, 620:9, 652:17
ἐν ὑποκειμένῳ 201:9
ὑποκιστίς 84:17, 23, 618:23
ὑποκοριστικόν 121:9
ὑπόκρισις 142:18?, 252:19
ὑπόλεπτον 1512:4?
ὑπόληψις 82:9, 85:2, 250:22, 618:27, 619:26, 620:26, 646:7
ὑπόλυσις 80:18–19, 85:8
ὑπόλυτος 85:6, 145:4
ὑπομνήματα 80:22, 618:10, 620:18, 621:14, 645:16
ὑπομνηστικόν 258:11, 618:14, 620:20
ὑπομονή 120:1
ὑποπόδιον 120:3
ὑπόπυον 81:12, 144:17
ὑπόστασις 120:7–9
ὑποστατικός 619:22, 619:25
ὑποστήσεται 120:11
ὑποστησόμεθα 120:11
ὑπόσφαγμα 79:3, 254:12
ὑπότασις 85:4, 142:14
ὑποφήτης 80:3?
ὑποχόνδρια 254:6, 463:18
ὑποχόνδριον 81:18–19, 141:9, 233:10, 254:6, 1160:27
ὑπόχυμα 81:21–3, 81:27, 255:13, 257:23
ὑποχύματα 80:15, 81:21, 27, 82:28
ὑπωθείς 64:3?
ὑπώπια 81:12, 81:14, 255:2, 639:6, 640:1
ὑπώπιον 144:17
ὑπώπτευσα 120:13
Ὑρκανία 94:20
ὗς 120:15
χοῖρος 139:18, 241:4, see χοῖρος
ὕσσωπος 78:3, 234:18?
ὑστερήσει 120:16
ὑψηλοῖς 120:22, 202:18 (ἐν ὑψηλοῖς)
ὑψηλός 120:18
Ὑψιστάριοι 85:5, 618:16
ὕψιστος 120:20, 141:22, 262:23
ὕψος 120:22, 202:18
ὕψωμα 141:20, 144:3
ὑψώθητε 121:1–3
ὑψωθήτω 121:1:3
ὑψῶν 121:5

Φ

φάγανον 909:1

φαγέδαινα 1471:20

φάγεται 1471:18

φάγομαι 1471:19

φάγρος 1471:16

ποῦ φάγωμεν 1542:25?

φαέθων 1472:12

φακός (-οί) 1479:7, 12, 1521:9

ὁ ἐπὶ τῶν τελμάτων 1479:12

Φακούση 1479:16?

φάλαγγες 1475:24

φαλάγγιον 957:9, 1475:15, 1629:1

φαλαγγίτης 689:11, 1475:20

φαλαγγίτιον 957:9, 1475:19

φαλακρός 1636:16

φαλαρίς 1475:21

φαλλός 1584:22?

φάναι 1576:14, cf. φάσις

φανός 586:18?, 1577:18

φαντασία 1476:16, 1579:8, 10 (φαντασίας), 1580:3

φαράγγιον 708:11

φαρέτρα 1484:9

φαρμακευτικόν 1482:5, 1628:3

φαρμακός 1484:11, 1627:21

φάρυγξ (-υγγα) 1614:13

φάσγανον 866:1

φάσηλος 1477:24

φασιανός 979:9, 1478:17

φασίολος 139:4–8

φάσις 1477:20, 1557:15, 1588:17, 21, cf. φάναι

φάσσα 1477:15

φαῦσις 1471:11

φέγγος 1494:1

φεῖσαι 1491:12

φελόνης 1545:11

φελόνιον 1545:11

φήνη 6:20, 1555:3

φθειρίασις 1647:19

φθινώδης 1647:14

φθισικοί 1648:21

φθίσις 1560:14, 1645:19, 1647:15, 1648:22, 1994:14

φθόη 1645:19

φθορά 269:15

φιάλη 241:2, 1007:20, 1544:1, 7, 1547:3, 15 (-ην)

φίβλα 1540:9, 1560:9

φιλάγαθος 1547:11

Φιλάγριος 1544:16

φιλαδέλφιον 1545:6, 1566:9

φιλάδελφος 1544:20, 1545:2

φιλαλήθης 1545:19

φιλάνθρωπος 272:6, 1545:10

φιλαργυρία 1548:6

φιλαρχία 1546:14

φίλαρχος 1547:4

φιλεταίριον 1511:26, 1547:13

Φίλιππος 1546:11

κολωνία 1546:19

φιλλυρέα 1554:3

φιλοδέσποτος 1544:15

φιλοδοξία 1547:9

φιλόζωος 1544:12

φίλοι 1546:2

ἐμοῦ 1546:2

φιλόθεος 1547:19, 1554:5

φιλόκαλος 1547:7

φιλόκτισις 1554:4

φιλολόγοι 1546:17

φιλομαθής 1548:1
Φιλόξενος 1546:7
φιλόξενος 1546:3, 1547:12
φιλοπάτωρ 1544:19
φιλόπονος 1544:13, 1545:12 (φιλόπονοι), 14, 1547:20, 22 (φιλόπονοι)
φίλος 1545:21
φιλόσοφος 1548:11
φιλοσοφία 1548:10
φιλούμενος 1567:3?
φιλόχορος 1568:7
φιλόχριστος 1546:21
φίλτατος 1544:22?
φιλωνεῖον (φάρμακον) 1545:16, 1546:10
φιμός 1554:12
Φλαβιανός 1568:5
φλεβοτόμον 315:8, 1566:15 (φλεβότομον)
φλέγμα 1565:20
φλεγμονή 589:22, 1176:14, 1347:8, 1497:12, 1566:10, 1567:13, 1624:22, 1634:7
φλέξ (-έβος) 1564:3, 1574:8
φλογός 1568:3
φλόμος 302:25, 372:19, 603:13, 1479:24, 1567:1, 1568:22, 1569:1 (φλόμοι), 1572:11, 1793:14
ἰδαῖος 1786:18
φλόξ 1568:3
φλύκταινα 1566:13, 1568:14
φλυκτίς 1508:13?
φοβερός 1499:21, 1505:15
φοβηθήσομαι 1499:24, 1505:20
φόβος 1499:21, 26, 1505:9, 15
φοινιγμοί 1517:10
Φοινίκη 1516:5
φοίνιξ 234:20, 1505:14, 1514:24, 28, 1518:3, 1542:8
ἡ βοτάνη 1514:25
κολλύριον 1516:3
φοινικίτης οἶνος 1516:16
μή φονεύσεις 1076:3
φόνιοι 1517:12
φόνιος 1517:12
φόνος 1517:12
φόρβιον 1523:21
φορεῖον 1522:25, 1523:7 (φορεῖον)
φορμίον 1523:26
φορτίον 1523:23
φοῦ 1499:10
φοῦρνος 1524:1, 9
φραγμός 1603:3
φρακτά 1636:10, 1637:13 (φρακτός)
φραφείδιον? 521:3
φρέαρ 1607:14
φρενῖτις 1497:16, 1607:3
φρενός 1606:23
φρήν 1606:23
φρόνησις 1518:12
φροντιεῖ μου 1610:15
φρύγανον 1628:12
Φρυγές 1035:1
Φρυγία 1608:14
φρύγιος (λίθος) 864:18, cf. Καππαδοκία (λίθος), λίθος (φρύγιος)
φρυκτὴ (ῥητίνη) 1616:4, 12
φρυκτωρία 1616:8?, 10?
φυγάς (-άδος) 1542:9
φύγεθλον (-λα) 1500:5, 10
φύκη 1521:22
φῦκος 1521:14, 22
θαλάσσιον 1522:1
φυλακή 1541:18
φυλακτήριον (-ια) 1510:15, 2063:14 (φυλακτήρια), 2079:20 (φυλακτήρια)

φύλαξ 1546:1,1547:6
φυλετικοί 1508:11, 1510:17
φυλή 1541:23, cf. φῦλον
φυλία 1510:3
φυλλῖτις 1510:23
φύλλον 932:16, 1087:15, 1276:17, 1509:8, 1511:11, 1542:1, 1568:16, 17
φῦλον 1508:10, cf. φυλή
φύματα 1513:9
φύραμα 261:14, 1541:6
φυσαλίς (-ίδος) 237:10, 1585:20
περὶ φύσεως 1497:25
φύσησις 906:18?
φυσικοί 1517:24
φυσιογνωμονική 1519:1, 1557:9, 1581:20, 1588:1
Πολέμωνος 1518:23
φυσιολογῆσαι 1517:21
φυσιολογία 1557:3
φυσιολογικόν 1557:4
φύσις 468:19–20?, 1518:9, 1555:13, 1588:15
φύτευμα 1513:28
(οἰνάνθη) τὸ φυτόν 59:9
φώκη 1521:20
φῶς 1129:8, 1504:15, 1518:11, 1541:16
ἐκ φωτός 1518:7
φῶτα 1503:23, 1504:15, 1504:26
φωτεινοί 1503:23
φωτίσω 1504:17
φωτός 1129:8

X

χαιρετισμός 1624:11
χαλάζιον 858:11, 1208:12
χαλβάνη 858:13, 894:15
χαλινάριον 1786:15
χαλινός 898:1
χάλκανθον 858:17, 859:7, 1099:4, 1797:9
χαλκεύς 1790:15, 1797:6
Χαλκηδών 898:23
χαλκητάριν 859:5, 898:25, 899:2, 1798:2, see καλκῖτις
χαλκίον 899:4
Χαλκίς 899:1
χαλκῖτις 859:5, 898:25, 899:5, 981:18
χαλκός 1792:15 (-οί)
κεκαυμένος 858:18, 898:21, 1381:7
χαλκοῦ ἄνθος 51:11–12, 859:1, 899:7
χαλκύδριον 899 n. 1, 1786:1, 1798:13
χαμαιάκτη 274:18
χαμαιδάφνη 859:23
χαμαιδρυΐτης οἶνος 860:6
χαμαίδρυς 395:25, 788:18, 796:12, 859:15, 900:13
χαμαίκισσος 860:8
χαμαιλεύκη 860:11
χαμαιλέων 292:5, 596:24, 726:24, 860:5, 898:10, 903:25 (-οντος), 904:6, 1455:14, 1457:17
λευκός 859:27
μέλας 860:2–3
χαμαίμηλον 215:15, 904:8
χαμαίπιτυς 859:17
χαμαιπίτυς 217:10–13, 303:2, 596:26, 898:10, 904:16, 1162:13
χαμαισύκη 859:19
χαμελαία 904:6, 2046:17
χαρά 865:23, 915:3
χαραδριός 211:25–6
χαράκωμα 1797:14
χάρις 865:19
χαριστίων 925:7, 1146:16

χάριτες 1037:23
χάρτης 920:2
χαρτουλάριος 896:26, 920:1
χάσκανον 909:1
χείλη 869:3
χειμάρρους 869:4, 888:8
χειμών 888:9, 1394:14
χείρ 683:26, 869:19, 891:4 (-ες)
χείρες 907:21
χειροπέδη 869:20, 907:19, 1559:10
χειροποιητοί 1719:10
χειροποίητος (χίτων) 1052:17
χειροτονία 891:6
χειρουργία 890:21
χειρώνεια 890:24
χελιδόνες 869:12, 888:1
χελιδόνιον 350:12, 869:8, 878:3, 887:21,
895:12, 897:4, 1100:12, 1785:19
χελώνη 156:21, 887:13
χηλός 857:16
χημεία 901:9, 904:10
χήμη 859:25, 1799:7 (-ῶν)
χήμωσις 888:13
χήρα, -ας 891:1
χθές 928:12
χία 886:20? 868:22
γῆ 868:22
χιακὸν (κολλούριον) 886:20?
χιλίαρχος 887:17, 1798:18
χιλιοδύναμιν 1511:27
χιλιόφυλλον 1509:9
χιμαιρίς, -ίδος 869:5
χιών 887:6
χλαμύδιον 897:24, 898:17
χλαμύς 810:19, 898:1
χλανίδιον 898:16
χλευασμός 895:14
χλόν 896:9
χλωρότης 896:16
χοεύς 879:19
χοῖνιξ, -κος 878:18, 879:9
χοιραδόλεθρον 909:1
χοῖρος 1957:8?, see ὗς χοῖρος
χολέρα 544:15, 876:5, 877:3
χολή 876:8, 877:14
χόνδρος 173:14, 878:27
χόος 879:19, 905:19
χοραύλης 917:8
χορδαψός 167:25–7, 869:1, 872:6
χορός 882:13
χόρτος 882:10, 882:15?
χοῦς 872:9, 879:19, 905:19
χρεία 915:24?
χρέος 915:10
χρῆσις 921:4, 925:9
χρηστότης 918:26, 921:6
χρίσμα 920:26
Χριστοῦ γενέα 885:25, 918:22
Χριστός 920:24, 924:26, 1169:9
Χριστόφιλος 921:2
χριστοφόρος 919:5, 925:11
χρονικόν 918:3, 924:4
χρονίσεις 918:1
χρόνος 917:21, 924:1
χρυσάνθεμον 634:12
Χρυσαόριος 918:16
χρυσῆν (ἕδραν) 918:23?
χρυσίον 920:18
χρυσῖτις 918:24
χρυσόγονον 919:9
χρυσοθήκη 919:3
χρυσόκολλα 918:9, 925:5, 1630:14

χρυσοκόμη 918:25, 919:6
χρυσολάχανον 918:5, 919:1
χρυσοποιός 921:8
χρυσός 918:15, 920:14
Χρυσόστομος 918:20
χρυσοῦ γλῶσσαι 924:23
χρυσοῦν (ἔριον) 427:5
χρῶμα 917:9
χυλάριον 876:3, 899:8
χυλός 553:6, 876:7, 877:8, 877:10, 887:3
χυμοί 877:15
χυμός 1565:20
χώνη 878:5, 878:25
χῶνος 879:6
χώραν 91:7
χωρεπίσκοπος 881:17, 887:1

Ψ

ψαλίδιον 99:8, 235:12, 237:6
ψάλλειν 263:12
ψαλίς, -ίδες 1590:12
ψάλλων 1583:20?
ψαλτήριον 263:16, 1590:9
ψάλτης 1589:18
ψαλῶ 1583:20?
ψάρες 1583:22
ψαρὸς κόπρος 673:25, 673:26
ψευδοβούνιον 1584:10
ψευδοεπής 1381:9?, 1381:13?, cf. 1383:5
ψευδοκασσία 1701:23–6, see κασσία
ψευδομάρτυς 1584:16
ψευδοπροφήτης 1584:21
ψεῦδος 258:4, 1383:5?, 1584:8, 1585:17
ψευδόχριστος 1584:14
ψήν 1590:17
ψήφισμα 1518:26, 1555:16, 1556:3, 1589:3
ψίλωθρον 86:5–7, 1573:20, 1587:20
ψιμύθιον 265:10, 1554:8, 1588:12
ψίξ 1585:12, 1587:24, 1589:5
ψιττακός 1578:15?, 1580:8?, 1582:11, 1586:24, see σιττακός
ψιχές 1585:12, 1587:24, 1588:7, 1589:5
ψόαι 1588:3
ψόγος 1585:19
ψυδράκια 1584:17, 1586:3
ψυκτήρ 1585:4
ψύλλιον 265:14, 1585:6
ψυχή 1488:12, 1557:13, 1588:5
ψῦχος 1488:13
ψυχότροφον 1816:4, see κέστρον ψυχότροφον
ψωλή 1584:22?
ψωμίον 284:18, 288:23, 408:3, 1541:13, 1586:1
ψώρα 1585:9
ψωρικὸν (φάρμακον) 1585:13
ψωροφθαλμία 1584:19, 1585:10, 1586:14

Ω

ὠά 11:1?, 115:26, 663:4, see ὠόν
ᾠα 47:13
ᾠδεῖον 53:18
ὡδήγησεν 53:6
ὠδῖνες 53:20
ὠθήσεις 76:3
ὠκεανός 77:24, 85:28, 86:1, 275:20
ὠκίμινον (μύρον) 667:11, see ὤκιμον
ὠκιμοειδές 86:10
ὤκιμον 86:14, 667:8, see ὠκίμινον
ᾠκίσθησαν 1272:3?
ὠλισθήσατο 64:25?
ὠμήρισα 616:4
ὦμος 66:8

ὠμοτάριχος 66:5
ὠμοτριβές (ἔλαιον) 65:26
ᾠόν 47:15, 55:18, see ᾠά
ὥρα 622:4
ὠράριον 87:10, 95:18
ὠράριος? 87:6
ὠργίσαντο? 87:28
ὡρεῖα 54:3, 55:25
ὤρθωσεν 121:15
Ὠριγενίσται 89:6, 91:2
Ὠριγένης 91:2
ὡρικός 92:27
ὡροσκόπος 91:14, 299:10
ὤρυξαν 70:24
ὤρυξε 53:17
ὠρυόμενος 90:10
ᾠός 75:19
ὡσαννά 78:15, 97:9
ὠτία 57:18, 228:17
ὠτίς 835:11, 835:25
Ὠφειρά? 82:5
ὠφέλεια 80:5
ὦχρα 61:20
ὦχροι 59:25, 61:18
ὦχρος 59:25, 61:18

Latin Words

accubitum? 272:9

adragantha 592:17, 676:1

Africanus 268:9

amentum 185:6?, 192:23?

ampulla 250:21, 263:10

Aprilis (menses) 261:23, 268:8

atramentum 1370:19?

axis 156:13

baculus 373:9

baptisma 1503:23

buccina 373:2, 10

buccinator 373:2

caballarius 1708:9

caeruleum 1719:14?

calidarius 1803:22

caliga 1788:7

caligarius 1788:6

Caligula 443:18

Campania 1700:9

camphora 1746:1

cancellarius 1812:12

cancelli 1812:13

canterinum (hordeum) 1580:16

carruca 1835:3

castrensianus 1816:11

castrensis 1816:13

casula 1741:23

Census 1009:2

census 1776:6

centenarium 1807:20

centuriones 806:14

Census 912:1, 1009:2

Chors 882:15

De cibis frumentariis 1362:25

Cibus 889:1?

circenses 1781:18

Circesium 1782:1

Claudia 1785:23

Claudius 1785:23

Cledonius 1788:19

Clemens 1790:8, 1794:2

creta 1847:4

culeadae 1698:8?

cultrum 1732:7?

curator 1752:10

custodia 1741:15

Dalmatia? 535:23

Danubius 1559:24?

Decius 528:11

Domnina 544:2

Domninus 544:2

ductores? 547:4

Dumachus 543:13

dux 540:24, 541:6

edictum 114:26

emancipatus 133:1

exceptores 1129:14?

exercitus 159:14, 163:19

exilium 55:15 (preferred to exsul)

exsul 55:15, 76:8

fabrica 1471:12

februarius 1491:18

funiculus 1517:19

furnus 1524:1, 9

galearii 486:20, 499:9

herba rubia 621:20, 656:7, 2029:7

Hispanica 234:20?

horreum 54:3, 55:5

Hospitia 67:4

Ianuarius 110:4

Ignatius 26:26, 29:3, 30:10, 111:27
ignem 111:16
ignes 111:16
indictio 100:1, 199:10
Iorarii 1363:10
janua 555:22
Latinus 1788:18?
lectica 935:18, 946:5, 980:8
(in) lectica? 402:11
Legatum 941:7
Libellum 576:17, 937:6
Libellus 964:7-8
Longina 948:20
Longinus 948:4
nauta 1225:8, see ναύτης
Novatiani 1225:13
Novatus 1225:17
Marcellus 994:1
Martius 993:21, 1621:15
Mauricia 1040:20?
Mauricius 1040:13
melissa 1070:15
mensis Maius 1074:21
mille 1068:6, 1071:9
moschatum 1045:12-14?
muria 1041:6
Mysia 1037:21
officialis 266:20
patriarcha 1473:15, 1539:1
Phrygia salutaris et Pactiana 1608:14
pontifex imperator 1516:19
pontonium 1578:13
praepositus 1602:6, see πραιπόσιτος
primus 993:22?, 1621:15
proemium 866:15
quaestionarius 1815:9
repudium 1900:8
Romulus 1888:5
Rufus 1890:19
sacristarium 114:16
scala 1385:8
scamnum regni? 242:10
scrinium 1378:22
Sergius 1295:8
Sextilis 1303:29
signum 1336:1
Silentiarius 1341:23
stabulum 219:13
statio 222:15
strata 224:16
tabellarius 787:2
talare 810:17
talentum 809:6
Taurus 785:1
tetracha 832:15
tetrarcha 801:6–9
tressis 784:7?, 830:7?
Tribuni 825:7
Tribunus 825:10
trulla 794:19
Valens 665:25
Valens Palaestinus 664:10
Valentinus 663:8
Valerianus 663:10
vela 663:13, 665:21
Veneti et Albati 382:25, 403:22, see Βένετοι καὶ Πρασινοί
Venus 244:19
victima? 352:17

Unknown Greek Words

64:25 (*ex verbo* λύω)

78:12

118:14

136:20

147:26

148:1

148:25, cf. 150:4

149:22, cf. 289:20

150:3

150:4

155:12

156:23, cf. 209:18

160:6, cf. 231:18

170:11

184:9, cf. 114:22

190:14, cf. 190:22,

199:2

209:18, cf. 156:23

220:25, cf. 222:9

235:3

238:6

240:18

254:16, cf. 257:2

255:4

258:14

258:27

263:17

265:26

266:19

268:16

269:16, cf. 1071:5

275:8

279:16

284:5

284:6 (ἀρνόγλωσσον), cf. 298:22

285:17

289:18

289:20

297:13 (ἀρωματικὸν [φάρμακον])

349:16

350:10

351:17

369:21 (παλαίστρα)

370:2

374:24

375:5

421:21

428:4

452:14

488:23, cf. 507:16

536:22

539:17

553:1

560:18

568:16

568:17

568:22

574:11

592:24

615:8

619:4

622:12

628:1

630:23

646:4

653:1

656:1

667:9

684:4

686:5

757:23
791:1
791:2
800:13
811:17
825:26
827:17
832:2
835:1
886:20
887:7
907:4
936:2
965:23
991:9
995:2
1007:11
1038:23
1038:24
1076:1, cf. 1082:26
1081:24
1083:8
1099:18
1106:8
1113:3-4
1208:8
1245:9
1245:13
1245:15
1245:18
1257:19
1300:16
1311:20, cf. 1385:19
1311:22
1329:20
1354:6, cf. 391:8
1365:1, cf. 1384:16
1373:5
1374:10
1374:25
1378:24 (... κιμωλία γῆ)
1384:16 cf. 1365:1
1385:19 cf. 1311:20
1387:23
1457:6 cf. 622:12
1479:25
1493:19
1495:26
1505:18
1511:19
1519:23
1523:20
1530:26
1532:6
1544:8
1546:15
1557:14
1567:16
1573:3
1576:19
1585:4
1587:5
1611:9
1621:18
1627:23
1637:16
1650:1
1698:7
1700:18
1702:22
1704:21
1727:18

Indices

A
ἀγαθός 14–16
ἄγειν 143
ἀγωγή 17, 47
ἀήρ 76–7, 90
ἀθληταί 63, 88, 90
αἰδοῖον 17–18
αἷμα 29–30, 85
αἱμορροΐδες 52, 88
ἀκμή 18–19, 111
ἀκρατής 19–20
ἀκριβής 30–1
ἀκροχορδόνες 77–8, 90
ἀλφοί 31–2
ἀλφός 32
ἅμα 32
ἁμάρτημα 7
ἁμαρτάνετε 7–10
ἁμαρτάνω 7
ἀμόργη 33–4
ἀναγκαῖον 21–3
ἀνάγκη 22
ἀνάληψις 23–4
ἀνδράσι 34
ἀνέλπιστος 24–6, 47
ἀνήρ 34
ἄνθραξ 34–6
ἀνταποδιδούς 26–7
ἀνταπόδοσις 26
ἄνυδρος 10–11, 14, 44
ἀποπληξία 64–7, 88, 89, 90, 179
ἀπόστημα 36–40, 73
ἀρθρῖτις 40
ἀριστερά 40
ἄρρην 41
ἀρχή 41–2, 44
ἄρωμα 67–8, 88
ἀσθενής 42–3
ἆσθμα 27, 28
ἀσθματικοί 27–8, 48
ἀσκαρίδες 78–9, 90
αὐτοματισταί 12
αὐτόματον 12–14, 44, 88, 89, 173
αὐχμηρός 10–11
ἀφρώδης 28–9
ἀχλύς 43–5

B
Βήχιον 122
βούλεται 96
βράγχοι 121
βραχύνει 154

Γ
γέροντες 42, 158
γνώμη 107–10
γυμναστικοῖσιν 144

Δ
δίαιται (-ης) 151–2
δυσεντερία 79–80, 90
δύσκριτα 154–5

Ε
εἰλεός 53–5, 88, 89
ἐλλεβόρους 102
ἐξανθήματα 131–3
ἐπιληψία 68–9, 88, 89
ἐπίπλοος 55, 88
εὐεξίαι 144
εὔκριτα 154–5
εὔροα 96

Θ
θανάσιμον 95

Κ
καιρός 137
καθαίρειν 96
καθίστημι 156
κατάρροος 120–1
κατάστασις 155–7, 181
καῦσος 69, 88
κίνδυνος 55–6, 88, 90
κιρσός 56–7, 88, 89
κόρυζα 118–21, 122
κρίσις 137, 138–41, 154, 175
κυνάγχη 117–18, 175

Λ
λείπεται 143
λειχήν 129–30
λέπρα 122–29, 133, 146, 173, 176, 179, 180
λήθαργος 57–8, 88
λογισμός 163
λόγος 163–7

λουτρόν 104–5
λυεί 104

Μ
μανία 116–7
μελαγχολία 58–61, 85, 88, 89
μηκύνει 154

Ν
νηστείην 158

Π
παρέχειν 137
παροξύνει 111
παροξυσμός 111–15, 133, 176
περιπλευμονία 80–1
ποδάγρα 81–2
πολέμιον 139

Σ
Σατυριασμοί 82–3
συμβεβηκός 161
σφάκελος 83–4
σῶμα 97–102
σώματα 97, 99

Τ
τάξις 156
τέτανος 70–3, 88, 90, 178, 179
τριταῖος 84

Υ
ὑποχόνδριον 170–2, 173

Φ
Φέρουσι 158
φίλιον 139
φθίσις 73–4, 88
φλεβοτομίη 105–6
φλέγμα 85, 90
φλεγμαίνω 85
φλεγμονή 7 –85
φρενῖτις 61–3, 88
φρενός 75, 88, 90, 179
φύματα 131–3
φύσις 144–9
φύω 145

Χ
χαρακτήρ 145
χολέρα 87

Ω
ὠφελῆ 95

الجمر 34–5
الجنون 68–9, 116–17
أجود 30
جيد 16
الجوهر 144

ح
الحجاب 75
حدّة 112, 115
حديد 137
التحدّب 71–3
الحزاز 130
الحمّام 104–5
احتمل 158
الحمى
الحدة 169
المحرقة 69
التي تدعى قوسوس 70
التي تعرض حين بعد حين 112
التي يكون معها اختلاط العقل 62
التي يكون معها السهر 58
التي مع ورم الدماغ 62
محمود 15–16
حالات الهواء 156
الحيات المتولّدة في البطن 79

خ
الخبطة 119
الخدر 20–1
الخربق 103
الخراج 36–7, 86, 131–2
خاصّة 163
خصب البدن 144
خطأ 7–10
الخطر 56
اختلاف 169
الدم 79–80
الأغرس 80
الخنازير 82
خير 15–16, 143

د
دبّر 151
التدبير 151–2
الدبيلة 37
الدليل 15
الدالي 56–7
الدم 29–30
دم النساء 16–17
الدود 78–9
الدور 111
التداول 26
الأدوية 67

ذ
الذبحة 117–18
الذكر 41
ذهب 20
الذهن 107, 109
إذابة 96
من ذاته 13
ذات الرئة 81

ر
الربو 27–8
المرتبة 156
رجا 24
الرجل 34
الإرخاء 21
الاسترخاء 65
المراقّ 55
الريح 67

ز
الزبد 28–9
الزكام 118–22
ازداد 143
الزيادة 19, 26–7
التزيّد 26

س
السبب 12
السبات 58
سحج الأمعاء 79
السوداء 59–60, 89
السودوية 60
السرسام (see البرسام)
السعال 122
السكتة 64–7
السلّ 73–4
سائر الحالّت 163

ش
ما دون الشرسيف 170–1
تشقّق 124
الإشكال 156
التشنّج 70–3
الشاف 139

ص
الصحة 144

الصرع 68–9
الصرّيع 63–4
المصارع 64
صَعِد 19
الصفاق 75
صالح 14–16
صار 19, 60
الصوم 159

ض
الضرورة 21–3
ضَعُف 42
ضعيفة 20, 43
الضمر 74
ضيق النَفَس 27

ط
طَبَع 145
الطبيعة 144–9
أطراف الأوتار 77–8
أطعم 151
الطعام 151
الأطعمة 151
طوعاً 12–13
أطوَل 31
طيّب 67
الطيب 67
أطيب 67

ظ
الأظفار 124

ع
عدم بغتة 21
عرق المديني 57
العضو 65, 97
العقل 107
علة
التي يقال لها سفقيلوس 83
التي يتقشّر منها الجلد 123–5, 128
النسيان 58
العلامة 15

غ
الغبّ 84
الغبّ
غذا 24
الغذاء 151
التغذية 23
الأغرس 80
غشاوة 43, 45

ف
فتح 20–1
انفتاح (أفواه العروق من أسفل) 52
الفرّج 17–18
الفَرَج 138
التفسّخ 21
فصد العروق 106
الانفصال (أوقات) 139
الفالج 65–6
الأفاويه 67–8

ق
من قبل نفسه 13
متقدّم 13
القرح 74
قروح الأمعاء 80
التقشّر 124
قصر 154
قصير 154
اقتصر 137
قضى 138
القضاء 139
قطع العروق 106
القوباء 130
القولنج المستعاذ منه 54
القياس 163–7

ك
الكزاز 70–3
التكشيف 144
التكميد 67
الكلية 75
كوّن 146–7
الكيموس 96

ل
لهيب 70

م
التمدّد 70–3
الامتداد 73
المرّة
السوداء 59–60
الصفراء 169
المرار 169
المطر 10–11
معاً 32
ملء 23
أمات 95
الميّت 95

مال 143

ن

نبغ 164–5

النزلة 122 ,118–20

الناسور/الناصور 38

النظام 156–7

من نفسه 13

النافض 84

النقرس 81–2

النقصان 74–5

انتقل 143

نقه 24

نَقِي 96

المنتهى 114 ,111 ,18–19

النوب 111

النار الفارسي 35

ه

الهزال 23–4

الهلاك 56

الهواء 77

هاج 114 ,111

الاهتياج 114–15 ,112

الهيضة 87

و

وَجب 165 ,22

وجّب 164

الواجب 22

وجع المفاصل 40

الورم 132 ,85–6

الوضح 128 ,123

التوقّد 70

توليد (الأمراض) 162

ي

يابس 10

الأيسار 40

i. 1 136–41
i. 2 12
i. 3 23, 141–8, 149
i. 4 30, 149–52
i. 5 7, 30
i. 6 30–1
i. 8 19
i. 9 19
i. 10 19
i. 11 111, 114
i. 12 26, 41, 152–7
i. 13 157–61
i. 15 63
i. 19 139
ii. 1 94–5
ii. 2 15
ii. 5 12
ii. 6 98, 106–10
ii. 7 98
ii. 9 95–102
ii. 13 112, 115
ii. 15 97
ii. 19 162
ii. 23 138
ii. 27 164
ii. 28 164
ii. 29 19
ii. 33 15
ii. 40 118
ii. 46 32
ii. 49 42
ii. 51 98
iii. 1 161–7
iii. 5 43
iii. 8 155
iii. 11 10, 79
iii. 12 10, 20
iii. 13 10
iii. 14 10, 59
iii. 15 155
iii. 16 40, 65, 79
iii. 19 110–15
iii. 20 31, 40, 60, 115–33
iii. 21 17, 84
iii. 22 54, 117
iii. 23 81
iii. 24 86
iii. 26 27, 77, 78
iii. 30 52, 58, 62, 70, 79, 81, 87
iv. 9 59
iv. 13 97, 102–3
iv. 25 15
iv. 27 24
iv. 43 56
iv. 54 69
iv. 59 30, 84, 139, 140
iv. 64 170
iv. 71 165–6
iv. 72 62
iv. 73 170
v. 9 74
v. 11 34
v. 16 20–1, 107
v. 22 17, 138
v. 23 86
v. 28 16, 67
v. 33 29
v. 46 55
v. 64 74, 164, 167–72
v. 69 34, 98
vi. 11 15, 61–2
vi. 16 81
vi. 18 75
vi. 21 56
vi. 23 60
vi. 31 103–6
vi. 34 56
vi. 37 15
vi. 44 54
vi. 56 65, 98
vi. 58 22, 55
vii. 5 15
vii. 10 54
vii. 11 81
vii. 12 62, 81
vii. 17 86
vii. 28 98
vii. 36 37
vii. 40 21, 65
vii. 41 15
vii. 45 33
vii. 47 24
vii. 49 15
vii. 50 83
vii. 55 55
vii. 60 98
vii. 61 98
vii. 74 98
vii. 78 37

Index of Entries from Bar Bahlul's Syriac Lexicon

Ref	Entry	Page
7:13		76
22:26		14
22:27		14
24:8	(ἀγαθοῦ)	14
24:12		16
33:17		14
57:18		12
58:1		12
58:2		12
67:21	(αἱμορροΐδες)	52
81:18	(ὑποχόνδριον)	170
98:25		40
106:18		12
128:17		53
132:10		29
133:15		84
135:14		29
143:11	(ἐπιληψία)	68
144:20		68
145:6		19–20
155:22		33
157:16		43
167:25		53
178:17		31
179:5		22
181:17		32
184:1		33
195:25		23
199:6		34
206:26		26
207:1		26
209:12		10
210:8		34
211:13		21
211:14		21
215:11		24
216:15		34
218:4		97
227:13		27
233:10	(ὑποχόνδριον)	170
241:10		78
245:20		42
251:6		64
251:23		36
251:24		36
253:21		36
253:25	(ἀποπληξία)	64
254:6	(ὑποχόνδριον)	170
263:8	(ἀποπληξία)	64
264:26		36
265:12	(ἀποπληξία)	64
268:26		28
276:13		18
277:25		30
278:5		77
278:7		77
278:14		77
278:19		30
293:5		41
293:19		41
299:22		40
303:12		41
304:1		41
330:20		63
361:28		32
365:8		140
394:22		105
399:20		105
403:1		105
408:25		68
444:8		83
445:10		170
447:4		34
453:19		159–61
466:20		35
476:6		99
477:3		99
494:23		11
496:2		11
504:3		107
512:15		125–6
536:19		120
537:4		152
559:16		151
574:24		41
577:2		57
579:8		17, 30
602:12	(αἰδοῖον)	17
606:8		38
616:7		52
628:18		131
636:27		29